Compliments of

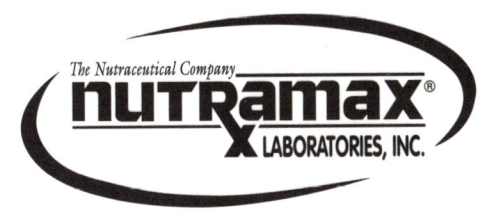

NUTRAMAX LABORATORIES, INC.
The Nutraceutical Company

www.nutramaxlabs.com

theclinics.com

VETERINARY CLINICS OF NORTH AMERICA

Small Animal Practice

Nutraceuticals and Other Biologic Therapies

GUEST EDITOR
Lester Mandelker, DVM

January 2004 • Volume 34 • Number 1

SAUNDERS
An Imprint of Elsevier, Inc.
PHILADELPHIA LONDON TORONTO MONTREAL SYDNEY TOKYO

W.B. SAUNDERS COMPANY
A Division of Elsevier Inc.

The Curtis Center • Independence Square West • Philadelphia, Pennsylvania 19106

http://www.vetsmall.theclinics.com

THE VETERINARY CLINICS OF NORTH AMERICA: Volume 34, Number 1
SMALL ANIMAL PRACTICE   ISSN 0195-5616
January 2004
Editor: John Vassallo

Copyright © 2004 by Elsevier Inc. All rights reserved. No part of this publication may be reproduced or transmitted in any form or by any means, electronic or mechanical, including photocopy, recording, or any information retrieval system, without written permission from the Publisher.

Single photocopies of single articles may be made for personal use as allowed by national copyright laws. Permission of the publisher and payment of a fee is required for all other photocopying, including multiple or systematic copying, copying for advertising or promotional purposes, resale, and all forms of document delivery. Special rates are available for educational institutions that wish to make photocopies for non-profit educational classroom use. Permissions may be sought directly from Elsevier Inc. Rights & Permissions Department, PO Box 800, Oxford OX5 1DX, UK; phone: (+44) 1865 843830, fax: (+44) 1865 853333, e-mail: permissions@elsevier.co.uk. You may also contact Rights & Permissions directly through Elsevier's home page (http://www.elsevier.com), selecting first 'Customer Support', then 'General Information', then 'Permissions Query Form'. In the USA, users may clear permissions and make payments through the Copyright Clearance Center, Inc., 222 Rosewood Drive, Danvers, MA 01923, USA; phone: (978) 750-8400, fax: (978) 750-4744, and in the UK through the Copyright Licensing Agency Rapid Clearance Service (CLARCS), 90 Tottenham Court Road, London WIP 0LP, UK; phone: (+44) 171 436 5931; fax: (+44) 171 436 3986. Other countries may have a local reprographic rights agency for payments.

The ideas and opinions expressed in *The Veterinary Clinics of North America: Small Animal Practice* do not necessarily reflect those of the Publisher. The Publisher does not assume any responsibility for any injury and/or damage to persons or property arising out of or related to any use of the material contained in this periodical. The reader is advised to check the appropriate medical literature and the product information currently provided by the manufacturer of each drug to be administered to verify the dosage, the method and duration of administration, or contraindications. It is the responsibility of the treating physician or other health care professional, relying on independent experience and knowledge of the patient, to determine drug dosages and the best treatment for the patient. Mention of any product in this issue should not be construed as endorsement by the contributors, editors, or the Publisher of the product or manufacturers' claims.

The Veterinary Clinics of North America: Small Animal Practice (ISSN 0195-5616) is published bimonthly (For Post Office use only: volume 34 issue 1 of 6) by W.B. Saunders Company. Corporate and editorial offices: The Curtis Center, Independence Square West, Philadelphia, PA 19106-3399. Accounting and circulation offices: 6277 Sea Harbor Drive, Orlando, FL 32887-4800. Periodicals postage paid at Orlando, FL 32862, and additional mailing offices. Subscription prices are $162.00 per year for US individuals, $240.00 per year for US institutions, $81.00 per year for US students and residents, $205.00 per year for Canadian individuals, $299.00 per year for Canadian institutions, $218.00 per year for international individuals, $299.00 per year for international institutions and $109.00 per year for Canadian and foreign students/residents. To receive student/resident rate, orders must be accompanied by name of affiliated institution, date of term, and the *signature* of program/residency coordinator on institution letterhead. Orders will be billed at individual rate until proof of status is received. Foreign air speed delivery is included in all *Clinics* subscription prices. All prices are subject to change without notice. POSTMASTER: Send address changes to *The Veterinary Clinics of North America: Small Animal Practice*, Elsevier, Customer Service Department, 6277 Sea Harbor Drive, Orlando, FL 32887-4800, USA; phone: (+1)(877) 8397126 [toll free number for US customers], or (+1)(407) 3454020 [customers outside US]; fax: (+1)(407) 3631354; email: usjcs@elsevier.com

The Veterinary Clinics of North America: Small Animal Practice is also published in Japanese by Gakusosha Company Ltd., 2-16-28 Nishikata, Bunkyo-ku, Tokyo 113, Japan.

Reprints. For copies of 100 or more, of articles in this publication, please contact the Commercial Reprints Department, Elsevier Inc., 360 Park Avenue South, New York, New York 10010-1710. Tel. (212) 633-3813 Fax: (212) 633-3820 email: reprints@elsevier.com

The Veterinary Clinics of North America: Small Animal Practice is covered in *Current Contents/Agriculture, Biology and Environmental Sciences, Science Citation Index, ASCA, Index Medicus, Excerpta Medica,* and *BIOSIS.*

Printed in the United States of America.

NUTRACEUTICALS AND OTHER BIOLOGIC THERAPIES

GUEST EDITOR

LESTER MANDELKER, DVM, Diplomate, American Board of Veterinary Practitioners; Community Veterinary Hospital, Largo, Florida

CONTRIBUTORS

BRIAN S. BEALE, DVM, Diplomate, American College of Veterinary Surgeons, Gulf Coast Veterinary Specialists, Houston, Texas

DAWN MERTON BOOTHE, DVM, PhD, Diplomate, American College of Veterinary Internal Medicine; Diplomate, American College of Veterinary Clinical Pharmacology; Associate Professor, Department of Veterinary Physiology and Pharmacology, Texas A & M University, College Station, Texas

SCOTT A. BROWN, VMD, PhD, Diplomate, American College of Veterinary Internal Medicine; Department of Physiology and Pharmacology, College of Veterinary Medicine, University of Georgia, Athens, Georgia

MICHAEL A. CEDDIA, PhD, The Iams Company Research and Development, Lewisburg, Ohio

SHARON A. CENTER, DVM, Professor, College of Veterinary Medicine, Cornell University, Ithaca, New York

DEBORAH J. DAVENPORT, DVM, MS, Diplomate, American College of Veterinary Internal Medicine (Small Animal Internal Medicine); and Director of Professional Education, Hill's Pet Nutrition Inc., Topeka, Kansas

MICHAEL G. HAYEK, PhD, The Iams Company Research and Development, Lewisburg, Ohio

ELIZABETH HEAD, PhD, Assistant Professor, Institute for Brain Aging and Dementia, University of California at Irvine, Irvine, California

NICHOLAS LARKINS, DSc, MRCVS, Nutritional Laboratories, Penrhos, Raglan, Monmouthshire, United Kingdom

LESTER MANDELKER, DVM, Diplomate, American Board of Veterinary Practitioners, Community Veterinary Hospital, Largo, Florida

STEFAN P. MASSIMINO, MS, The Iams Company Research and Development, Lewisburg, Ohio

BRUCE J. NOVOTNY, DVM, Helios Communications, LLC, Shawnee, Kansas

PAUL D. PION, DVM, Diplomate, American College of Veterinary Internal Medicine (Cardiology); Veterinary Information Network, Davis, California

ROBERT C. ROSENTHAL, DVM, PhD, American College of Veterinary Internal Medicine (Small Animal Internal Medicine, Oncology), Diplomate, American College of Veterinary Radiology (Radiation Oncology); SouthPaws Veterinary Referral Center, Springfield, Virginia

PHILIP ROUDEBUSH, DVM, Diplomate, American College of Veterinary Internal Medicine (Small Animal Internal Medicine); and Veterinary Fellow, Technical Information Services, Hill's Pet Nutrition Inc., Topeka, Kansas

MAUREEN L. STOREY, PhD, Director, Center for Food and Nutrition Policy, Virginia Polytechnic Institute and State University, Alexandria, Virginia

SUSAN WYNN, DVM, Private Practice, Woodstock, Georgia

STEVEN C. ZICKER, PhD, DVM, American College of Veterinary Internal Medicine, Diplomate, American College of Veterinary Nutrition; and Veterinary Clinical Nutritionist, Science and Technology Center, Hill's Pet Nutrition, Inc., Topeka, Kansas

NUTRACEUTICALS AND OTHER BIOLOGIC THERAPIES

CONTENTS

Preface xi
Lester Mandelker

Evidence-based Medicine Concepts 1
Robert C. Rosenthal

> Today, the busy clinician will benefit from a philosophy of practice that brings together the best applicable evidence and the experiences of clinical work in an effort to provide the best care for individual patients. Evidence-based medicine (EBM) provides a structured approach that recognizes the contributions of both. An EBM practice will be efficient and effective in meeting the goal of assuring optimum care. The concepts of EBM make sense for veterinary medicine, even if there are limited numbers of randomized, blinded studies, and they can be applied by clinicians in all types of practice.

Balancing Fact and Fiction of Novel Ingredients: Definitions, Regulations, and Evaluation 7
Dawn Merton Boothe

> Veterinarians have an opportunity to help educate their clients regarding the safety and efficacy of novel ingredients used by their clients. This is no small task because of the lack of acceptable information. Clients should be counseled regarding the lack of scientific evidence and be encouraged to discriminate fact from fiction, including many testimonials. Safety should be of primary concern, and clients should be encouraged not to neglect traditional therapies in lieu of novel ingredients unless clinical evidence of efficacy exists. Quality assurance is equally important and cannot be underestimated. Although skepticism is encouraged regarding any unknown product with medicinal indications, open mindedness should also guide the veterinarian as these products are considered. Indeed, veterinarians should take actions to ensure that the use of these compounds is accomplished within the confines of

the veterinary-client-patient relationship, thus ensuring the role of the veterinarian in the health and well-being of animals, regardless of the modality of therapy. The veterinary profession should support the development of standards that might guide manufacturers of novel ingredients to meet criteria that protect the consumer. Likewise, we should encourage manufacturers and agencies to fund veterinary clinical trials to provide evidence for the use of these potentially exciting compounds. Above all else, the veterinarian needs to become a credible resource of information about the possible role of these products. The lack of a regulatory mechanism that establishes the safety and efficacy of these products is not justification for ignoring the potential therapeutic benefit of some of these products.

The Natural Activities of Cells, the Role of Reactive Oxygen Species, and their Relation to Antioxidants, Nutraceuticals, Botanicals, and other Biologic Therapies 39
Lester Mandelker

There is a strong probability that cellular functions and cellular responses that pertain to inflammation, disease, and life and death activity can be modulated with supplementation; however, what works well in one individual or species might work differently in another. The cellular effects of antioxidants and other supplements are well defined and meaningful, and their clinical application looks promising despite individual variations. Combinations of antioxidants are best suited for clinical application in modulating disease and reducing premature aging when caused by excessive free radical accumulation. Clinicians should approach clinical application of these supplements based on the best available scientific research and species-specific information available.

Metabolic, Antioxidant, Nutraceutical, Probiotic, and Herbal Therapies Relating to the Management of Hepatobiliary Disorders 67
Sharon A. Center

Many nutraceuticals, conditionally essential nutrients, and botanical extracts have been proposed as useful in the management of liver disease. The most studied of these are addressed in terms of proposed mechanisms of action, benefits, hazards, and safe dosing recommendations allowed by current information. While this is an area of soft science, it is important to keep an open and tolerant mind, considering that many major treatment discoveries were in fact serendipitous accidents.

Functional Foods and the Urinary Tract 173
Scott A. Brown

There is no universally accepted definition of a commonly used term for a functional food: nutraceutical. For the purposes of this article, a nutraceutical is any ingredient found in foods that has a demonstrated (or proposed) physiologic benefit. Although a nutraceutical is generally taken to be an ingredient that can be isolated or purified from food, plants, or marine products and made available in medicinal form, this article also considers claims of benefit to the urinary tract for foods or food supplements in which the active ingredient has not yet been characterized or isolated.

Traditional and Nontraditional Effective and Noneffective Therapies for Cardiac Disease in Dogs and Cats   187
Paul D. Pion

In this article, the author's perspective of the current state of knowledge addressing the role of traditional and nontraditional therapeutics is presented. The focus is on the nontraditional therapeutics. Among these, the only ones the author currently considers to have any documented value are taurine and, less commonly, L-carnitine. The role of taurine (and likely carnitine) remains limited to cases of documented deficiency. In the case of cats with taurine deficiency–induced myocardial failure, it is now clear that most cases are the result of formulation errors by owners and manufacturers. In dogs, it is less clear if the causes of taurine deficiencies represent manifestations of pathologic conditions or dietary formulations errors. Increasingly, it seems the latter may prove to be the case in most, if not all, circumstances.

Nutraceuticals, Aging, and Cognitive Dysfunction   217
Elizabeth Head and Steven C. Zicker

Decline in cognitive function that accompanies aging in dogs might have a biologic basis, and many of the disorders associated with aging in canines might be preventable through dietary modifications that incorporate specific nutraceuticals. Antioxidants might be one class of nutraceutical that benefits aged dogs. Brains of aged dogs accumulate oxidative damage to proteins and lipids, which might lead to dysfunction of neuronal cells. Reducing oxidative damage through food ingredients rich in a broad spectrum of antioxidants significantly improves, or slows the decline of, learning and memory in aged dogs; however, determining which compounds, combinations, dosage ranges, when to initiate intervention, and long-term effects constitute critical gaps in knowledge about this subject.

Modulation of Immune Response through Nutraceutical Interventions: Implications for Canine and Feline Health   229
Michael G. Hayek, Stefan P. Massimino, and Michael A. Ceddia

Mounting research demonstrates that certain nutraceutical compounds interact with the immune system. These interactions may be positive or negative depending on the compound or dose administered to the individual. Understanding the mechanisms by which these compounds work should provide opportunities to design nutritional interventions to bolster the health of dogs and cats.

The Use of Nutraceuticals in Cancer Therapy 249
Philip Roudebush, Deborah J. Davenport, and Bruce J. Novotny

> The high prevalence of nutraceutical use among human patients with cancer suggests that the use of nutraceuticals in pet animals with cancer is probably common. Dogs with a wide variety of malignant diseases have significant alterations in carbohydrate, protein, and fat metabolism. These metabolic alterations may be ameliorated by using functional foods relatively low in soluble carbohydrate, moderate amounts of protein that includes sources of arginine, and moderate amounts of fat supplemented with ω-3 long-chain polyunsaturated fatty acids. Well-controlled clinical studies in a variety of species with cancer, including rodents, people, and dogs, have documented that increased dietary and serum levels of ω-3 fatty acids are associated with a number of health benefits, including improved disease-free interval, survival time, and quality of life. Other nutraceuticals of interest in patients with cancer include antioxidant vitamins, trace minerals, glutamine, protease inhibitors, garlic, tea polyphenols, vitamin A, and shark cartilage.

Use of Nutraceuticals and Chondroprotectants in Osteoarthritic Dogs and Cats 271
Brian S. Beale

> Chondroprotectants and nutraceuticals have become attractive adjunctive or alternative treatments for cats and dogs suffering from osteoarthritis. Osteoarthritic patients can be managed satisfactorily in most situations with optimization of body condition, exercise modification, anti-inflammatory therapy, and the use of chondroprotectants agents. Presently, recommendations cannot be made as to which chondroprotectant is best for each dog and cat afflicted with osteoarthritis. Head-to-head comparisons of these products have not been made, and it is not known when the different mediators of osteoarthritis play an important role. Currently, the best recommendation is to use products that have well-designed experimental and clinical research evaluating efficacy and safety, and products that are manufactured under the high quality standards practiced by the pharmaceutical industry.

Pharmacognosy: Phytomedicines and their Mechanisms 291
Nicholas Larkins and Susan Wynn

> Phytochemicals, archetypal plant constituents, are recognized as secondary plant metabolites that do not appear to be necessary to sustain life. However, they have functions that increase the ongoing survival prospects of the plant in its natural environment. Do these secondary plant metabolites have biologic activity in animals? Enzymes, for example, in animals can share a common ancestry with enzymes and proteins in plants. This evolutionary relationship, when combined with the multiple structural similarities between plant and animal substrates for such constituents,

helps explain the hormone-like or hormone-modulating effects of several phytochemicals in animals. Phytomedicines from these phytochemicals provide valuable therapeutic tools in disease management and control.

Regulatory Issues of Functional Foods, Feeds, and Nutraceuticals 329
Maureen L. Storey

> The United States has a sophisticated and complex infrastructure of policymaking that regulates the food, drug, and cosmetics industries. The Federal Food, Drug, and Cosmetic Act of 1938 gave the US Food and Drug Administration (FDA) the authority to develop and enforce rules governing these industries. There is no separate regulatory category for functional foods or nutraceuticals; this industry is regulated in the same way as foods and dietary supplements by the FDA, which operates within the Department of Health and Human Services. Several recent laws now allow the food industry greater latitude to make several types of claims about food, ingredients, or nutrients that may promote health or prevent disease. The future of the functional foods and nutraceuticals industry will depend on regulations that are flexible enough to (1) protect the public health, (2) encourage research and development of innovative food products, and (3) communicate the benefits of those products to the public.

Cellular Effects of Common Nutraceuticals and Natural Food Substances 339
Lester Mandelker and Susan Wynn

> Tabular information of proposed cellular effects regarding the use of certain nutraceuticals (including antioxidants, phytonutrients, and other biological therapies) and herbs, compiled from scientific sources and experimental research, is provided.

Cellular Effects of Various Herbs and Botanicals 355
Lester Mandelker and Susan Wynn

> Tabular information of proposed cellular effects regarding the use of certain nutraceuticals (including antioxidants, phytonutrients, and other biologic therapies) and herbs, compiled from scientific sources and experimental research, is provided.

Index 369

FORTHCOMING ISSUES

March 2004
Ear Disease
Jennifer Matousek, DVM, MS,
Guest Editor

May 2004
Ocular Therapeutics
Cecil Moore, DVM, MS, *Guest Editor*

July 2004
Clinical Urology
India Lane, DVM, MS, Shelly Vaden, DVM,
and S. Dru Forrester, DVM, MS,
Guest Editors

RECENT ISSUES

November 2003
Hematology
Joanne B. Messick, VMD, PhD, *Guest Editor*

September 2003
Gastroenterology
Michael D. Willard, DVM, MS,
Guest Editor

July 2003
Emerging and Re-emerging Infectious Diseases
Douglass K. Macintire, DVM, MS and
Edward B. Breitschwerdt, DVM, *Guest Editors*

The Clinics are now available online!

Access your subscription at:
www.TheClinics.com

Preface

Nutraceuticals and other biologic therapies

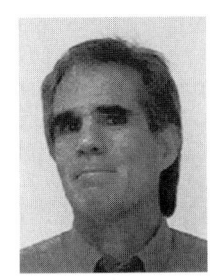

Lester Mandelker, DVM
Guest Editor

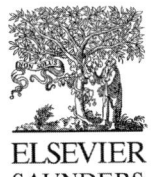

The purpose of this issue of the *Veterinary Clinics of North America: Small Animal Practice* is to present the veterinary profession with current information on the theories and scientific studies concerning the cellular effects and application of nutraceuticals, antioxidants, and botanical and other biological therapies. The issue is controversial—as it should be. As would be expected, the authors have differing opinions on the clinical relevancy of these agents. Some are very skeptical and others less so. One thing is commonly understood—the body is a very complex system of biochemical reactions influenced by many events; therefore, it is extremely difficult to acknowledge something you cannot easily prove. Many practitioners may unwittingly credit nutritional supplementation without significant proof simply because of the body's response from illness. This credit is in contrast to pharmaceutical therapy, where proof is evident because drug therapy can be measured by blood and tissue studies as well as direct clinical evidence. In addition, the source of evidence comes from both independent scientific and clinical studies as well as corporate-funded research; therefore, equally important mechanisms can be both overestimated and underestimated with regard to their clinical benefits. Additionally, there is not an exact science to evaluate such therapies. We have a long way to go before scientific knowledge and effectiveness of individual or combinations of nutrients is known. This issue is a beginning.

Most of us are familiar with the damaging effects of oxygen-free radicals. The rationale for the application of many antioxidant supplements involve the free radical theory of aging and disease. Several authors discuss the relevancy of this theory and some do not. Most of us are also familiar with many of the botanicals and herbs mentioned herein and how they claim to impact our health. Nature has put these chemicals in many different forms that appear to compliment their biological function. Processing these compounds from natural sources tends to concentrate one chemical in lieu of others that may have promoted additional synergy. While the effectiveness of individual compounds can be concentrated manyfold, it may lack the completeness of the intended natural source. In addition, there is a relative paucity of clinical applications of these botanical supplements. As more practitioners incorporate these supplements into their practices, more information regarding their clinical effectiveness will be known. We hope to see more scientific and clinical studies result from this increased interest by practitioners.

The information in this issue excited me and enhanced my own opinions about nutraceuticals and antioxidants. This enthusiasm is tempered by some of the authors who have more clinical experience and knowledge in their specialities than I do, and rightly so. We should not jump from theory to clinical relevancy in one leap. Cellular effects may or may not equate with clinical healing. The body's reaction to supplementation is quite complicated, and we need to learn more about these cellular reactions; this issue initiates that process.

I would like to commend the superb authors who contributed articles to this issue; they are daring and progressive educators and veterinarians who undertook this task not knowing what to expect. There is no doubt that the clinical relevancy of nutritional supplements needs more "hard science" and less anecdotal information to substantiate clinical applications. I would especially like to thank Paul Pion for all his input and skepticism that kept me grounded in reality. In addition, I thank Nick Larkin for all his assistance and his superb efforts in editing several of the articles and John Vassallo, Associate Publisher, for being exceptionally patient in allowing us extra time to complete this issue. Finally, I thank my wife and children for putting up with an invisible husband and father for the 18 months it took to research, organize, and publish this issue.

Lester Mandelker, DVM
Community Veterinary Hospital
1631 W. Bay Drive
Largo, FL 33770, USA

E-mail address: lestervet2@aol.com

Evidence-based medicine concepts

Robert C. Rosenthal, DVM, PhD

SouthPaws Veterinary Referral Center, 6136 Brandon Avenue, Springfield, VA 22150, USA

By definition, evidence-based medicine (EBM) is the conscientious, explicit, and judicious use of current evidence in making decisions about specific patients. The practice of EBM integrates an individual's clinical expertise with the best available external clinical evidence from systematic research. Individual clinical expertise encompasses the proficiency and judgment that individual clinicians acquire through clinical experience and clinical practice. The best available external clinical evidence includes clinically relevant research about the accuracy and precision of diagnostic procedures, the power of prognostic tests, and the safety and efficacy of preventive and therapeutic regimens. The practice of EBM is a process of lifelong self-directed learning that recognizes the need for the application of new information about diagnosis, prognosis, and therapy.

Several points demonstrate the need for bringing EBM into practice. New types of evidence are being generated that will change the way that clinicians care for patients; it is no longer sufficient to understand the pathophysiology of an ailment and to apply interventions shown to interrupt that process. Action based on evidence from clinical trials and other published evidence is now a critical benchmark for the modern clinician. Although patients would benefit from this evidence, clinicians often fail to obtain it. With time, up-to-date clinical knowledge and clinical performance deteriorate. Traditional continuing education programs have not addressed the problem of keeping up, but a different approach to clinical learning, EBM, has been shown to be effective. Asking a well-formulated clinical question is the beginning of this process.

E-mail address: rcr@southpaws.com

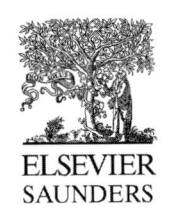

Well-formulated clinical questions

Origins of clinical questions

Clinical questions can arise from any juncture of a clinician's interaction with a patient. Most clinical questions arise from the core tasks of the clinical encounter. Recognizing the areas that give rise to the need for more information allows the clinician to focus on the development of good clinical questions. Eight such domains focus on the central work that a clinician performs:

1. Clinical findings—how properly to gather and interpret findings from the history and physical examination
2. Etiology—how to identify causes for disease, including iatrogenic disease
3. Differential diagnosis—how to rank the possible causes of a patient's problems
4. Diagnostic tests—how to select and interpret diagnostic tests to confirm or exclude a diagnosis
5. Prognosis—how to estimate the patient's clinical course and anticipate likely complications
6. Therapy—how to select treatments that do more good than harm and are worth the effort and cost
7. Prevention—how to reduce the chance of disease by identifying and modifying risk factors
8. Self-improvement—how to keep up-to-date, improve clinical skills, and run a better, more efficient practice

Remembering these eight areas of questioning will aid the clinician in developing a set of well-formulated clinical questions.

Building the clinical question

It is not enough that a question addresses a pertinent issue. The well-formulated clinical question must also be phrased in a way that will direct the clinician's search to relevant and precise answers. Practically speaking, a well-built clinical question includes four elements: (1) the patient or the problem, (2) the intervention being considered, (3) a comparison intervention when relevant, and (4) the clinical outcomes of interest. Clinical questions can be constructed with these components in mind as a means of specifying the best search for the most useful evidence.

Using the domain and element approach to develop well-formulated clinical questions

When a patient's presentation is so puzzling that the clinician is at a loss regarding where to begin, it might be useful to ask, for each of the eight domains, whether or not there are any uncertainties. If the clinician cannot quickly and confidently answer no, there is a knowledge gap. Identifying such a gap is an excellent starting place. When a clinician has trouble stating the question, it might be helpful to write the question down, stressing the inclusion of all four elements. Thus, a question that should be answerable in a meaningful way can be developed in two steps—identification of the domain of the question and completion of the four elements.

When there are more questions than time to answer them, it is helpful to remember that EBM is characterized by learning in small increments over time. Trying to learn everything at once—trying to answer all possible questions now—is impossible and, therefore, frustrating. Clinicians can avoid that trap by asking themselves the following queries to decide which question to answer now:

- Which question is most important to my patient's well being?
- Which question is most feasible to answer within the time I have available?
- Which question is most interesting?
- Which question will I most likely encounter repeatedly in my practice?

The careful and repeated application of these strategies to develop well-formulated clinical questions is the first step in the use of EBM as a means to improve clinical work. These well-formulated clinical questions open the door to better care and better service.

Quality of evidence and strength of recommendations

Several schemes have been used to define quality of evidence and categorize the strength of recommendations defined from various types of studies. Although there is no formalized, objectified grading system applied to these criteria, it is helpful for the clinician to have such standards in mind when evaluating evidence and recommendations. Guidelines have been published in human and veterinary medicine. Integrating these concepts into daily thinking and evaluation of the clinical literature in any attempt to bring new evidence—evidence that will change clinical practice in a meaningful way—is a worthwhile goal. Polzin, Osborne, and James have proposed the following system, which provides a useful construct.

Grades of quality of evidence

I. Evidence from at least one properly randomized, controlled study
II. Evidence from at least one well-designed clinical trial without randomization; evidence from controlled studies using experimental models; evidence from cohort or case–control analytic studies; evidence from dramatic results in uncontrolled studies

III. Evidence from respected authorities on the basis of clinical experience, descriptive studies, findings in other species, or pathophysiologic rationale

Strength of recommendations

A. Good evidence to support recommendations for use
B. Moderate evidence to support recommendations for use
C. Poor evidence to support recommendations for or against use
D. Moderate evidence to support recommendations against use
E. Good evidence to support recommendations against use

These simple guidelines will help the clinician evaluate evidence in a consistent, if not totally objective, manner and should be kept in mind as part of the process of critical appraisal of evidence used to make clinical decisions in practice.

Literature appraisal in an evidence-based medicine practice

General guidelines for critical appraisal of an article

There are a number of reasons why clinicians read the literature, and not all of them are applicable directly to a case in hand at the moment. In a busy practice, clinicians need an efficient strategy to screen articles to determine if the information is valid and applies to their clinical situation. In general, in an evidence-based practice, the clinician seeks articles that provide patient-oriented evidence that matters in an effort to streamline the process and improve clinical care. The following three-step process applies to this appraisal:

Step 1

An initial validity and relevance screen answers the question "is this article worth taking the time to review in depth?" Eight important questions help the reader make this decision: (1) Is the article from a peer-reviewed journal? (2) Is the location of the study similar to mine so that results, if valid, would apply to my practice? (3) Is the study sponsored by an organization that might influence the study design or results? (4) If the results are true, will there be a direct impact on the health of my patients? (5) If there is an impact on the health of my patients, will the owner of the animal care? (6) Is the problem addressed one that is common in my practice? (7) Is the test or intervention feasible and available to me? (8) If it is true, will the information require me to change my practice?

Step 2

Determine the intent of the article and identify the clinical question that is asked. These tasks can usually be accomplished by reading the abstract and skimming the introduction.

Step 3

Evaluate the validity of the article based on the author's stated intent. The questions asked in this step vary depending on the author's intent. Evaluation can usually be accomplished by reading the abstract, reviewing tables, graphs, and illustrations, and focusing on the methods section. Of the eight domains, most of the articles important to clinicians are in the realm of etiology, diagnostic tests, therapy, or prognosis. Space and time allow elaboration on only one of these. See the suggested readings for much more complete treatments of these subjects and in-depth explanations of other topics such as diagnostic strategies and statistical evaluation.

Critical appraisal of an article on therapy

For an article on therapy, the following questions should be considered:

- Is the study a randomized, controlled trial?
- Are the study subjects similar to my patients?
- Are the study subjects all accounted for at the end of the study?
- Was the study properly blinded?
- Were groups similar at the start of the trial?
- Other than the experimental intervention, were the groups treated equally?
- If the results are negative, is the study powerful enough for proper analysis? Were other factors present that might have affected the outcome?
- Are the treatment benefits worth the potential costs or adverse effects?

The answer to these questions will help determine whether or not the article is likely to be valid and useful in practice.

Summary

Today, the busy clinician benefits from a philosophy of practice that brings together the best applicable evidence and the experiences of clinical work in an effort to provide the best care for individual patients. EBM provides a structured approach that recognizes the contributions of evidence and clinical experience. An EBM practice is efficient and effective in meeting the goal of assuring optimum care. The concepts of EBM make sense for veterinary medicine (even if there are limited numbers of randomized, blinded studies), and clinicians in all types of practice can apply them.

Further readings

Dixon RA, Munro JF, Silcocks PB. The evidence based medicine workbook—critical appraisal for clinical problem solving. Oxford (UK): Butterworth-Heinemann; 1997.

Geyman JP, Deyo RA, Ramsey SD. Evidence-based clinical practice: concepts and approaches. Boston: Butterworth-Heinemann; 2000.

Polzin DJ, Lund E, Walter P, Klausner J. From journal to patient: evidence-based medicine. In: Bonagura JD, editor. Kirk's current veterinary therapy. XIII edition. Philadelphia: WB Saunders; 2000. p. 2–8.

Polzin DJ, Osborne CA, James KM. Medical management of chronic renal failure in cats: current guidelines. In: August JR, editor. Consultations in feline internal medicine. 3rd edition. Philadelphia: WB Saunders Company; 1997. p. 325–36.

Sackett DL, Haynes RB, Tigwell P. Clinical epidemiology: a basic science for clinical medicine. Boston: Little, Brown and Company; 1985.

Sackett DL, Richardson WS, Rosenberg W, Haynes RB. Evidence-based medicine—how to practice and teach EBM. 2nd edition. New York: Churchill Livingstone; 2000 [the first edition of this book, published in 1997, is also highly recommended].

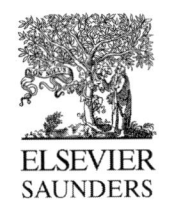

Balancing fact and fiction of novel ingredients: definitions, regulations and evaluation

Dawn Merton Boothe, DVM, PhD

Department of Veterinary Physiology and Pharmacology, Texas A & M University, College Station, TX 77843-4466, USA

Throughout the history of medicine, novel ingredients, such as herbs and nutraceuticals, have had a major role in human and veterinary medicine [1–3]. Herbal medicine has been practiced for more than 60,000 years [2]; indeed, effective compounds, such as salicylates, cardiac glycosides, quinine, and morphine, remain important therapeutic agents today [4]. Novel ingredients are enjoying a resurgence of importance. From 1990 to 1997, the use of herbs and other ingredients in human medicine grew close to 400%, with current growth approximating 15% per year. To date, more than 20,000 human herbal products contribute to an approximate $37 billion market [5,6]. Use in veterinary medicine has paralleled that in human medicine. Close to 30% of pet owners have used or considered the use of novel ingredients in their animals. Approximately 90% of veterinarians sell some type of novel ingredient, and the current market of veterinary novel ingredients is between $20 and $50 million per year [5–9]. The American Veterinary Medical Association (AVMA) recognizes the importance of these medicaments through its guidelines regarding complementary or alternative medicine, which includes veterinary nutraceutical therapy. Despite the impact of the products, however, their use is controversial. Much more than drugs, the use of novel ingredients is complicated by issues regarding their safety, efficacy, and manufacturing.

Definitions and laws

Assessing the rationale use of novel ingredients is complicated by the lack of clear definitions. The term *nutraceutical* is not a legal term but was coined

E-mail address: dboothe@cvm.tamu.edu

in the 1980s by a physician referring to oral compounds that were neither nutrients nor pharmaceuticals. The initial list of products, such as minerals (calcium and magnesium) and vitamins (vitamin A, niacin, and pyridoxine), grew to include products, such as β-carotene, fish oil, garlic, cranberry juice, and antioxidants [1,2]. Today, the category of "nutraceuticals" is broad and includes selected nutrients, dietary supplements, functional foods, genetically engineered designer foods, hypernutritious foods, pharmafoods, phytochemicals [including herbs], and processed (human) foods [3,10]. The commonality among these products is that they are neither foods nor drugs as recognized by the US Food and Drug Administration (FDA), and as such, they undergo no premarket approval process. A brief history of the FDA enhances the understanding of the current regulations that apply to these compounds.

The FDA was formed with Congressional passage of the Federal Food, Drug, and Cosmetic Act (FDCA) of 1938. Because this was a period during which pharmaceutical manufacturing was emerging, the original intent of this act (law) was to ensure the safety of human drugs [11]. It was not until the 1962 amendment that assurance of drug efficacy was included in the missions of the FDA. With passage of the Animal Drug Amendment in 1968, the FDA finally discriminated between human and animal drugs. This amendment provided for the formation of the Bureau (now Center) of Veterinary Medicine (CVM) and directed the CVM to ensure safety to humans of drugs used in animals [12]. As such, the resources of the CVM must include prioritization of regulatory activities that ensure public health. This prioritization may preclude FDA regulation of activities related to veterinary novel ingredients that clearly are illegal. Actions taken by the FDA toward regulation of drugs or related products must be explicitly defined by the acts defining the administration of foods and drugs [13].

The FDCA and its amendments have defined foods, drugs, and feed additives; a review of these definitions is necessary to understanding the complexities of novel ingredient regulation. A food is defined as "an article used for food or drink for man or other animals" and includes any article that provides taste, aroma, or nutritive value [9,14]. Foods are considered by the FDA as "GRAS," that is, generally recognized as safe. The GRAS designation requires a consensus among experts regarding the safety of the product. A company seeking a GRAS designation for an ingredient must provide a history of the product used as a food rather than as a medicinal. Nutraceuticals are not recognized as foods for several reasons: they are not GRAS; their nutritive value generally has not been established; and whereas the primary role of nutrition is in the prevention of diseases, nutraceuticals target prevention and treatment of medical illnesses [2]. Nutraceuticals also cannot be marketed as food additives. These articles, also defined by the FDCA, are substances that directly or indirectly become a component of or affect the character of food [14,15]. In contrast to foods, but as with nutraceuticals, food additives are not GRAS and are considered unsafe unless a regulation specifically exists that provides for their safe use. Thus, for a product to be marketed as a food additive, it must undergo a premarket approval process. Drugs are defined by the FDCA as any "substance, food or non-food used to treat, cure, mitigate or prevent a disease; and any non-food substance that is intended to affect the structure or function of the animal" [14–16]. As with a food additive, a product to be sold as a drug must undergo premarket approval for safety, efficacy, and assurance in manufacturing. Generally, each ingredient in a combination product must be individually evaluated by the FDA. Thus, for the same reasons, a neutraceutical may not be marketed as a drug. However, legally the FDA perceives veterinary neutraceuticals as unapproved drugs if their intended use is as a drug. However, because nutraceuticals are not labeled or marketed as drugs, foods, nor feed additives, the FDA generally does not regulate these products unless they become unsafe or are associated with labels that claim a drug use. Any product is considered by the FDA to be a drug, however, if it is sold with a label (including advertisements) that indicates use for the treatment or prevention of disease or the ability to alter body structure or function. Such a label claim is considered by the FDA to render the product an unapproved drug, thus subjecting it to FDA regulatory action. However, many nonapproved products are in fact sold with medicinal claims, however; their presence reflects FDA prioritization of other issues for regulation. Those that are more likely to have a negative impact on human health are the first to be regulated.

The designation of botanicals, or medicines of plant origin (including herbs), not surprisingly, is complicated and depends on intended use [17–19]. Despite the fact that botanicals historically have been used for medicinal purposes, the product is considered by the FDA as an unapproved drug and can be regulated if it is sold with a label claim that reflects a medicinal purpose. A botanical can be recognized as a food, that is, GRAS, if it has a history of use in food before 1958 as long as the history supports its use as a food or food ingredient without medicinal intent and information supporting a GRAS request for a botanical or herb is submitted to and approved by the FDA. The amount of a botanical or herb consumed is important to interpretation of GRAS. Whereas a little may be good or safe, consumption of a large amount of a botanical or extracting its contents and marketing a concentrated form of its ingredients may be hazardous and thus may preclude a GRAS designation by the FDA [17–19].

Animal foods (in particular, dog and cat foods) often are accompanied by health claims. The FDCA grants the CVM regulatory authority over pet food claims [16,20], and the definitions of food, food additives, and drugs apply to veterinary foods as well. The FDA allows labels of pet foods to claim a reduction of disease as a result of consumption of the food, but the claim must generally apply to all similar foods and not solely to the food bearing the claim. Thus, labels of foods low in salt can claim a health benefit for cardiovascular disease, but a label cannot claim efficacy only for that brand. Likewise, diets can be formulated and marketed with a claim to reduce weight, decrease the incidence of stones, or decrease the progression of renal disease as long as the claim applies to the same pet diet in general.

Human dietary supplements

In 1994, the regulation of human dietary supplements changed. The FDA historically had held dietary supplements to the same standards applied to foods, requiring evidence of safety as well as evidence that labeling was truthful and not misleading. Human nutraceutical interest groups sought leniency from the FDA that would allow marketing of products with label statements that might otherwise lead to interpretation as drug claims by the FDA, allowing the FDA to require full premarket approval of the product [1]. The dietary supplement industry was successful in lobbying Congressional passage of the Dietary Supplement Health and Education Act of 1994 (DSHEA), which amends the FDCA to address the regulation of these products specifically. The act effectively restricts the FDA's ability to regulate dietary supplements [11]. The act legally defines a dietary supplements as a "non-tobacco product intended to supplement the diet, that bears or contains one or more of the following dietary ingredients: a vitamin, mineral, herb or other botanical, amino acid, or dietary substance for use by man to supplement the diet by increasing the total daily intake, or a concentrate, metabolite, constituent, extract, or combinations of these ingredients" [1,11]. The act amends the FDCA, with several provisions that apply only to human dietary supplements or dietary ingredients. Whereas a dietary ingredient not marketed as a dietary supplement before October 1994 is considered adulterated (unapproved) unless information is provided ensuring that it does not present a significant or unreasonable risk of illness or injury, premarket safety evaluation is no longer required of new dietary supplement products. The manufacturer of the dietary supplement is responsible for ensuring that a dietary supplement is safe before it is marketed, although it is up to the manufacturer to determine what constitutes assurance of safety [5,6]. The act also provides for the use of various types of statements on the label of dietary supplements that refer to effects on structure or function of the body [2]. Dietary supplement labels still cannot claim to diagnose, prevent, mitigate, treat, or cure a specific disease, however, unless the product is an approved drug. For example, a product cannot claim to cure cancer or treat arthritis. Nevertheless, general claims can be made that link an ingredient to the prevention of selected diseases such as might occur as the result of a nutritional deficiency as long as the deficiency and its incidence are stated on the label. Manufacturers also may describe the supplement's effects on "structure or function" of the body or the "well-being" that follows consumption of the ingredient. Manufacturers must have substantiation that the statements are truthful and not misleading. The product label also must bear the statement: "This statement has not been evaluated by the Food and Drug Administration. This product is not intended to diagnose, treat, cure, or prevent any disease" [1,11]. The act requires that products be labeled with the name and amount of ingredients; if the product is a botanical, the label must specify the part of the plant as well as the designation "dietary supplement." Additionally, the DSHEA grants authority to the FDA to establish good manufacturing practice regulations that govern the preparation, packing, and holding of dietary supplements under conditions that ensure their safety. The FDA recently has released its plan for implementing its responsibilities toward manufacturing [21]. Good manufacturing processes are not necessarily guaranteed simply because FDA resources to prosecute offenders are limited, however. Finally, the DSHEA directs postmarketing responsibilities of the FDA to include monitoring of safety through voluntary adverse event reporting and monitoring of product information, such as labeling, claims, package inserts, and accompanying literature. The FDA is responsible for taking action against any dietary supplement product that proves to be unsafe after being marketed. The burden of proof of lack of safety lays with the FDA, however [2,6,8]. The FDA has published a Dietary Supplement Strategy that describes a 10-year plan for implementing a science-based regulatory program as provided for in the DSHEA, including an adverse event reporting program and a good manufacturing practice. Unfortunately, funding for agencies regulating dietary supplements may limit effective regulation [11].

Two other mechanisms exist for some level of regulation of human dietary supplements. The Federal Trade Commission (FTC) works closely with the FDA in monitoring advertising associated with dietary supplements [11]. Additionally, individual states can restrict the sale of products. For example, several states have banned or restricted the sale of herbal products containing herbal fen-phen [11].

Veterinary nutraceuticals

Not surprisingly, the FDA's approach to nutraceuticals intended for human consumption differs from its approach to those intended for animal consumption. The CVM of the FDA has determined that the DSHEA does not apply to animals or animal feeds and thus not to veterinary nutraceuticals [22,23]. As such, the term *dietary supplements* does not apply to veterinary products and is not used in this article to refer to products marketed for veterinary use. The CVM believes that public health is better served if the special concessions given to human dietary health supplements by the DHSEA do not apply to those given to food-producing animals [22,23]. Such a stance is considered by the CVM to be paramount to their mission of ensuring that harmful residues from either the compound or its metabolite do not reach food intended for human consumption. The CVM has offered several reasons for their decision [22,23]. Although much information exists regarding human dietary components (eg, vitamins, minerals) and supplements, little information exists regarding veterinary dietary supplements, particularly in food-producing animals. Further complicating extrapolation of information among species receiving novel ingredients are the different nutritional requirements and function in the body among species. A final concern of the CVM is that should the act be considered applicable to animals, current "production drugs" (ie, those that increase the production of food) might be considered to "fit" under this act, thus increasing the risk of human exposure to unapproved products. The more lenient approval process afforded human dietary supplements might cause drugs that currently undergo rigid scientific review to bypass restrictions intended to protect the human food consumers [22,23]. Because the DSHEA has legally defined dietary supplements and the act does not apply to veterinary products, the term *dietary supplement* should not be used when referring to veterinary novel ingredients.

The lack of a clear mechanism by which the CVM regulates veterinary nutraceuticals does not mean that these products do not fall under some regulatory jurisdiction. In fact, these products are regulated to some degree at the state level. Both state and federal officials are responsible for implementation of federal or state policies that regulate foods, feed additives, or other oral animal products. Unfortunately, state laws that guide the marketing of nonfederally regulated products are variable. In an attempt to provide conformity among the states, federal and state feed officials have organized the American Association of Feed Control Officials (AAFCO; www.aafco.org). The stated goal of this nonregulatory organization is to "provide a mechanism for developing and implementing uniform and equitable laws, regulation, standards, and enforcement policies for regulating the manufacture, distribution, and sale of animal feeds" such that the use of these products is "safe, effective and useful." The organization has stated its intent to cooperate with members of industries producing the products to promote their effectiveness and usefulness.

Although nonregulatory, the AAFCO nonetheless influences regulation and thus the marketing of oral products administered to animals in many (although not all) states. For those states that follow the AAFCO's guidelines, a manufacturer seeking the sale of an unapproved oral product in a state must provide information necessary for the product to be recognized as an "ingredient" that has been "defined" by the AAFCO [24]. For an ingredient to become defined, information regarding its manufacture as the raw product (eg, synthesis, concentration, extraction) and information regarding safety of the product must be submitted for review by an AAFCO "ingredient investigator." Although the criteria on which an ingredient is approved by the AAFCO are similar to those required for FDA approval of feed additives (manufacturing chemistry, human and animal food safety, utility, labeling, and environmental safety), the extent of information required is not as great (S. Jordre, CVM, FDA, personal communication, October 2002). On approval by the AAFCO investigator, the information is then submitted to the FDA, which then either asks the manufacturer for additional supportive information or approves the ingredient as being "defined" by the AAFCO. This "approval" is not a drug approval; rather, it is a recognition by the FDA that regulatory discretion will ordinarily be followed by the FDA regarding the sale of the product, meaning that under normal circumstances, the FDA will not take regulatory action against the product. Circumstances under which the FDA might change its discretionary approach to a defined ingredient would include but not be limited to mislabeling of the product such that it becomes an unapproved drug and evidence of harm to human beings or animals. Sale of a product that is not a drug, food, or feed additive is more likely to be denied by a state feed official if the product is not listed in the AAFCO publication. It is not clear how many states implement the AAFCO guidelines, which are published annually along with a list of defined ingredients [25]. Although AAFCO's actions toward a product do seem to enhance the safety of the product, it is important to note that veterinary influence on these decisions may be questionable. The veterinary profession might be wise to seek input into AAFCO decisions that require interpretation of medical response (ie, safety, efficacy). Additionally, it is not clear how evidence of AAFCO "approval" as an ingredient will be manifested to the consumer unless states make an effort to communicate the importance of the AAFCO's influence.

The dramatic increase in veterinary nutraceutical use in the last 5 years led the AAFCO to focus specifically on the regulation of these products. Recently, the AAFCO announced a regulatory program entitled "Enforcement Strategy for Marketing Ingredients" (ESMI), which will address unapproved ingredients and ingredients with unapproved claims [26]. The ESMI is intended to encourage and facilitate marketing of novel ingredients in compliance with current state and federal laws regulating animal feeds. State feed regulatory officials will be encouraged to implement a uniform enforcement event coordinated by the AAFCO and FDA. The goals of the strategy are to increase consumer awareness, minimize the availability of unapproved feed ingredients, provide a uniform regulatory approach for animal feeds, assess the success of the strategy, and provide a "level playing field with fair competition among the feed industry." Actions will include prioritizing a focus on those products that present a concern regarding food safety, animal health, and consumer fraud and gathering reputable published information on animal feeds distributed in the marketplace. When the ESMI was initially announced in January 2002, public concern regarding possible regulation of glucosamine led the AAFCO to re-evaluate the first focus of their strategy. The first target of ESMI (2002) was comfrey; in August of 2003, kava became the second target.

The veterinary profession and manufacturers of veterinary nutraceutical products have been proactive in the recognition of the importance of nutraceuticals to animal health. The North American Veterinary Nutraceutical Council was formed in 1996 by interested persons in industry, practice, and academia [4,27]. The primary mission of this organization was to promote and enhance further the quality, safety, and long-term effectiveness of nutraceutical use in veterinary care. Although the Council never effectively implemented a strategy, it defined a veterinary nutraceutical as "a [non-drug] substance which is produced in a purified or extracted form and administered orally to a patient to provide agents required for normal body structure and function and administered with the intent of improving the health and well-being of animals." More recently, two groups have formed in North America with an interest in veterinary nutraceuticals: the Nutraceutical Alliance (www.nutraceuticalalliance.com) based in Canada and the National Animal Supplement Council (NASC; www.nasc.cc) based in the United States. The latter group has taken an aggressive approach in working with the AAFCO to implement voluntary actions among nutraceutical manufacturers that will cause the AAFCO to respond to their products in a positive fashion. The NASC has submitted to the AAFCO and FDA a plan referred to as "Compliance Plus" in the hope that voluntary implementation of the plan by manufacturers of novel ingredients might minimize the need for wide enforcement by state feed officials [28]. The goals of the program are to establish a reporting system for adverse events that might occur in an animal receiving a supplement, require its members to establish manufacturing and quality controls, and fund research that would cause ingredients to meet the AAFCO's definition program. Members also would initiate a self-policing enforcement program to ensure that supplement labels are accurate and void of a drug claim. As such, the proposed Compliance Plus program would surpass the requirements of the AAFCO for ingredient definition. Thus far, the FDA and AAFCO have responded favorably to the ideas set forth in the Compliance Plus program. The proposal identified five ingredients currently not defined by the AAFCO that the Council intends to bring into regulatory compliance: three nutraceuticals—glucosamine, chondroitin sulfate (CDS), and methylsulfonylmethane—and two herbs—garlic and rehmania. The AVMA supported and encouraged regulatory discretion of glucosamine by state feed officials. However, in September of 2003, the Iowa Department of Agriculture and Land Stewardship (IDALS) issued a letter to all pet supplement distributors stating that non-FDA approved pet supplements would no longer be sold in Iowa, including selected products containing glucosamine, since doing so would be a clear violation of Iowa feed regulations. Products containing labels without claims of contents as dietary or nutritional supplement, or with nutritional guarantees will be considered for sale. It is likely that other states will follow suit.

In summary, a manufacturer of a veterinary novel ingredient currently has several options to pursue in the marketing of a product: through FDA approval as either a New Animal Drug Approval (NADA), a Food Additive Petition, or GRAS; through the AAFCO as a defined ingredient; or as an ingredient that is so commonly used in feed that the AAFCO does not require a definition (eg, salt, sugar, water, corn) [24]. In contrast, the only option that can be pursued for a veterinary product with a medicinal intent or claim is through FDA approval of an NADA. Economic recovery of a company that seeks FDA approval for a product would markedly increase the cost of the product; this cost would be passed to the consumers. For veterinary products, the addition potentially could render the cost of the products prohibitive, causing animal owners either not to use the products at all or to use (human) dietary supplements instead. Veterinarians should be reminded that because the DSHEA specifically applies only to human beings and neither dietary supplements nor veterinary nutraceuticals are approved drugs, use or prescription of neither veterinary nor human dietary supplements is protected by the Animal Medical Drug Use Clarification Act of 1994, which otherwise legalizes veterinary extralabel drug use.

Evaluation of novel ingredients

Novel ingredients often are used without doctor supervision; up to 70% of people do not report herbal use to physicians, in part because of their failure to recognize the products as drugs [3]. Likewise, pet owners often do not cite nutraceutical or herbal use when queried regarding drug therapy for their pet. Users of novel ingredients often are not aware of their lack of premarket approval or of the implications that lack of approval might have regarding the safety and efficacy of the products. Indeed, the availability of these products on shelves in pharmacies, health food stores, and groceries as well as on the Internet and advertisements in scientific journals, lay magazines, and newspapers often lead the consumer to assume efficacy and safety. Yet, the lack of regulations and guidelines regarding nutraceutical use in veterinary medicine should lead the buyer to beware.

The FDA's guidelines for new (human) drug approval offer a basis of comparison for the expectations of novel ingredients [11,29]. For drug approval, phase 1 establishes safety in a small number (20–100) of human subjects; phase 2 establishes efficacy in a controlled blind design; and phase 3 further addresses benefits and risks in a much larger population of targeted patients. Good manufacturing procedures are verified through premarketing studies, whereas postmarketing surveillance studies offer insight to long-term effectiveness and safety as well as comparisons to similar marketed products. It is only through similar evidence of manufacturing quality assurance, safety, and efficacy that the veterinary profession can help consumers to gain confidence in the use of these products.

Labeling

The novel ingredient that is inappropriately labeled has a negative impact on safety and efficacy. Drugs that are approved by the FDA undergo intensive evaluation regarding ingredients. Evaluation begins with the raw product: the source (national or international) of ingredients must be an FDA-approved site, and proof of potency and freedom from contamination must be provided. The manufacturing process is examined in depth. Evidence of quality control ensures accuracy in labeled content from tablet to tablet, bottle to bottle, and lot to lot.

Manufacturers of novel ingredients should be held to similar standards and queried about the company's quality assurance programs. Strong consideration should be given to purchasing those products for which assurance in manufacturing can be obtained. Whereas selected manufacturers have been proactive in sharing information regarding their manufacturing procedures (eg, in the author's experience, Nutramax Laboratories), most have not. Manufacturers should be queried about the accuracy of their label and all aspects of their manufacturing program, with an emphasis on which good manufacturing program they follow as outlined in Box 1 (www.dietarysupplementinitiative.com). The manufacturer also should be queried regarding its participation in any of the programs that offer evidence of quality assurance, such as ConsumerLab's certification seal or programs offered by the Institute for Nutraceutical Advancement or trade associations (eg, the NASC when available).

Several sources of scientific information indicate the need to focus on those products whose quality assurance can be verified. CDS offers an example of consistent mislabeling. A University of Maryland study, funded in part by Nutramax Laboratories, found deviations from label claims for CDS in 84% (9 of 11) of the products studied; the amount by which products were mislabeled ranged from 0% to 115% [30]. Further, the study found that products costing less than or equal to $1 per 1200 mg of CDS were seriously deficient (less than 10% of the label claim), suggesting that cheaper products should be avoided. Expense did not guarantee accuracy, however. Several of the most expensive products also were found in this study to be mislabeled. In contrast to CDS, the glucosamine of only 1 of 14 products was mislabeled in this study. Another study found products containing glucosamine sulfate to vary from the label claim, however, with contents ranging from 60% to 140% of the label claim [31].

Independent analysis by commercial laboratories provides evidence of accuracy for some products. ConsumerLab (www. Consumerlabs.com) is a for-profit laboratory that offers a seal of "validation" for dietary supplements that are appropriately labeled. The efforts of the laboratory reflect either a request from a paying manufacturer or a nonmanufacturer-sponsored investigation. In either case, the products to be tested are obtained from commercial sites (grocery or health food stores) rather than from the manufacturer, thus avoiding manufacture-induced bias through product selection. The "pass" criteria vary for each ingredient but include labeling of ingredients by proper name (for herbs, this includes the part of the plant); a match between the listed and measured ingredients; and lack of

Box 1. Questions for manufacturers of nutraceutical products addressing quality assurance

Regarding raw ingredients
1. What are the sources of your ingredients, and what criteria are used in the selection of sources?
2. What methods are used to assure the potency of ingredients, whether active or fillers, and that they are free of impurities, contaminants, or toxins? Are testing methods independent of the manufacturer?
3. How does the label indicate the presence of potential allergens in the formulation?
4. What assurances can be made regarding the proper shipment and storage of raw ingredients, including environmental temperature and humidity, storage containers, and time limits (shelf life)?

Regarding the manufacturing processes
5. Do you employ degreed industrial, chemical, or production engineers?
6. Is a lot-tracking system used that can identify all the ingredient sources of a particular bottle?
7. If multiple production lines are active, what assurances are made to prevent mixing?
8. How is consistency of ingredient content from batch to batch or tablet to tablet assured?
9. What level of accuracy of individual ingredient amount do you aim for (eg,1%, 5%, 10% of the labeled amount)?
10. How is consistency of ingredient content from batch to batch or tablet to tablet assured?
11. If multiple production lines are active, what assurances are made to prevent mixing?
12. What are the nature and scope of cleaning programs? This includes the duration of machine or other device use between cleanings, the types and strengths of cleaning substances used, and the precautions and tests used to ensure products are free of cleaning substances?
13. What assurances can be made regarding the proper shipment and storage of finished products, including environmental temperature and humidity, storage containers, and time limits (shelf life)?

(continued on next page)

14. Do product labels provide information about proper storage conditions? Are expiration dates provided on the label; if yes, on what is the date based? How is the useful shelf life specifically determined?
15. What type of overall good manufacturing practice (GMP) program(s) is (are) followed, and do they meet or exceed any food, drug, dietary supplement, over-the-counter, or other GMP standards?
16. Does the company participate in a program that establishes eligibility through certification (eg, ConsumerLab certification, Institute for Nutraceutical Advancement botanical testing, NNFA's TruLabel program, Paracelsian's BioFIT certification, United States Pharmacopeia (USP) disintegration and/or dissolution standards, or USP Dietary Supplement Verification Program?)

Regarding testing for quality assurance
17. What is the nature of testing programs that guard against or test raw ingredients or final products for the presence of heavy metals, including lead; herbicides, pesticides, and other agricultural chemicals; microbial contaminants; organic and petroleum chemical contaminants; and steroids and antibiotics?
18. Are materials and product testing performed in-house or by independent laboratories, and what kind of testing is performed?
19. At what stages of the manufacturing is testing performed: raw products, after manufacturing, after packaging?

Regarding evidence of efficacy and safety
20. What is the scientific basis for the formulations or substances included in a product?
21. What is the scientific basis for the clinically effective and safe dose?
22. What are the qualifications of the product development group?
23. How does the company remain knowledgeable of the scientific data relevant to the product?
24. Are customers provided with scientific information about the clinical eectiveness of specific ingredients in your products?
25. What scientific clinical studies regarding the product have been published, and are the publications available for distribution to the public?

> 26. Do the studies include comparative analysis of the product? Does the information include negative as well as positive findings? Have the health benefits of the ingredients in the products been published in a monograph or peer-reviewed journal?
> 27. Have the toxic levels been identified for the product, and is this information available on the label?
> 28. Do product labels carry contraindications?
> 29. What system is used for receiving/investigating/reporting adverse events associated with the administration of the product? Are adverse events reported to a national compiling/reporting group?
>
> *Regarding the manufacturing company*
> 30. Does your company belong to any trade associations; if yes, which ones and for how long?
> 31. Is the company independently owned or part of a larger organization? If the latter is the case, what is the nature of the owning company's business?
> 32. What is the overall size of the company (eg, approximate number of employees, number of products, gross annual sales) and is the company publically held or a private company?
>
> *Data from* McAlindon T. Glucosamine for osteoarthritis: dawn of a new era? Lancet 2001;357:247–8.

contaminants, including toxicants (heavy metals, cleaning agents, and, particularly for herbs, pesticides or insecticides), metabolites, and other degradative products of the active ingredient. Products that pass analysis are allowed to place the ConsumerLab seal on the product label.

The public can access selected information from the ConsumerLab web site for a fee ($20 annual fee at the time of this printing) for ingredients that have been tested. Criteria for passing and failing and reasons for failure for specific ingredients can be accessed, as can a list of proprietary products that have passed. A review of the web site reveals disconcerting issues regarding accuracy in labeling. Ten of the ingredients studied by ConsumerLab and listed on their web site have been used in veterinary medicine (although none of the products are veterinary); yet, products of only 4 ingredients (glucosamine, co-enzyme Q, iron, and methosulfonylmethane [MSM]) were accurately labeled at least 80% of the time (Fig. 1). Reasons for failure ranged from unacceptable inaccuracy in labeling of product content to contamination (with heavy metals or pesticides). Among the passing

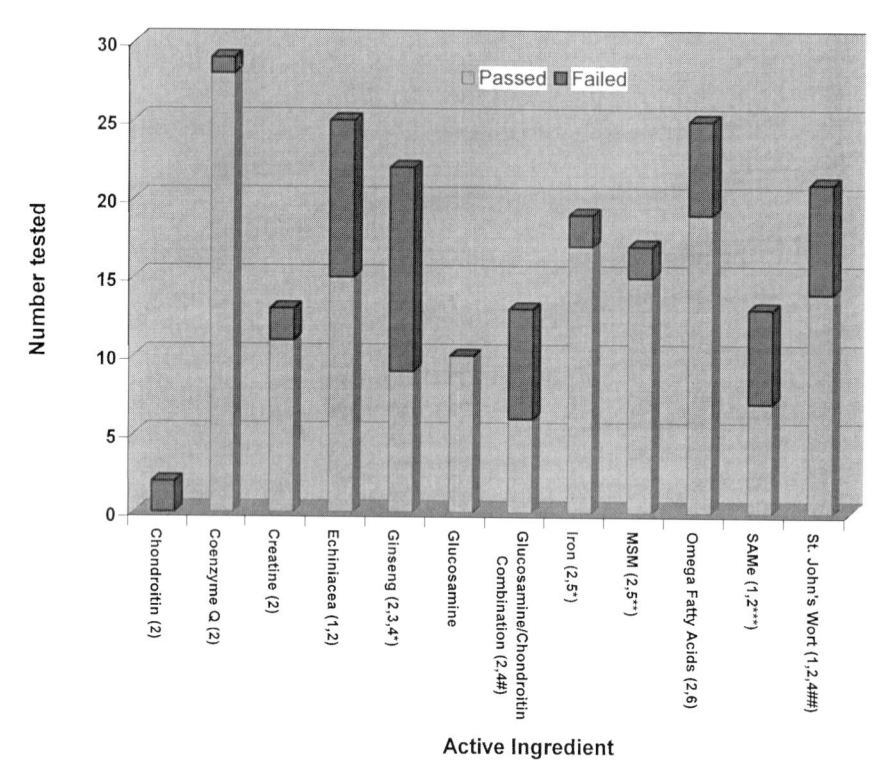

Fig. 1. Accuracy in labeling of selected novel ingredients as measured by ConsumerLab (www.consumerlab.com). 1, inadequate ingredient labeling; 2, mislabeled concentration; 3, pesticide contamination, 4, heavy metal contamination; 5, other contamination; 6, degradation of product; *lead; **DMSO concentration; ***average amount was 50% of labeled claim in failing products; #failure reflected chondroitin portion; ##cadium.

products was Cosamine, the human version of Cosequin DS for dogs, manufactured by Nutramax Laboratories, Inc., Edgewood, MD. Recently, ConsumerLab reported on results of pet products containing novel ingredients. Two of the three products labeled to contain chondroitin sulfate contained no detectable chondroitin sulfate; the third product, Cosequin DS, was found to be accurately labeled. Both products tested for glucosamine (Arthramine and Nutrivet Nutritionals) were accurately labeled, as was the one product tested to contain glucosamine and MSM (DVMSyboviMSM).

The United States Pharmacopeia (USP), whose history dates back to 1820, functions to establish standards and analytic methods for therapeutic agents (USPNF) [32]. Although its activities are nonregulatory, their criteria are recognized in the FDCA and its amendments, including the DSHEA. The USP has recently implemented the Dietary Supplement Verification Program (DSVP) [33], which is a voluntary program intended to protect consumers through accuracy in labeling. As with other volunteer programs (eg, ConsumerLab), the success of the USP program is dependent on voluntary participation by the manufacturers. Consumer purchase power can pressure manufacturers toward compliance, however. Unfortunately, the USP does not intend to address veterinary products. The NASC Compliance Plus program offers a potential mechanism for assurance of accuracy in labeling in veterinary products; however, their program must be held to criteria of independent analysis and the use of ingredients that meet USP standards.

Common sense should guide assessment of labels; indeed, some labels can provide limited evidence of accuracy. The presence of a seal from an unbiased validating laboratory provides variable evidence of accuracy. ConsumerLab, USP, and Good Housekeeping are examples of seals that offer credibility. Note that some manufacturers offer "seals of verification," which mean little and are misleading. The presence of a lot number and expiration date offers some evidence of accuracy in labeling. Labels should contain a list of ingredients and the intended use of the product. Ingredients should be listed by their common name in decreasing order of magnitude based on weight [20]. Note that for selected herbs, the total constituents may not be known. Additionally, the number of constituents in herbs can be overwhelming: garlic contains more than 200 active ingredients [34]. Because the ingredient content can vary with the portion of the plant, the source of the plant (leaf, flower, root, or stem) should be included. Depending on state feed regulations, guarantees must be given for specific feed contents, such as protein, fiber, fat, and selected vitamins and minerals. Adequate directions for use also should be provided [20]. Absence of any of this information should cause the user of the product to look for alternative products. Products whose labeling is accompanied by scare tactics, exaggerated claims, and testimonials should be avoided, as should products whose label includes medical claims, such as "for use in the prevention or treatment of" or "intended to change a body structure or function." The FDA has become somewhat proactive in this regard; its Center for Food Safety and Applied Nutrition (CFSAN) recently warned several web site operators that their promotion of dietary supplements with claims of prevention or treatment of disease may be an illegal activity.

Safety of novel ingredients

"Above all else, do no harm" should be the primary directive regarding the use of novel ingredients. Harm to the patient from the use of novel ingredients can reflect adverse reactions to the active ingredient, excipients, contaminants [7,34], or therapeutic failure, particularly if traditional therapy is overlooked or not pursued in the belief that the novel ingredient will be sufficient. Of these, adverse reactions are the most likely to contribute to harm. Lack of adverse event reports in the literature for a novel ingredient should not be interpreted as evidence of safety, particularly in light of the absence of an effective adverse event reporting system.

Studies that establish safety of novel ingredients can be implemented relatively easily [35]. The outcome measures of toxicity (ie, clinical signs, clinical laboratory changes, evidence of histopathology in organs of excretion, teratogenicity) are more discreet and easily defined than are criteria of efficacy [3]. Toxicity studies can be costly, however, particularly if chronic dosing studies are implemented, and the cost of such studies is likely to be transferred to the consumer. Nonetheless, the profession should demand and expect evidence of safety in the target species of any product marketed for animal use. Unfortunately, the safety of a marketed product is not assured even if evidence of safety, such as acute or chronic dosing toxicity studies, is provided before marketing. Even for FDA-approved drugs, which undergo extensive premarket safety review, it is only during widespread use of the product (ie, phase 4) that many adverse reactions are detected. For example, to establish a real incidence of 2%, several hundred subjects probably should be studied, which is prohibitively expensive. Thus, it is only during postmarket surveillance that evidence of some adverse reactions is realized.

Despite their endogenous (and thus truly "natural") origin, nutraceuticals may be associated with adverse events. For example, creatine, a popular (presumed) ergogenic compound, is consumed by up to 28% of college athletes [18]. It is metabolized to potentially toxic aldehydes, however, including formaldehyde, which may reach sufficient concentrations with chronic dosing to cause undesirable effects [36]. Creatine also may be contaminated during industrial production. Creatine is produced by synthesis from sarcosine (often originating from bovine tissues) and cyanamide, which may result in the presence of contaminants, such as creatinine and dicyanidiamide. These contaminants should be delineated on the label [37]. Androstenedione is a popular product used by athletes because of its potential (perceived) conversion in the body to testosterone. Neither the efficacy nor safety of this product has been demonstrated, however, despite the potential adverse effects documented for other anabolic steroids [18]. L-tryptophan is an example of a natural yet endogenous amino acid that is not necessarily safe. It is approved for use when added to proteins in small quantities to improve the quality of nutrition. In this form, it is presumably safe; yet, when used as a sedative in the free amino-acid form, more than 1500 users developed an eosinophilic myalgia syndrome, probably because of a contaminant during the manufacturing process. Close to 40 people died as a result of this effect [11]. Phenylalamine is another amino acid that has been used in its free form. Essential in the diet, phenylalamine has been added to improve the quality of food; however, when used in large doses as an analgesic, it can cause severe amino acid imbalances [38].

As with drugs, novel ingredients may cause side effects that, although not dangerous, certainly are undesirable. Examples in veterinary patients might include odor as a result of fish oil administration and diarrhea and flatulence with products containing fiber or probiotics. Finally, products may include materials to which an animal may be intolerant, such as lactose, or antigens that might contribute to an allergy [25]. A final point to consider is the source of the raw ingredients. For example, evidence of ingredient purchase from countries free of transmissible spongiform encephalopathies (TSE) should be established.

The FDA is explicitly prohibited by the DSHEA from requiring manufacturers to test dietary supplements for safety or efficacy before sale [11]. Standardize doses or strengths are not required of these products. Legislation currently regulating dietary supplements has been described as dangerously inadequate; although intended to be a compromise that reduced regulatory burdens on the manufacturer, in practice, the DSHEA has allowed dangerous products to remain on the market [11]. Thankfully, some manufacturers have proactively provided evidence that supports product safety. For example, the assumed safety of glucosamine and CDS has been scientifically demonstrated when the compounds are administered according to the labeled dose for several weeks in human beings [26] and animals [39–41].

Of the novel ingredients, herbal/botanical products may present a greater risk compared with nutraceuticals, although the incidence of adverse reactions does not seem to be as high in human medicine as that for either prescription or over-the-counter drugs [6]. Although herbal products are described in advertisements as "mild" because they are "natural," the prudent user of herbal products recognizes that the products are natural to plants rather than to animals [11,34]. One only has to consider the poisonous yet "natural" mushroom. Indeed, animals have developed sophisticated mechanisms (eg, efflux pumps, drug-metabolizing enzymes) to prevent the absorption and accumulation of plant chemical products in the body. Further, many drugs originally were discovered because of their presence in plants; because ingestion of the plant to consume the chemical of interest often was associated with ingestion of undesirable compounds, chemicals of interest have been extracted and concentrated or synthesized to minimize the risk of contaminants [6].

Herbal products may be unsafe for several reasons. Active ingredients, whether the intended ingredient or another chemical within the plant, may not be safe, particularly when used in excess. Pet owners assuming these products to be natural and safe may not hesitate to dose their pet beyond the labeled recommendations. Five broad classes of active chemicals exist in plants: volatile oils (eg, catnip, garlic, citrus), fixed oils, resins, alkaloids, and glycosides. Of these, fixed oils, often used as emollients, demulcents, and bases for other agents, are among the least toxic. Alkaloids are among the most pharmacologically active plant chemicals and include a wide range of potentially harmful products. Resins can be strong gastrointestinal irritants [6,17,34].

The risk of adverse effects to herbs is increased by the presence of many active ingredients in the same plant. Indeed, herbalists often used unpurified plant extracts because of the belief that different chemicals interact synergistically [6]. The portion of the plant (ie, leaf, flower, stem, root, seed) may influence safety. Whereas one portion of the plant might be safe, another portion might not. Herbalists often administer the whole plant in the belief that, in contrast to the purified extract, toxicity is reduced by a buffering effect of the whole herb [6]. During growth of the plant, environmental contaminants may become unintended residues during the manufacturing process. Microorganisms, including bacteria, fungi, and molds, can either directly contaminate the product or produce contaminating toxins. Bacterial contamination is more likely with root products as opposed to flower or leaf products. Heavy metals, such as lead, cadmium, or mercury, increasingly are contaminating plants exposed to environmental pollutants. Further, unless organically grown, insecticides and pesticides can contaminate herbal products. Consumers are often unaware that legislation regulating exposure to environmental contaminants vary and that foreign sources of herbal products may present a greater risk to the consumer than domestic sources [17]. Factors during production and storage, such as storage length and conditions, can alter herbal potency and quality [11]. Finally, herbal products might be supplemented with active ingredients (often referred to as herbs), such as ephedrine, caffeine, or fenfluramine (the latter ingredient being one of the two ingredients in the notorious phen-fen dietary supplements). Health Canada recently has issued a warning to Canadians not to use selected herbal products that contain undeclared prescription drugs, including indomethacin, diethylstilbestrol, and alprazolam (an antianxiety drug).

An often unrecognized contribution to adverse effects are interactions among active ingredients in herbs or between herbs and drugs that the patient also might be using (Table 1) [3]. The risk of drug interactions in persons consuming herbs has caused the American Society of Anesthesiologists to generate a brochure for its members entitled "What You Should Know About Your Patients' Use of Herbal Medicine." Examples of potential interactions involving the central nervous system (CNS) include enhanced stimulation by caffeine, ephedra, yohimbine, guarana, and ginseng as well as enhanced sedation by valerian, kava, and St. John's wort. Drug-induced hemostasis defects may be potentiated by garlic, ginger, gingko, ginseng, chamomile, feverfew, and bromelain, whereas the effects of hypoglycemia may be exacerbated by bilberry, bitter melon, dandelion, and garlic. Echinacea and astragalus may offset the immunomodulatory effects of corticosteroids or other immunosuppressants.

Labeling techniques may contribute to the advent of adverse effects. The lack of quality control already has been addressed. Those products that contain more than the labeled dose present a risk of overdose; those with less present a risk of therapeutic failure. Manufacturers may improperly

Table 1
Drug interactions of selected popular herbs

Herb	Side effect	Drug interactions	Effect
Ephedra	Hypertension, cardiac arrest, seizures, respiratory depression	Cardiac glycosides, halothane	Arrhythmias
Feverfew	Interference with hemostasis, mouth ulcers	Warfarin and other coumarin derivatives, aspirin and other antiplatelet drugs	Prolonged bleeding time
Garlic	Nausea, flatulence, stomach irritation	Aspirin and other antihemostatics	Prolonged bleeding time
Ginger	Heartburn	Aspirin and other antihemostatics	Prolonged bleeding time
Ginseng	Hypertension, tachycardia	Hypoglycemics, cardiac stimulants, warfarin	Hypoglycemia, enhanced hypertension and tachycardia, decreased efficacy
Gingko	Abnormal bleeding, hemorrhage		
Licorice	Hypertension, hypokalemia, fluid retention		
Senna	Abdominal cramping, electrolyte disturbances	Oral drugs, diuretics	Decreased absorption, enhanced hypokalemia
St. John's wort	Photosensitivity, peripheral neuropathy, serotonergic crisis	Anesthetics, other behavior-modifying drugs	Prolonged effects, enhanced side effects
Valerian	Headache, nausea	Anesthetics	Prolonged effects

Data from Flanagan K. Preoperative assessment: safety considerations for patients taking herbal products. J Perianesth Nursing 2001;16:19–26.

identify plants [11]. Even if properly identified, the consumer may have difficulty in identifying a product as potentially dangerous, because an herbal agent may be referred to by many different names (Table 2) or an herbal name may be used in lieu of the more easily recognized chemical name (eg, guarana for ephedrine or ma huang for caffeine). The FDA has become more proactive in directing manufacturers to list generic drug names in lieu of or in addition to herbal names; however, consumers may have to look closely. For example, the label of a dietary herbal product reveals the ingredients to include multiple herbs, including guarana and ma hung (Fig. 2). Closer examination of the label at the bottom reveals the product to contain ephedra and caffeine. The recent recognition of herbal medications containing ephedrine as a cause of adverse cardiovascular reactions (including death) in human beings underscores the need for caution in using herbs. In one study, 54% of persons taking dietary supplements containing ephedrine reported agitation and 21% dropped out because of side effects [2]. The FDA has proposed rules that limit

Table 2
Side effects of selected herbal or botanical products

Source of warning	Novel ingredient	Type	Common names or ingredient	Perceived risk
Text (Springer 1993)		Food	Laurel berry oil	Sesquiterpene is a potent allergen with topical use
		Food	Mustard (black)	Topical allergy
		Food	Nutmeg (seed)	Nausea, vomiting, tachycardia, convulsions, miosis, mydriasis, euphoria, hallucinations
		Food	Nutmeg (oil)	Safrol is mutagenic and carcinogenic
		Food	Oregano	Gastrointestinal irritation, uterine contractions
		Food	Sage	Oil (thujone) with chronic intake of 15 g per dose
US Food and Drug Administration Medwatch (www.fda.gov)	*Aristolochia* sp	Herbal/botanical	Fang chi, fang ji, guan mu tong, guang fang ji, kou-boui, kwangbanggi, ma dou ling, mil homens, mokuboi, qing mu xiang, sei-mokkou, tian xian teng, birthwort, Dutchman's pipe, oval leaf, serpentaria, ukulwe, Virginia snakeroot, yellowmouth	Contains aristolochic acid, which is a potent nephrotoxin as well as a carcinogen
	Ascarum	Herbal/botanical	Do-saishin, tanyou-saishin, xi xin, colic root, false coltsfoot, wild ginger, ginger, snakeroot (eg, Canada, Southern, Vermont)	Contains aristolochic acid, which is a potent nephrotoxin as well as a carcinogen
	Akebia trifolita caulis	Herbal/botanical	Mu tong	Contains aristolochic acid, which is a potent nephrotoxin as well as a carcinogen

Combinations	Herbal/botanical	Ba zheng, san, dang gui si ni tan, dao chi san, fu fang di hu tang, gan lu xiao du dan, kou yan ning, long dan xie gan tang, pai shi tang, xiao ji yin zi, xin yi san, yang yin xoao yan tang	Product may contain aristolochic acid; which is a potent nephrotoxin as well as a carcinogen
Piper methysticum	Herbal/botanical	Kava	Hepatotoxicity
Lipokinetix	Herbal/botanical	Norephedrine (phenylpropanolomine), caffeine, yohimbine, diiotothyroine, sodium usniate	Hepatotoxicity
Pericum perforatum	Herbal/botanical	St. John's wort	Drug interactions as a result of induction of drug-metabolizing enzymes
Triiodothyroacetic acid (TRIAC)	Herbal/botanical	Tiratricol	Potent thyroid hormone that may cause heart attack and strokes
Ephedra sinica	Herbal/botanical	Ephedrine alkaloids, ma huang	Exacerbation of hypertension and other cardiac conditions, complications in pregnant women
Gamma hydroxybutyric acid (GHB), gamma butyrolactone(GBL), and 1,4 butanediol		GHBs	"Party drugs" or sleep aids can cause low respiratory rates, bradycardia, seizures, vomiting, unconsciousness, death

(continued on the next page)

Table 2 (continued)

Source of warming	Novel ingredient	Type	Common names or ingredient	Perceived risk
Text (Springer 1993)		Food	Laurel berry oil	Sesquinterpene is a potent allergen with topical use
		Food	Mustard (black)	Topical allergy
		Food	Nutmeg (seed)	Nausea, vomiting, tachycardia, convulsions, miosis, mydriasis, euphoria, hallucinations
		Food	Nutmeg (oil)	Safrol is mutagenic and carcinogenic
		Food	Oregano	Gastrointestinal irritation, uterine contractions
		Food	Sage	Oil (thujone) with chronic intake of 15 g per dose

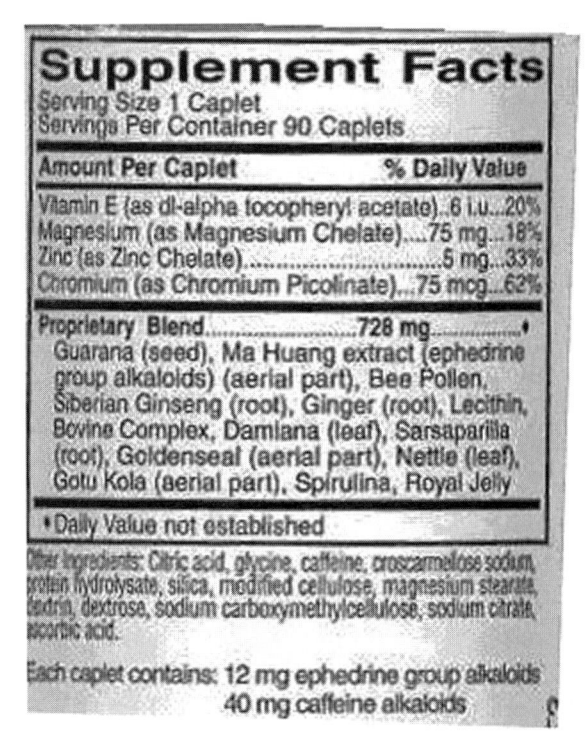

Fig. 2. This herbal dietary supplement used for weight loss contains multiple ingredients. Closer examination of the bottom of the label reveals the product to include caffeine and ephedrine, two compounds that share similar side effects on the central nervous and cardiovascular systems. Toxicity after ingestion of this or similar products has been reported in dogs.

the amount of ephedrine alkaloids in products (not more than 8 mg in a 6-hour period or 24 mg in a 24-hour period) and require labeling and marketing measures that make clear the risks associated with the use of such products [42].

A number of other herbs have been associated with adverse effects (see Tables 1 and 2). In 1975, the FDA reported more than 30 herbs prepared as teas to be unsafe [43]. Excessive consumption of herbal teas containing senna, aloe, buckthorn, and other laxatives has been associated with the death of four women. The FDA also is currently investigating the potential association of hepatotoxicity and the administration of kava (kava kava, Piper methysticum), an herbal product used for a variety of disorders, including stress and anxiety. Recent regulatory actions offer evidence of the risks that can be associated with the use of these unapproved products.

Adverse events have also occurred in veterinary patients receiving novel ingredients as is exemplified by the Society for Prevention of Cruelty to Animals Poison Control Center (APCC) at the University of Illinois at

Urbana. The APCC recently published a report of adverse reactions in 47 dogs that ingested a popular weight loss dietary supplement containing guarana (caffeine) and ma huang (ephedrine) [44]. Seventeen percent of the dogs died after the appearance of clinical signs expected from these central and cardioactive compounds.

The importance of reporting adverse reactions to any product, drug or nondrug, used to treat animals cannot be overemphasized. Unfortunately, the existence of an adverse reaction to a product does not guarantee that the profession or pet owner will become aware of the adversity. The users of the product (pet owners and veterinarians) must be able to recognize the clinical sign as an adverse reaction and then associate the reaction with the administration of the product. The reaction must be reported in a manner that is likely to lead to evaluation of cause and effect between the product and reaction. Finally, the reaction must be analyzed using appropriate statistical methods and then reported back to the profession. Consumers should be encouraged to report adverse events associated with novel ingredients to the product manufacturer as well as to their veterinarian. Although mechanisms for reporting adverse events in human or veterinary medicine are currently limited, effective mechanisms are evolving. Among the FDA's postmarket responsibilities toward (human) dietary supplements is the monitoring of product safety [34], although the FDA may remove a dangerous or supplement only when and if the product presents an "imminent hazard to public health or safety" [11]. The burden of proof is on the FDA. The FDA CFSAN recently implemented the Adverse Events Reporting System (CAERS) to be used as a monitoring tool for dietary supplements as well as other medicinal products. Adverse events also can be reported for human products through the FDA's MedWatch program [42]. Some of the recent FDA actions taken to address safety of dietary supplements can be reviewed at ConsumerLab.com [45] or at the FDA's Medwatch program or the FDA's Center for Drug Evaluation and Research (CDER) [42]. Information regarding herb use also is available at the ConsumerLab.com site [46].

Unfortunately, the current FDA sites for reporting adverse events to dietary supplements do not pertain to veterinary products. Until currently, the only program that addressed veterinary adverse events was the USP Veterinary Reporting Program, which addresses adverse events with any therapeutic agent used in veterinary patients (eg, drugs, nutraceuticals, herbs, vaccines, insecticides) [47]. An advantage to this program is the relatively rapid turnaround regarding reporting to the profession for products associated with adverse events. Unfortunately, because of funding issues and underuse by the veterinary profession, this program was discontinued recently. The AVMA and NASC have recognized the importance of reporting animal adverse events to novel ingredients and individually are striving to develop effective reporting mechanisms for the veterinary profession. An important component of the NASC Compliance

Plus program, should it be implemented and widely used by veterinary nutraceutical manufacturers, will be adverse event reporting by manufacturers to the FDA. The NASC should be encouraged to ensure that reporting mechanisms are easily used by consumers and veterinarians, that manufacturers be thorough in their reporting to the FDA, and that effective and accurate statistical analysis of the events be reported back to the users of these products in a timely fashion.

Efficacy of novel ingredients

With a multibillion dollar industry at stake, the plethora and variety of advertising and labeling claims or testimonials that accompany novel ingredients are not surprising. Unfortunately, consumers often are not trained to discern fact, fiction, or wishful thinking. Indeed, veterinarians often do not realize that advertisements and labels for these products are misleading if not illegal. Consumer confidence in the scientific process and in the health care professional's input is subsequently undermined.

Evidence of efficacy for drugs generally is supported by pharmacokinetic and pharmacodynamic information [13,29]. Pharmacokinetic data establish the time course of drug movement through the body and serve as the basis for the design of a dosing regimen. Such data are of little relevance without pharmacodynamic data that establish plasma (tissue) drug concentrations necessary to induce the desired therapeutic response, however. Defining the outcome measures for a therapeutic response may be difficult, depending on the target illness, particularly for novel ingredients. Whereas heart rate can easily be measured as an indicator of cardiac slowing attributable to a drug, defining response to a product intended to treat osteoarthritis is hampered by the lack of discreet measurements of improvement.

Collecting each of these pieces of evidence of efficacy may be more difficult for novel ingredients, particularly for nutraceuticals as compared with drugs. Pharmacokinetic analysis of a compound requires that the compound be measured in a body tissue (usually blood, serum, or plasma) across time after administration of a dose. The data can describe individual drug movements important to establishing efficacy: absorption from the gastrointestinal tract, distribution from blood to the targeted site of action, and elimination from the body through metabolism or excretion. Because nutraceuticals also exist in the body, discriminating an exogenously administered product from the endogenous product can be difficult and is likely to require a radiolabeled product. In addition, many nutraceuticals are marketed as a mixture of compounds; herbs naturally contain multiple ingredients. The disposition of each compound should be established in support of product efficacy. Among the movements that define disposition of exogenously administered compounds, evidence of absorption might be the most critical; efficacy does not exist if the product cannot be orally absorbed.

As with drugs, many factors can alter the oral absorption of a novel ingredient. Product formulation, destruction of the active ingredient in the gastrointestinal tract, the molecular weight of the ingredient, and the impact of hepatic first-pass metabolism are among the most important. The extent of oral absorption of a compound is described by bioavailability, or the percentage of an oral dose that reaches systemic circulation. Bioavailability is the ratio of the intravenous concentration (100%) compared with the oral concentration of the ingredient in plasma across time [13]. The marketed oral preparation should be studied in the target animal. Bioavailability studies for herbs are compounded by the number of active ingredients in a preparation, each of which should be studied independently. For nutraceuticals, although fewer active ingredients are present, the endogenous chemical is often impossible to discern from the exogenous product. Radiolabeling of the compound of interest may allow discrimination. For example, using radiolabeling, the bioavailability of glucosamine hydrochloride in humans is 84%, suggesting that most of the oral dose reaches systemic circulation. In contrast, the oral bioavailability of the sulfate salt is only 47%, indicating that only half of the oral dose of this salt reaches systemic circulation [21,48]. Thus, the oral dose of the sulfate salt should be approximately twice that of the hydrochloride salt. Labeling often may not provide doses adjusted for differences among the forms of the active ingredient or preparations. Extrapolation of oral bioavailability data among species should be made carefully. Recently, the oral bioavailability of glucosamine in dogs was reported to be 10% [49], suggesting that the oral milligrams per kilograms dose of glucosamine should be much higher in dogs compared with people. Another example of differences in bioavailability exists for CDS, an ingredient whose oral bioavailability markedly decreases with an increase in molecular weight. The permeability of CDS varies inversely with molecular weight, with CDS with a low molecular weight of 17,000 having the most favorable permeability coefficient. Unfortunately, product labels are not likely to include the molecular weight of the product, and manufacturers might be queried about the size of the CDS included in the product. Nutramax Laboratories can provide evidence that molecular weight of the CDS in their product is predominantly less than or equal to 17,000 [30].

Distribution of the product to the target site should be demonstrated whenever possible. As an endogenous product, however, metabolism to basic molecules and incorporation into tissues may not easily be discriminated from incorporation of the intact molecule. Metabolism to building parts does not necessarily preclude efficacy if synthetic efficiency is improved during diseased-induced states of deficiency. Determining routes of excretion may help to predict and assess potential organ toxicity.

Collection of pharmacodynamic information that describes clinical response may be difficult for novel ingredients, because the diseases being studied often are complex and characterized by outcome measures that are neither easily measured nor discreet. For the same reasons, establishing the most effective dosing regimen (dose and interval) may be difficult. As with drugs, experimental models must be developed that allow assessment of the product under conditions that are clinically relevant or spontaneously diseased animals must be studied [50]. For the latter group, variability in the type of disease may either preclude detection of significant or clinical differences or necessitate a prohibitively expensive study group size. Studies of spontaneously diseased animals also may be influenced by ethical constraints that require the continued use of traditional therapies in addition to the treatment being studied.

When assessing the validity of scientific information supporting the safety and efficacy of nutraceuticals, criteria that apply to clinical trials for drugs should apply to clinical trials for novel ingredients [51–53]. The report must include a description of the study design and methods, such as random assignment of treatments, placebo controls, and blinding techniques that reduce the risk of scientific bias. The need for placebos in veterinary medicine cannot be overemphasized. In human beings, the placebo effect in studies evaluating pain can be profound, ranging from 30% to 40% or more [2]. A similar if not higher placebo effect should be expected in veterinary medicine. Handling of animals during treatment with a novel ingredient (or drug) is likely to make the pet feel better. Additionally, the owners themselves may interpret a placebo effect because of the expected improvement. The requirements for randomization, a placebo group, and the avoidance of traditional therapies are examples of reasons why evidence of informed consent (not simply permission but provision of truthful information) must be provided in the report [52]. Other criteria of a well-designed study should include methods to standardize treatment groups and appropriate statistical analysis. In addition to the level of type I error (the percent error allowed for identifying a significant difference when one does not truly exist, generally 5% or $P \leq 0.05$), the power (type II error; percent error allowed for failing to detect a significant difference when one truly does exist, generally 80%) of the study should be given [54]. The larger the variability in the outcome measures, the greater is the number of animals that must be studied to detect a significant difference. Care should be taken not to interpret the lack of a significant difference as an indication that the groups are the same unless the study investigators demonstrate that the study design provided sufficient power. Credence might be given to the results of a study that demonstrates a clinical difference despite the lack of statistical difference. Likewise, a significant difference may not be relevant if the difference is not clinically relevant [51]. For example, products containing glucosamine and CDS cause a significant decrease in the indices of red blood cells or platelet activity in dogs and cats, but these differences are within clinical normals and thus are not clinically relevant [41,55]. Negative clinical trials also should be reported; manufacturers should be queried about their inclusion in distributed information (see Box 1) [56]. As with drugs, care should be taken when extrapolating information from studies in a species other than the one in which the compound is to be used. Differences in pharmacokinetics and pharmacodynamics among species may be too great to allow accurate extrapolations.

For selected novel ingredients, scientific evidence of efficacy is becoming available. For herbs, historical use has contributed to a level of efficacy not enjoyed by nutraceuticals. Not surprisingly, herbal therapy is well established in European and Asian countries, as evidenced by the numbers of texts originating from these countries supporting their use [17,34]. Manufacturers, academicians, and independent laboratories are increasingly contributing to the pool of credible scientific data on herbs and nutraceuticals. Glucosamine offers an example of the types of studies that can support nutraceutical safety and efficacy. Surprisingly, scientific data supporting the efficacy of glucosamine in the treatment of osteoarthritis have existed for some time. McCarty [40] noted in 1994 that "Osteoarthritis...causes misery and disability to tens of millions of...Americans" and that "there is no truly rational and well tolerated drug therapy for this disorder..." He notes further, however, that "every published clinical study [of glucosamine] reports significant...efficacy without side effects." Indeed, a review of the literature reveals interest and support for glucosamine since the 1950s and 1960s. McCartney [40] suggests that the fault lies with the medical community by allowing research to be guided by the pharmaceutical companies that have chosen the drug options for approval. Much of the more recent data regarding the efficacy of glucosamine in treating osteoarthritis reflects the efforts of Nutramax Laboratories, a major manufacturer of a patented glucosamine-CDS product. The path of their efforts offers a model as to how scientific evidence in support of a nutraceutical use might be addressed. Evidence of efficacy has been provided using in vitro models (eg, chondrocyte cultures to cartilage cores [57]), experimental animal models (eg, rabbit surgically induced joint instability [58], chemically induced canine synovitis), and studies in patients with spontaneous disease, including questionnaire-based assessment of clinical response [49], and well-defined syndromes in human beings and dogs [5,59,60]. Care must be taken to avoid the bias that might be associated with industry-supported data, although credibility can be maintained if the study design includes methods to prevent bias. The addition of nonbiased data generated by nonindustry-sponsored research should be sought, however, as has occurred for glucosamine sulfate [60]. The scientific evidence of efficacy for glucosamine in the treatment of osteoarthritis is sufficient to cause the Arthritis Foundation to state that "The notion that glucosamine and chondroitin might have disease-modifying effects in OA is highly appealing and supported by preliminary data" [61]. The role of novel ingredients in veterinary medicine is a two-edged sword. Clearly, these products can provide a rational, safe, and effective approach for the prevention or management of selected disorders. However, the lack of approval places the burden of scientific assessment solely on the veterinary community.

Summary

Veterinarians have an opportunity to help educate their clients regarding the safety and efficacy of novel ingredients used by their clients. This is no small task because of the lack of acceptable information. Clients should be counseled regarding the lack of scientific evidence and be encouraged to discriminate fact from fiction, including many testimonials. Safety should be of primary concern, and clients should be encouraged not to neglect traditional therapies in lieu of novel ingredients unless clinical evidence of efficacy exists. Quality assurance is equally important and cannot be underestimated. Clients are likely to resort to less expensive products. Clients should be directed to the advice offered by the Arthritis Foundation as follows: "When a supplement has been studied with good results, find out which brand was used and buy that." Although skepticism is encouraged regarding any unknown product with medicinal indications, open mindedness should also guide the veterinarian as these products are considered. Indeed, veterinarians should take actions to ensure that the use of these compounds is accomplished within the confines of the veterinary-client-patient relationship, thus ensuring the role of the veterinarian in the health and well-being of animals, regardless of the modality of therapy. The veterinary profession should support the development of standards that might guide manufacturers of novel ingredients to meet criteria that protect the consumer. Likewise, we should encourage manufacturers and agencies to fund veterinary clinical trials to provide evidence for the use of these potentially exciting compounds. Above all else, the veterinarian needs to become a credible resource of information about the possible role of these products. The lack of a regulatory mechanism that establishes the safety and efficacy of these products is not justification for ignoring the potential therapeutic benefit of some of these products. Veterinarians should follow the advice of the Arthritis Foundation, which notes: "Since glucosamine is self-prescribed...health care professionals are not regarded [to have] objective advice. This situation must change. It is time for the profession to accommodate the possibility that many nutritional products may have valuable therapeutic effects" [61].

Further readings

Abdel Fattah W, Hammand T. Chondroitin sulfate and glucosamine: a review of their safety profile. Am Nutraceut Assoc 2001;3:16–23.

Ask the supplier. Supplement Quality.com. Available at: http://www.supplementquality.com/ask/index.html Accessed November 15, 2002.

Current Good Manufacturing Practice in Manufacturing. Package or Holding Dietary Supplements: Proposed Rule. 21 CFR Ch. 1, Docket No. 96N–0417 RIN 0910–AA59.

Department of Health and Human Services, Food and Drug Administration. Federal Register 1997;62(25):1–21.

Fetrow CW, Avilta JR. The professional's handbook of complementary and alternative medicines. Springhouse, PA: Springhouse; 1999.

Graham AS, Hatton RC. Creatine: a review of efficacy and safety. J Am Pharm Assoc 1999;39: 803–10.
Gruenwald G, Brendler T, Naenicke C, editors. The physicians' desk reference for herbal medications. 2nd edition. Montvale, NJ: Medical Economics Company; 2000.
Guidelines for alternative and complementary veterinary medicine. J Am Vet Med Assoc 1996; 209:1027–8.
Guyatt GH, Sackett DL, Cook DJ. User's guides to the medical literature: what were the results and will they help me in caring for my patients? JAMA 1994;271(1):59–63.
Lund EM, James KM, Neaton JD. Veterinary randomized clinical trial reporting: a review of the small animal literature. J Vet Intern Med 1998;12:57–60.
Nutraceuticals. Hope or hype? CATNIP: a newsletter for caring cat owners. Tufts University School of Veterinary Medicine. 1996;4(4).
Pecci MA, Lombardo JA. Performance-enhancing supplements. Phys Med Rehabil Clin North Am 2000;11:949–60.
Varga J, Himenez SA, Uitto J. L-tryptophan and the eosinophilia-myalgia syndrome: current understanding and pathogenesis. J Invest Dermatol 1993;100:975–1055.
Vickery G. Safety of herbal remedies. Ann Pharmacother 1999;33:1359–62.

References

[1] DeFeice SL. The nutraceutical revolution: its impact on food industry R & D. Trends Food Sci Technol 1995;6:59–61.
[2] Filmore CM, Bartoli L, Back R, et al. Nutrition and dietary supplements. Complementary therapies. Phys Med Rehabil Clin North Am 1999;10:673–703.
[3] Flanagan K. Preoperative assessment: safety considerations for patients taking herbal products. J Perianesth Nurs 2001;16:19–26.
[4] Nutraceutical maker calls for industry standards. J Am Vet Med Assoc 1995;207:1399.
[5] Deal CL, Moskowitz RW. Nutraceuticals as therapeutic agents in osteoarthritis. Rheum Dis Clin North Am 1999;25(2):379–95.
[6] Poppenga RH. Risks associated with the use of herbs and other dietary supplements. Vet Clin North Am Small Anim Pract 2001;17(3):455–77.
[7] Bauer JE. Evaluation of nutraceuticals, dietary supplements and functional food ingredients for companion animals. J Am Vet Med Assoc 2001;208:1755–60.
[8] Boothe DM. Nutraceuticals in veterinary medicine: part I. Definitions and regulations. Compend Contin Educ Pract Vet 1997;20:1248–55.
[9] Boothe DM. Nutraceuticals in veterinary medicine: part II. Safety and efficacy. Compend Contin Educ Pract Vet 1998;19:15–21.
[10] Nutraceuticals "set to outstrip drug markets". Marketletter 1994;December 12:26.
[11] Sardina J. Misconceptions and misleading information prevail—less regulation does not mean less danger to consumers: dangerous herbal weight products. J Law Health 1999/2000;14:107–32.
[12] Boothe DM. Regulatory issues [Appendix 1]. In: Boothe DM, editor. Small animal clinical pharmacology and therapeutics. Philadelphia: WB Saunders; 2001. p. 693–705.
[13] Boothe DM. Principles of drug therapy. In: Boothe DM, editor. Small animal clinical pharmacology and therapeutics. Philadelphia: WB Saunders; 2001. p. 3–17.
[14] Nutrition Labeling and Education Act (amendments). 21 USC 343, 1990.
[15] Food labeling: requirements for nutrient content claims, health claims, and statements of nutritional support for dietary supplements. 21 CRF Part 101, Docket No. 95–0282. Department of Health and Human Services, Food and Drug Administration. Federal Register 1995;60:249.

[16] Troutman LM, Vaughn SD, Schmerfield G, Beaulieu AJ. Impact of the Animal Drug Availability Act on veterinary practitioners and the animal health industry. J Am Vet Med Assoc 1997;210:1597–600.
[17] Bisset NG, Wichtl M, editors. Herbal drugs and phytopharmaceutics. Ann Arbor: MedPharm Scientific Publishers, CRC Press; 1994.
[18] Metzle JD, Smale E, Levine SR, et al. Creatine use among young athletes. Pediatrics 2001;108:421–5.
[19] Wagner AB. Herbal foods. Texas food processor. Texas Agricultural Extension Service 1996;XVV(3):1–3.
[20] Siegel H. When is a dog food really a drug? Good Dog 1995; November/December:8–9.
[21] Conte A, Volpi N, Palmieri L, et al. Biochemical and pharmacokinetic aspects of oral treatment with chondroitin sulfate. Arzeimittelforschung 1995;45:918–25.
[22] Department of Health Human Services. Inapplicability of the Dietary Supplement Health and Education Act to animal products. Federal Register 1996;61:17706–8.
[23] FDA's view of dietary supplement legislation. FDA Veterinarian 1995; May/June:5–6.
[24] Anderson MA, Slater MR, Hammand TA. Results of a survey of small animal practitioners on the perceived clinical efficacy and safety of an oral nutraceutical. Prev Vet Med 1999;38:65–73.
[25] Association of American Feed Control Officials. 2002 official publication. Sharon Senesac, Assistant Secretary-Treasurer, PO Box 478, Oxford, IN 47971.
[26] AAFCO Enforcement Strategy for Marketed Ingredients (ESMI) Working Group. American Association of Feed Control Officials. Available at: http://www.aafco.org. Accessed November 15, 2002.
[27] Nutramax calls for nutraceutical standards. DVM Newsmagazine 1995; August:34.
[28] Compliance Plus. National Animal Supplement Council. Available at: http://www.nasc.cc. Accessed November 15, 2002.
[29] Mathieu MP. New drug development: a regulatory overview. 3rd edition. Waltham, MA: Parexel International Corporation; 1994.
[30] Adabowale AO, Cox DS, Liang Z, et al. Analysis of glucosamine and chondroitin sulfate content in marketed products and the caco-2 permeability of chondroitin sulfate raw materials. Am Nutraceut Assoc 2000;3:37–44.
[31] Russell AS, Aghazadey-Habashi A, Jamali F. Active ingredient consistency of commercially available glucosamine sulfate products. J Rheumatol 2002;29:2407–9.
[32] United States Pharmacopeia National Formulary (USPNF). The official compendia of standards. Rockville, MD: United States Pharmacopeia Convention; 2000.
[33] United States Pharmacopeia Dietary Supplement Certification Program. Frequently asked questions. United State Pharmacopeia. Available at: http://www.usp.org/dietary/faq.htm. Accessed November 15, 2002.
[34] De Smet PAGM, Keller K, Hansel R, et al, editors. Adverse effects of herbal drugs. New York: Springer-Verlag; 1993.
[35] Walum E. Acute oral toxicity. Environ Health Perspect 1998;106:497–503.
[36] Yu PH, Deng Y. Potential cytotoxic effect of chronic administration of creatine, a nutrition supplement to augment athletic performance. Med Hypotheses 2000;54:726–8.
[37] Benzi G, Ceci A. Creatine as a nutritional supplementation and medicinal product. J Sports Med Phys Fitness 2001;41:1–10.
[38] Venevenga NJ, Steele RD. Adverse effects of excessive consumption of amino acids. Annu Rev Nutr 1984;4:157–81.
[39] Echard B, Talpur NA, Funck KA, et al. Effects of oral glucosamine and chondroitin sulfate alone and in combination on the metabolism of SHR and SD rats. Mol Cell Biochem 2001;225:85–91.
[40] McCarty MF. The neglect of glucosamine as a treatment for osteoarthritis: a personal perspective. Med Hypotheses 1994;42:323–7.

[41] McNamara PS, Barr SC, Erb HN, et al. Hematologic, hemostatic and biochemical effects in cats receiving an oral chondroprotective agent for thirty days. Vet Ther 2000;1: 108–17.
[42] Food and Drug Administration Safety Information and Adverse Event Reporting Program. Food and Drug Administration Med Watch. Available at: http://www.fda.gov/medwatch/. Accessed November 15, 2002.
[43] Safe and unsafe herbs in herbal teas. Washington, DC: Department of Health, Education and Welfare, Public Health Service, Food and Drug Administration; 1975.
[44] Ooms TG, Kahn SA, Means C. Suspected caffeine and ephedrine toxicosis resulting from ingestion of an herbal supplement containing guarana and ma huang in dogs. J Am Vet Med Assoc 2001;218:225–9.
[45] Laboratory test results. ConsumerLab.com. Available at: http://www.consumerlab.com/result/index.asp. Accessed November 15, 2002.
[46] Natural products encyclopedia. ConsumerLab.com. Available at: http://www.consumerlab.com/tnp.asp. Accessed November 15, 2002.
[47] United States Pharmacopeia Veterinary Practitioner Reporting Program. United States Pharmacopeia. Available at: http://www.usp.org. Accessed November 15, 2002.
[48] Setnikar I, Rovati LC. Absorption, distribution, metabolism and excretion of glucosamine sulfate. A review. Arnzeimettelforschung 2001;51:699–725.
[49] Adebowale AO, Du J, Liang Z, et al. The bioavailability and pharmacokinetics of glucosamine hydrochloride and low molecular weight chondroitin sulfate after single and multiple doses to Beagle dogs. Biopharm Drug Dispos 2002;23:217–25.
[50] Reeve-Johnson L. Use of disease models in the development and evaluation of therapeutic agents. Vet Rec 1998;142:638–42.
[51] Bonnett B, Reid-Smith R. Critical appraisal meets clinical reality: evaluating evidence in the literature using canine hemangiosarcoma as an example. Vet Clin North Am Small Anim Pract 1996;26:39–61.
[52] Boothe DM, Slater M. Proper implementation of clinical trials. In: Dodds WJ, editor. Veterinary medical specialization: bridging science and medicine, advances in veterinary science and medicine, vol. 39. Orlando: Academic Press; 1995.
[53] Guyatt GH, Sackett DL, Cook DJ. Users' guide to the medical literature. are the results of the study valid? JAMA 1993;270(21):2598–601.
[54] Pulver AE, Bartko JJ, McGrath JA. The power of analysis: statistical perspectives. Part 1. Psychiatry Res 1998;23:295–9.
[55] McNamara PS, Barr SC, Erb HN. Hematologic, hemostatic and biochemical effects in dogs receiving an oral chondroprotective agent for thirty days. Am J Vet Res 1996;57: 1380–94.
[56] Cleophas RC, Cleophas TJ. Is selective reporting of clinical research unethical as well as unscientific? Int J Clin Pharmacol Ther 1999;37:1–7.
[57] Noyszewski EA, Wroblewski K, Dodge GR, et al. Preferential incorporation of glucosamine into galactosamine moieties of chondroitin sulfates in articular cartilage explants. Arthritis Rheum 2001;44:1089–95.
[58] Lippiello L, Woodward J, Karpman R, Hammadm TA. In vivo chondroprotection and metabolic synergy of glucosamine and chondroitin sulfate. Clin Orthop 2000;381:229–40.
[59] McAlindon T. Glucosamine and chondroitin for osteoarthritis? Bull Rheum Dis 2001;50: 1–4.
[60] Reginster JY, Deroisy R, Rovati LC, et al. Long-term effects of glucosamine sulphate on osteoarthritis progression: a randomized, placebo-controlled clinical trial. Lancet 2001;357: 251–6.
[61] McAlindon T. Glucosamine for osteoarthritis: dawn of a new era? Lancet 2001;357:247–8.

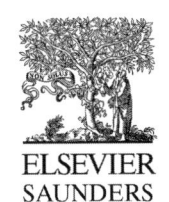

The natural activities of cells, the role of reactive oxygen species, and their relation to antioxidants, nutraceuticals, botanicals, and other biologic therapies

Lester Mandelker, DVM

Community Veterinary Hospital, 1631 W. Bay Drive, Largo, FL 33770, USA

As the basic unit of life, the cell is a very complex biologic system. To understand the role played by antioxidants, nutraceuticals, botanicals, and other biologic therapies, an understanding of cell structures, signaling pathways, and biologic processes involving life and death mechanisms is necessary [1]. In addition, identifying certain cellular structures and cellular activities is helpful in demonstrating the appropriate function that these therapies have in modulating specific biologic pathways. The focus of attention will be directed toward the activities of mitochondria and those signaling molecules and transcription factors altered by antioxidants and other biologic supplements, particularly those involving the process of physiologic cell death referred to as 'apoptosis.' The ensuing information on biologic processes relies heavily on the premise known as the "free radical theory of aging." This theory presents as the most compelling scientific explanation for the degenerative changes associated with cellular aging and disease [2]. The role of free radicals and reactive oxygen species (ROS), and their relationship to scientific information presented is based on Evidence Based Medicine (EBM). EBM stresses the consideration of evidence based data from clinical scientific research as an important basis for the practice of medicine [3]. Specific clinical applications of nutraceuticals, antioxidants, botanicals, and other biologic therapies will be addressed in the proceeding chapters.

E-mail address: lestervet2@aol.com

0195-5616/04/$ - see front matter © 2004 Elsevier Inc. All rights reserved.
doi:10.1016/j.cvsm.2003.09.014

Free radical theory

Oxidative damage from free radicals injures DNA, proteins, and lipids and has been implicated as a contributor to aging and various chronic diseases [4]. Oxidative damage first occurs from an accumulation of free radicals in tissues and cells. Most free radicals in the body are derivatives of oxygen. Free radicals, which have two unpaired electrons, are always looking to stabilize their own molecular structure [5]. ROS often grab or take electrons from any stable molecule that they encounter. This electron stealing leads to unstable tissues and could evoke a chain reaction that can destroy the delicate structure of cells. If the molecular alterations that occur from ROS are severe enough, oxidative damage and cellular injury result.

Free radicals (ie, ROS) are diverse and exist wherever there is disease and cell damage and under normal conditions [6]. They are formed continually during normal physiologic conditions such as mitochondrial respiration. Appropriate levels assist many critical functions in our bodies and low levels function as signaling molecules; however, excessive amounts of ROS initiate cell damage by playing havoc on cells' reduction–oxidation (redox) state. The redox state is a consequence of the balance between the levels of oxidizing and reducing equivalents. A reducing environment is often associated with cell survival, whereas an oxidizing environment is associated with oxidative stress and cell damage [7]. In a classic reduction–oxidation reaction, the ROS takes a proton (not electrons) from the donor (ie, antioxidant), reducing the radical potential and making it less radical in a stepwise progress until it is neutralized. If enough cellular antioxidants are available, they can then act by taking up/delocalizing the excess electrons, which has the effect of making the species less reactive than before while the free radical form of the antioxidant molecule (now itself a free radical but far less aggressive) can react with another free radical species to form stable molecules (N. Larkin, personal communication, 2002). Antioxidants, known as quenchers of free radicals, act by disarming ROS before they can attack and damage cells [8]. The cellular role afforded by the application of certain nutraceuticals, antioxidants, and botanicals is defined in this manner. Information on cell structures, cellular activities, signaling molecules, and biologic pathways follows.

Cell structures

Cells come in different sizes and shapes but have similar cell structures (Fig. 1). The outer membrane or cell membrane consists of two layers of fatty molecules (phospholipids) in which protein is embedded [9]. The embedded protein provides various biologic pathways for the transport and regulation of the flow of materials into and out of the cell, which commonly include proteins and fatty acids. The uptake of fatty acids (FA) involves two components: (1) passive diffusion through the lipid bilayer, and (2)

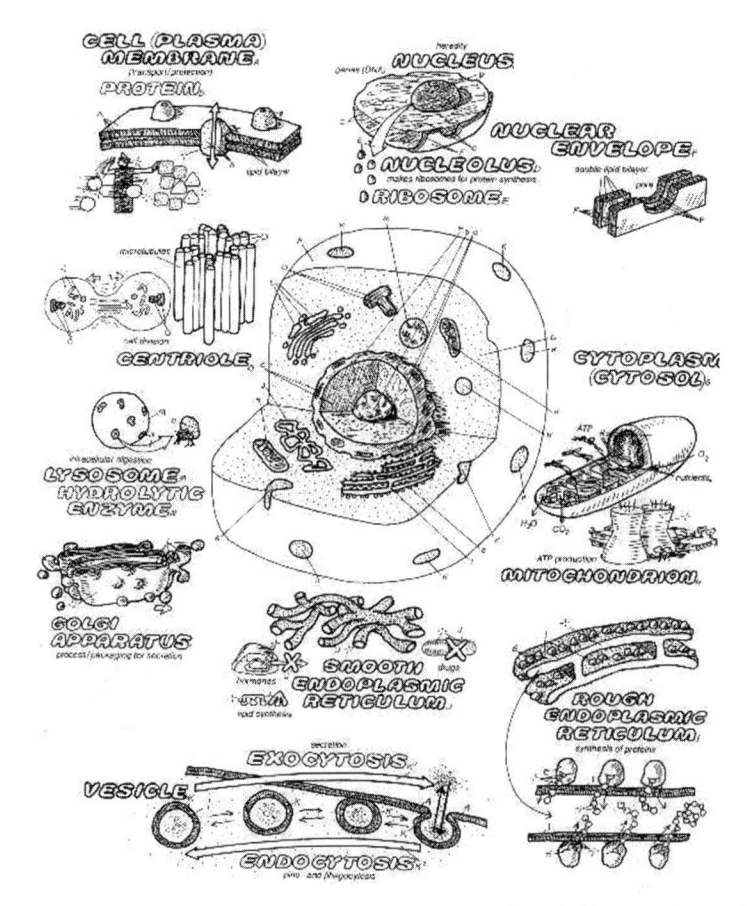

Fig. 1. Structures and organelles common to all cells. Cells are bounded by a continuous double layer sheet of lipid molecules containing embedded proteins called the plasma membrane. The space between the plasma membrane and the nucleus is called the cytoplasm. Membrane-bound organelles are suspended within the cytoplasmic fluid (cytosol). (*From* Kapit W, Macey R, Meisami E. The physiology coloring book. Menlo Park (CA): Harper Collins Publishers; 1987; p. 2; with permission.)

protein-facilitated transfer. The latter component appears to play the major role in mediating uptake by cells [10]. After uptake, cytoplasmic fatty acid binding proteins are involved in diffusion of FA from the plasma membrane to the intracellular sites of conversion such as the mitochondrial outer membrane. This long-term regulation of FA uptake and use is regulated by alterations in the rate of expression of genes [11].

Membrane proteins also serve as receptors for chemical signals coming from other cells [12]. These receptor proteins contain a variety of molecules that mediate the action of specific chemicals such as cytokines, chemicals, or hormones [13]. Typically, when cytokines or other chemicals interact with their corresponding specific cell surface receptor, the activation of intracellular signaling pathways is triggered, which ultimately programs the cellular response through genetic changes and activation of nuclear transcription factors [14].

One such family of protein molecules, tyrosine kinases, relay their effects on the transcription of genes for cell growth, differentiation, and transformation [15], which are accomplished through the recognition of receptors and associated intracellular signaling molecules. These signaling molecules can be latent in the cytoplasm but become activated through tyrosine phosphorylation, which is itself activated by certain cytokines initiated by oxidative stress. Signal transducers and activators of transcription (STAT) have long been recognized as crucial intracellular signaling molecules [16]. In contrast with other cellular signaling cascades, the STAT pathway is direct. STATs bind to receptors at the cell surface and translocate into the nucleus, where they function as transcription factors that trigger gene activation. Extracellular hormones, growth factors, or cytokines commonly relay effects on the transcription of genes through STAT signaling molecules [17]. Some antioxidants have been shown to modulate the activity of STATs. For example, antioxidants such as α-tocopherol and N-acetylcysteine have been shown to reduce the tyrosine phosphorylation of the signal transducer STAT, which, in turn, reduces genetic transcription and gene expression [17].

The cytoplasm occupying the space between the nucleus and the outer membrane consists of a semifluid substance that contains many thousands of distinct structures or membrane-bound organelles and ribosomes for synthesizing cytoplasmic proteins and the cytoskeleton. The cytoskeleton, located in the cytoplasm, consists of a complex network of protein filaments and tubules. The fluid portion of the cytoplasm between the structures is called the cytosol [18]. Many protein enzymes or catalysts are located here. These proteins also play a vital role in maintaining intracellular calcium (Ca^{2+}) homeostasis, which is essential to the health of a cell [19]. In a variety of experimental systems, an imbalance of intracellular Ca^{2+} homeostasis caused by increased Ca^{2+} influx or inhibition of Ca^{2+} extrusion has been found to be an early event in the development of cell injury and cell death [20]. These changes in cystolic calcium concentration finally result in an activation of the nuclear proteins (ie, endonucleases). Activation of endonucleases customarily initiates the cascade of cellular activity leading to physiological cell death (apoptosis) [21].

The Golgi apparatus is a dynamic organelle through which secretory and transmembrane proteins are transported, post-translationally modified, and finally packaged into carrier vesicles for transport along the cytoskeleton to a variety of destinations [22]. The Golgi apparatus appears to act as a sorting station for the cellular secretory pathway [23]. The endoplasmic reticulum (ER) represents the cell's quality control site for accurate folding of secretory and processing of membrane proteins [19]. Accumulating evidence suggests that, in addition to responsibility of protein processing, the ER is also an important signaling compartment and a sensor of cellular stress [24].

An accumulation of unfolded or damaged proteins in the lumen of the ER leads to this cellular stress [25]. There are also many proteins that cycle between the Golgi and the ER. Membrane traffic between the ER and Golgi has been recognized as a carefully regulated process controlled by distinct pathways. These pathways link two organelles that have different morphologies, structures, and localizations within the cell to common factors such as cellular stress [26].

The lysosome serves as a "biologic garbage dump" and a site for delivery of materials targeted for removal. It also functions as a source of enzymes that can digest natural particles, damaged organelles, and bacteria [19]. During phagocytosis and internalization, invagination of the plasma membrane occurs when the degradation of the phagocytosed material is completed [27]. Dysfunction of the lysosomal system can occur and results in incomplete degradation of molecules. A genetic defect in a protein responsible for maintaining the lysosomal system results in the accumulation within lysosomes of partially degraded molecules. This dysfunction is commonly called lysosomal storage disease [28]. The nucleus is perhaps the most prominent intracellular organelle, and it contains the genetic material DNA. DNA composes genes, by way of transcription and translation, that are responsible for the synthesis of proteins that control all cellular functions. These sequences of proteins comprising DNA modulate gene expression. By expressing information stored in these genes, the nucleus can direct its everyday activity and its own reproduction. The nucleolus, the smaller body inside the nucleus, consists of densely packed chromosomes, protein molecules, and RNA. RNA is the messenger of these genetic codes that are transcribed from DNA to be performed to the cytoplasm. The regulation of genes and their continued expression is accomplished through mRNA [19].

Mitochondria

One of the most important structures inside the cell is the mitochondrion. It functions as the powerhouse of the cell; it produces the energy that is required for life. Depending on the metabolic activity of the tissue, there can be few or many mitochondria in each cell. Generally speaking, the more metabolically active the cell, the more mitochondria it has. Mitochondria produce the energy of the body in the form of high-intensity molecules called adenosine triphosphate (ATP) [29]. Because mitochondria serve as the powerhouse of the cell, their proper function is essential to the integrity and optimal performance of living organisms. The outer mitochondrial membrane is the interface between the mitochondria and the cytoplasm. It is here where altered permeability involving the outer and inner membranes occurs, called mitochondrial permeability transition (MPT) [30]. The inner mitochondrial membrane is folded inward and forms a series of layers (cristae) that extend into the fluid located in the mitochondria. It is along these cristae that much of the cell's energy (ie, ATP) is produced [31]. Mitochondria undergo aerobic metabolism, called oxidative phosphorylation, and use glucose and fats selectively to produce ATP. The cell in homeostasis is capable of maintaining a steady-state flux of energy between mitochondrial oxidative phosphorylation producing ATP and the cytoplasmic protein enzymes performing work [32].

Mitochondria are the most redox-active organelles, and they are affected significantly by oxidative stress. During the course of normal metabolism, mitochondria in general (and the respiratory chain of mitochondria in particular) are active in the continuous generation of ROS, which must be neutralized [33]. During illness and pathologic conditions, the antioxidant mechanisms are unable to combat the excessive production of ROS; hence, antioxidant levels can deplete, which results in an increase in oxidative stress proceeding to oxidative damage and inflammation [34]. Quenching ROS, or neutralizing, is controlled by the cellular redox buffer involving intracellular glutathione (GSH) [35]. Combinations of antioxidants such as ascorbic acid, tocopherols, and retinoids act in conjunction with the redox enzymes, GSH reductase, GSH peroxidase, catalase, and superoxide dismutase to neutralize ROS [36].

Not all ROS are harmful; they can also function as signaling molecules [10]. The signaling by ROS does not appear to be random, but targeted at specific metabolic and signal transduction cellular components. The presence of ROS does not appear to be just an unwarranted byproduct of primary oxidation; it is necessary to regulate cellular processes such as mitosis and apoptosis [37]. This idea of ROS as signaling molecules as opposed to toxic metabolites has been partly substantiated by findings that relate to its interaction with antioxidants. For example, intracellular antioxidants, which promote intracellular GSH, not only serve to regulate ROS levels but also have been shown to modify catalase function by way of the redox pathway by altering ROS production [36]. In this regard, catalase is an important part of the cellular redox buffer. Hence, antioxidants such as N-acetyl-L-cysteine (NAC) and α lipoic acid, which are known to increase intracellular GSH, appear to be effective in modulating cellular redox status as well [38].

While mitochondria are recognized as the powerhouse of the cell by virtue of their functions of oxidative phosphorylation and the production of energy, they also have other critical functions. Mitochondria participate in the sequence of rapid aging, and it is not surprising that this activity involves the oxidative machinery. The decline in mitochondrial energy production resulting in increased oxidative stress and cellular damage plays a significant role in degenerative diseases and aging. New scientific research regarding aging emphasizes just how ROS and other reactive species damage biomolecules. This damage then invokes a rapid induction of senescence and premature cell death. Rapid aging occurs with tissues inundated with these ROS [39].

Recent information has revealed that certain chemicals can act on a specific cell type's mitochondria but not others. For example, increasing pyruvate to fibroblast cells (mitochondria) caused them to intensify their metabolic activity and undergo induction of cellular senescence or aging following a rise in mitochondrial oxidant production and a fall in intracellular GSH levels. There appears to be a cause and effect relationship in which these cells exhibit a rapid rise in growth arrest associated with an elevation of protein death regulators such as p53 [40], which is a definite pro-death succession. Conversely, pyruvate added to liver tissue cells during shock improves the redox status of tissue and decreases cell death in hepatic cells. Pyruvate effectively maintaines an adequate NADH/NAD redox state and prevents loss of intracellular antioxidants such as GSH. In addition, pyruvate significantly increases levels of antiapoptotic (anti-death) molecules and decreased pro-apoptotic (pro-death) molecules [41], which is a definite pro-survival posture. Emerging evidence suggests that the tissue source of the mitochondrial receptors might be a determinant for pro-life or pro-death occurrences. Perhaps applying nutraceuticals, antioxidants, and other biologic therapies that bind to a certain tissue's cellular mitochondrial receptors in this capacity has significant merit. In the author's opinion, tissue-specific mitochondrial antioxidant therapies might have significant merit and might offer clinical medicine specific biologic modulators in the future.

Mitochondrial permeability transition

Permeabilization, or opening of the mitochondrial membrane pores (ie, MPT), is often an early and decisive feature of cell death. This activity is regulated by members of the Bcl-2, a family of cell death regulatory proteins that interact with the permeability transition pore complex [42]. The permeability of the mitochondrial transition involves pores or channels located along the outer mitochondrial membrane that participate in the regulation of the $Ca2^+$ influx, pH, voltage, and redox of antioxidants. In the mitochondrial membrane these pores open when exposed to elevated influx of $Ca2^+$, especially when the mechanism is accompanied by oxidative stress. The opening of the MPT causes massive swelling of in the mitochondria, rupture of the outer membrane, and release of intermembrane components such as cytochrome c, a protein that initiates the cell death mechanism. Pore opening appears to be a critical event of the apoptotic process. Mitochondria are also endowed with multiple $Ca2^+$ transport mechanisms by which they take up and release $Ca2^+$ across their membranes. They play a pivotal role in the regulation of cytosolic calcium ($Ca2^+$) signals, which are crucial in the control of most physiological processes including cell injury, mitochondrial permeability transition, pore opening, and cell death mechanisms.

In the daily activity of cells there are cell death molecules and cell survival molecules that are constantly at odds with one another. Cell death molecules are well represented in cells. Bax and Bid are proapoptotic, pro-death members of the Bcl-2 protein family that reside in the outer mitochondrial membrane. It is controversial whether or not Bax or Bid promote cell death directly through their putative function as channel proteins versus indirectly by inhibiting cellular regulators of the cell death proteases (caspases) [43]. Bax, for example, does not induce swelling of mitochondria and permeability transition changes to the mitochondrial membrane, but instead uses an alternative mechanism for triggering release of cytochrome c. The release of cytochrome c from mitochondria is associated with activation of cell death proteins (caspases), which ultimately leads to apoptosis [44]. Other members of the Bcl-2 family contain antiapoptotic members including the individual Bcl-2 protein, which can be antagonistic to other family members. The cellular effects of Bcl-2 are considered to be cytoprotective because they act to stabilize the mitochondrial transition pore membrane opening by inhibiting calcium influx. This effect demonstrates that alterations in the composition of the mitochondrial MPT relate directly to the pathophysiology of cell life and death [45]. As an example, cyclosporine A, which is a specific inhibitor of MPT, has a mitochondrial specific effect that can be applied in clinical cases to improve mitochondrial integrity and reduce cell death [46].

Increasing amounts of ROS are associated with increased pore opening, an effect that also has clinical indications. Extracts of Chinese mushrooms (sophoranone) increase the formation of mitochondrial ROS. These mushrooms act as pro-oxidants and initiate the opening of Ca^{2+}-selective channels in the inner mitochondrial membrane in selective cancer tissues. This effect, coupled with Ca^{2+} movement, leads to the increase in mitochondrial permeability transition pore opening and tumor cell death [47]. There are perhaps many applications of specific molecules, antioxidants, or biologic therapies that alter the mitochondrial MPT. They might be useful as therapeutic interventions to modulate ROS and oxidative stress, thereby altering cell life and death.

Cell communication

Cells carry on their daily activities by using signaling molecules, which are specialized protein molecules that act on receptors located internally or externally that are generated by their release. The molecules of the transduction pathways guide internal signaling. These intracellular signaling pathways mediate the main events of the cell, including growth, differentiation, proliferation, specialized functions, and apoptosis [48]. One such molecule is the transcription factor nuclear factor-κ B (NF-κB), which upon activation translocates into the nucleus, where it modulates the expression of a variety of genes. Activator protein-1 is another redox-sensitive transcription factor that acts through protein kinase-based pathways. NF-κB is a ubiquitous transcription factor and pleiotropic regulator of numerous genes involved in the immune and inflammatory response [49]. NF-κB activation is initiated by persistent cellular exposure to certain chemicals and events, including toxins, hormones, hyperglycemia, lipopolysacharrides, and various inflammatory cytokines. Intracellular redox imbalances and subsequent oxidative stress also appear to activate NF-κB. NF-κB in particular plays a central role in regulating the genetic transcription and encoding of inflammatory cytokines, growth factors, acute phase response proteins, cell adhesion molecules, transcription factors, and cell death regulators These NF-κB–regulated genes are important in modulating genetic activity during critical illness, inflammatory diseases, and cancer [50]. Specific biologic constituents that can modulate NF-κB activation would be immensely important in controlling inflammation and appear to have multiple applications in prevention and treatment of many diseases. Apparently, this reduction in inflammation might also be associated with a reduction in neoplastic transformation. Further studies will be necessary to elucidate specific mechanisms and selectivity of NF-κB function and its role in modulating different diseases (including cancer).

The I-κ B (IκB) proteins are inhibitory proteins that modulate NF-κB. They are sequestered in the cytoplasm as an inactive form bound to IκB proteins [51]. Upon stimulation of certain receptors, IκB is phosphorylated, eventually leading to its degradation and thus releasing NF-κB for translocation to the nucleus. During excessive oxidative stress and accumulation of ROS, IκB is destroyed, encouraging the enhancement of NF-κB. Certain antioxidants such as NAC, which can suppress IκB degradation, might influence inflammatory activity indirectly by its control of NF-κB [52]. Clinical research revealed recently that vitamin E and its acetate analogs can modulate the cellular response to NF-κB activation. Additionally [53], selenium, through its modulation of GSH peroxidase activity, can inhibit NF-κB activation and upregulate IκB [54]. Presently, it is not known whether or not this finding is clinically relevant. The fact that pretreatment with certain antioxidants can inhibit NF-κB activation for extended periods of time adds probability, but no assurances. Such is the case with other drugs. Dehydroepiandrosterone (DHEA), a nutraceutical with hormonal activities, has been demonstrated to inhibit NF-κB activation. This activity of DHEA can modulate oxidative imbalance and reduce the activity of NF-κB translocation before it acts to upregulate inflammatory genes [55]. Inhibition of NF-κB can also occur with the use of pharmaceuticals. Anti-inflammatory agents such glucocorticoids antagonize NF-κB binding to DNA and induce gene transcription and protein synthesis of the inhibitor IκB. This immune-modulating effect is especially significant clinically when the main effector is the T cell [56]. T cell lymphocytes play a most important role in immune disorders and inflammation. Nonsteroidal anti-inflammatory drugs (NSAIDs) also inhibit activation of NF-κB by blocking IκB kinase, a key enzyme in NF-κB activation [57]. NSAIDs have repeatedly been shown to be beneficial not only for their analgesic effects but also for their cellular effects. Recent studies revealed that NF-κB activation can also be reduced with the addition n-3 polyunsaturated fatty acids (PUFA) [58]. The process of downregulating the activity of NF-κB by three PUFAs (ie, omega-3 FAs) has been shown to reduce symptoms in animal models involving chronic inflammatory disease. This new information establishes a strong link between inflammation and the activities and regulation of NF-κB.

The activation of NF-κB is not always a detriment, however; NF-κB activation is the primary method that mediates cell growth and protection from activation-induced cell death [59]. Many signaling molecules act directly or indirectly through NF-κB, including transforming growth factor-β (TGF-β), ROS, prostaglandins (PGs), leukotrienes, nitric oxide, protein kinases, and certain hormones and growth factors. These molecules are involved in some way with regulating genes and enhancing/binding the transcription factors that modify or modulate cell growth and cell death. There are also signaling molecules that can upregulate NF-κB then activate antiapoptotic proteins that suppress cell death. The simultaneous expression of these signaling molecules often results in the biologic transformations known as cancer [60]. In some leukemia cells, death receptor ligation can lead directly to NF-κB activation and protection from or resistance to apoptosis [61].

The application of biologic therapies during inflammation that inhibit NF-κB might have clinical merit and application in a vast array of diseases. NSAIDs, for example, have been shown to inhibit NF-κB, which might explain the recent finding that NSAIDs reduce carcinogenesis. Calorie restriction has also been associated with suppression of NF-κB. Caloric restriction also acts to block the dissociation of IκB, the inhibitory protein of NF-κB [62]. A nutraceutical Genistein, a prominent isoflavonoid, has been shown to inhibit the activation of NF-κB, inhibit cell growth, and induce apoptosis in certain cancer lines [63]. Many other specific chemical constituents can modulate or modify NF-κB activation, and this reduced activity is desirable in subsequent genetic transcription. Modulation of this cellular activity would be welcomed for cellular applications involving inflammation and cancer. The application of certain specific antioxidant and botanical supplements in this regard seem to have significant merit in a variety of clinical cases.

Intercellular communication

Cells must communicate with neighboring cells to survive. Cellular communication appears to be a coordinated effort by individual cells to serve the entire body. Intercellular signaling (between cells) is accomplished through small pores between cells called gap junctions. Gap junctions are specialized areas of the plasma membranes of opposed cells where the membranes are 2 to 4 nm apart. They are penetrated by a connection channel that bridges the extracellular space [64], which provides a means of communication between the cytoplasm of the cell and that of another cell. The communication between cells is so important that the lack of intercellular communication often results in cell death or cancer. This communication between cells is called gap junctional intercellular communication (GJIC).

GJIC is one of the most important functions of cells; it allows them to survive in tissue. It is also required for completion of embryonic development, tissue homeostasis, and regulation of cell proliferation and cell death [65]. Gap junction channels form a conduit between cells for the exchange of ions, second messengers, and small metabolites. The sharing of these molecules can be rather selective and might be involved in growth control processes. Certain proteins reside along the small pores located at the gap junctions [66]. There they act to control chemical activity and communication between cells. This family of transmembrane proteins is called connexins. Connexins assist in forming gap junction channels, allowing metabolic and electrical coupling of cellular networks. There are different connexin molecules for different tissues, and they serve as receptors for chemical signals from other cells and contains genes that act to modify cellular activities [67]. These connexin molecules are likely targets for the development and discovery of chemical tools and supplements that specifically alter or influence intercellular communication. Several specific chemicals have been reported to modulate connexin molecules and alter their genetic expression. Studies in human and animal cells have identified a gene, connexin 43, whose expression is upregulated by chemopreventative carotenoids, which, by that activity, promote GJIC [68]. In addition, the chemical DMSO and the hormone melatonin can markedly induce gap junction protein expression and improve GJIC in liver cells [69,70]. Taurine, which is known to be cytoprotective, is used clinically to improve liver function through GJIC [71]. Moreover, damaging radicals like H_2O_2 decreased GJIC in liver cells, which taurine was shown to inhibit. This effect is mediated through the oxidative mechanism where there is apparently a significant link between oxidative stress and GJIC [72]. β carotene and related carotenoids such as lycopene cause enhancement of GJIC, but only at certain levels and at certain doses [73]. Transient up or down gene regulation of gap junctions can also be promulgated by many endogenous or exogenous biochemicals. Modulation of GJIC should be viewed as a scientific basis for genetic toxicology because alterations of intercellular communication alter the biophysiological state of the cell. Improving and increasing GJIC is important in cell and tissue survival. These mechanisms are associated with genetic changes through the gap junctions induced by connexin molecules. Restoring normal gap junction function to cells that have dysfunctional intercellular communication could be the basis for a new approach to therapeutic intervention.

The dysfunction of gap junctions appears to play a role in the actions of various signaling molecules that have cell type/tissue/organ specificity. For example, tumor cells often display dysfunctional GJIC as evidenced by their erratic cell growth. Malignant cells show aberrant expression of connexins, which suggests that connexin proteins and their derived dysfunctional gap junctions are critical determinants of the invasiveness of cancer cells [74]. The continued inadequate regulation and dysfunction of GJIC has also been associated with activated oncogenes, which further promote neoplastic transformation [75]. Moreover, scientific evidence has shown that healthy tissues with normal GJIC regulation have been associated with tumor suppressor genes [76]. With the recent discovery of a tumor suppressor gene lacking or missing in certain cancers, one might contemplate that this lack of expression is directly related to missing or damaged connexin molecules and dysfunctional GJIC.

Inflammatory chemicals such as cytokines can also disrupt gap junction channels. This inflammation leads to a disruption of the plasma membrane's identifiable gap junctions, which renders them dysfunctional. Carcinogens such as phenobarbital inhibit GJIC in a reversible fashion. Various oncogenes (tumor genes) downregulate GJIC, whereas several tumor suppressor genes (eg, p53) can upregulate GJIC. Antitumor promoters (eg, retinoids, carotenoids, green tea components) and antioncogene drugs (eg, lovastatin) can upregulate GJIC [77]. The restoration of normal gap junction function to cells that have dysfunctional intercellular communication could also be the basis for a new approach to supplemental therapies.

Cellular injury

Stress inducers cause oxidative stress, with the intensity and duration determining the mode of injury. At high concentrations, ROS are hazardous for all living organisms and can damage many major cellular constituents [78]. The cellular injury or necrolytic cell death that often follows induces a well-orchestrated series of cellular and biochemical events that often provoke a strong inflammatory response. Inflammation consists of a series of physiologic reactions by the body that brings cells and molecules of the immune system to the site of tissue damage and cell death [79], an effect that is made possible by certain signaling molecules that attract cells by the secretory products they release. The net result might appear in the form of increased blood supply, increased migration of leukocytes, and increased vascular permeability. Immediate biologic mediators such as PGs, leukotrienes, histamine, serotonins, platelet activating factor, and others released during cell death also act as signaling molecules in the acute phase of inflammation [80]. During sustained release, other biologic signaling molecules perpetuate cellular inflammation by activating additional chemical mediators such as tumor necrosis factor-α (TNF-α), interleukins, interferons, colony stimulating factors, and acute phase proteins. This chronic response involves a more extensive and complex commitment to inflammation. This phase of inflammation can occur from continued, acute, nonspecific stimulation or from sustained, specific immunologic stimulation [81].

Mediators of cellular inflammation: prostaglandins

The most abundant molecules produced during cell damage are PGs, which are signaling molecules and pronounced mediators of inflammation. They are formed from the breakdown of arachidonic acid in response to various stimuli involving cell injury and death. These stimuli activate phospholipases, which then act on the phospholipids derived from linoleic acid to form arachidonic acid (AA) [78]. AA is an inflammatory molecule, and upon oxidative stress its metabolism results in the formation of eicosanoids and ROS. The eicosanoids, like the PGs, leukotrienes, and related compounds, are important as signaling molecules in addition to their known proinflammatory activity [81]. Synthesis of PGs from AA is accomplished by the enzyme PG G/H synthase, also known as cyclo-oxygenase. Two isoforms have been identified, cyclo-oxygenase 1 (Cox1) and cyclo-oxygenase 2 (Cox2). Perhaps more isoforms exist as well. Cox1 enzyme is expressed constitutively in most cells and tissues. It expression is controlled by physiologic or pathologic conditions that relate directly to its function as regulator of homeostatic functions [82]. Cox2 is inducible in certain cells in response to injury or inflammatory stimuli. PGs formed by the Cox2 enzyme primarily mediate pain and inflammation and appear to have numerous activities that favor carcinogenesis. This carcinogenesis effect is evident by its activation of NF-κB, which promotes cellular proliferation and reduces apoptosis. Furthermore, the fact that many cancers have high levels of the inflammatory PG, prostaglandin E (2) (PGE2), and upregulated Cox2 genetic expression is conclusive that PGs play a significant role in carcinogenesis [83].

Biologic chemicals that inhibit Cox2 enzymes confer a mechanism for the treatment and prevention of many forms of cancer. Vitamin E has been demonstrated to inhibit cyclo-oxygenase activity in macrophages by reducing peroxynitrite formation [84]. Supplementation with highly polyunsaturated fatty acids (PUFA) such as docosahexaenoic acid (DHA) and eicosapentaenoic acid (EPA) added to the diet would shift metabolism away from the highly proinflammatory AA pathway [85]. This dietary application is well known to reduce inflammation at the cellular level and change the lipid composition of cell membranes. Clinical applications of this activity are well established; omega-3 FAs (PUFAs) have found a niche in human and veterinary therapeutics. In addition, age-associated tissue appears to have higher levels of inducible PGE2, which might be amenable to treatment with antioxidants [86,87]. Thiol antioxidants such as NAC can also reduce the oxidative stress that contribute to Cox2 activation. Additionally, polyphenol compounds found in black tea (theaflavin-3-monogallate, epigallocatechin gallate) have also been shown to inhibit Cox2 gene expression at mRNA and protein levels [88]. The modulation of Cox2 is especially important in cases in which the tumor suppressor gene (p53) is lacking, because the lack of p53 gene influence can lead to an increase in carcinogenesis [89].

Genetic manipulation in the future through dietary supplementation appears to be a promising modality for cancer treatment and prevention. Several specific chemical compounds have been demonstrated to induce genetic manipulation by initiating DNA repair [90]. Free radicals and reactive species that cause cell damage and DNA aberrations are especially responsive to dietary antioxidants, which can trap these molecules and limit their damage; however, there are currently few proven clinical applications that use these therapies.

Research has revealed inconsistencies with the effects of many antioxidants, especially in regards to carcinogenesis. For example, β carotene and vitamin C can act as pro-oxidants. The mechanism involves the ability of these compounds to induce oxidative stress by impairing mitochondrial respiration. The net effect might increase carcinogenesis [91,92]. Vitamin E has been shown to decrease effectiveness of some chemotherapeutic agents that act through the ROS mechanism. Certain chemotherapeutic agents acting as pro-oxidants induce apoptosis, leading to increase tumor death. Vitamin E has been found to blunt these effects in some cases [93]. The results of numerous trials on the preventative role of antioxidants and nutraceuticals (ie, β carotene, α tocopherol, vitamin C) are far from conclusive regarding carcinogenesis. Multiple primary and secondary intervention trials currently underway should fully assess the role of some vitamins and antioxidants in the prevention of various cancers. It is important not to extrapolate generalities regarding biologic therapies such as antioxidants and phytochemicals to cancer treatment. Each chemical constituent should be tested before any valid claims can be made. Each and every chemical compound should be substantiated scientifically to avoid misinterpretation of benefits that occurred with the general claims of β carotene and vitamin C with regard to cancer.

Leukotrienes

Leukotrienes belong to a family of pharmacologically active substances derived from PUFAs, notably AA. They are considered to be local hormones because they are not stored but synthesized in response to local stimuli. As mediators of inflammation they are immediately activated during cell injury. The biologic pathway includes enzymatic interaction of AA by lipoxygenase, which results in the formation of 5-hydroperoxeicosatetraenoic acid (5-HPETE), an intermediate compound, which is further metabolized to form leukotriene A4 [94]. Further metabolic steps can convert the intermediate LTA4 into LTB4 by hydrolysis and into LTC4 by conjugation with GSH. These intermediate leukotrienes are important signaling molecules. LTB4 formed in the absence of GSH has potent chemotatic properties, attracting neutrophils, eosinophils, and other inflammatory cells. With the cellular presence of GSH, the metabolism of LTA4 proceeds to form LTC4, LTD4, and LTE4, which are commonly called the cysteinyl leukotrienes. Leukotriene LTB4 and cystinyl leukotrienes have impressive systemic effects aside from their activity as signaling molecules, including stimulation of stem cell activity and their cellular precursors. Leukotrienes have also been shown to decrease apoptosis during inflammatory conditions and increase cell survival [95]. Such inflammation is associated with the expression and distribution of the proteins that characteristically transform cells [96]. This transformation often involves signaling mechanisms that actively reduce apoptosis. Therefore, when leukotriene activation combines with Cox2 PG expression, cellular activities display a definite pattern leading to neoplastic transformation [97]. Leukotriene-induced inflammation has also been shown to be inhibitory to the normal activity of gap junctions, which renders them dysfunctional. Dysfunctional GJIC have also been linked to cancer [98]. The clinical use of leukotriene antagonists has made only modest inroads in the treatment of asthma and atopy, particularly in veterinary medicine. Perhaps as more is learned about the activity of leukotrienes, future applications will focus on their effects on cellular diseases and oxidative stress. Many supplements demonstrate inhibitory activity to the formation of leukotrienes. For example, antioxidants such as flavonoids (eg, procyanidins [cocoa] and polyphenols [green tea]) decrease the blood levels of proinflammatory cysteinyl leukotrienes by inhibitory action on LTA4 synthase [99]. Botanicals such as Boswellia have been found to inhibit the release of leukotrienes LTB4 and LTC4 from activated white blood cells [100]. Few if any veterinary clinical studies to date have confirmed the effectiveness of these substances.

Tumor necrosis factor

Among prominent signaling molecules, tumor necrosis factors (TNFs) belong to a class of cytokines that bind the receptors that are important in mediating inflammation and cytotoxic reactions. The TNF family of protein molecules is a potent and versatile group. TNFs can activate cell survival and the cell death mechanism simultaneously [101]. Cell survival is activated by NF-κB, a transcription factor acting through a set of genes to regulate proliferation of cells. TNF-α can also induce cell death by initiating caspases, apoptotic death effectors [102]. TNF-α is considered to be perhaps the most pleotrophic of the group, and it can act as a host defense mechanism in immunologic and inflammatory conditions [103]. TNF-α has been implicated in the pathophysiology of a number of acute diseases in which it can contribute to cellular death by way of apoptosis and organ dysfunction. TNF-α can be generated under septic and ischemic–reperfusion conditions by activation of cell mitogen protein kinases and the nuclear protein NF-κB [104]. Unregulated TNF-α is harmful and accounts for wasting disease, cachexia, and various other inflammatory responses associated with cancer and autoimmune diseases [105]. Moreover, TNF-α has been found to act jointly with other cytokines such as interleukin (IL)-1 and IL-6 to potentiate adverse biologic activity [106]. In addition, the cellular redox state constitutes a potential signaling mechanism for the regulation of inflammatory signals that activate TNF-α. The presence of TNF-α, an oxidant, depletes intracellular GSH, and concomitant with an increase in oxidized GSH leads to an increase in oxidative stress. Targeting TNF-α in these circumstances to modify disease has ample merit. One mechanism of protection against TNF-α–induced ischemic–reperfusion injury has been demonstrated by the blockage of caspase activation, the pro-death regulator, which occurs because of the upregulation of Bcl-2, an antiapoptotic protein compound. The result is the inhibition of oxidant-induced cell death by interference with the production of oxygen free radicals. Certain antioxidants such as coenzyme Q10 and N-acetylcysteine have been shown to reverse (at appropriate levels) the destructive processes of TNF-α generated by ROS [106]. In the future, additional clinical applications of nutraceuticals and antioxidants might be a valuable therapeutic modality for modulating damage afforded by TNF-α.

Matrix metalloproteinases

Matrix metalloproteinases (MMPs) are a family of about 20 zinc-containing proteases [107] (enzymes) that are secreted into the extracellular matrix by most cell types. They act to cleave structural proteins, growth factors, adhesion molecules, and other proteins of the extracellular matrix [108]. MMPs degrade tissue in health and disease. They have significant roles in many disease states such as cancer, emphysema, arthritis, and in several other inflammatory diseases [109]. Oxidative stress can induce MMP activation, which contributes to physiologic conditions such as angiogenesis, tumor growth, metastasis, wound healing, uterine involution, and bone remodeling [110]. Pathologic conditions such as inflammatory bowel disease, peridontal disease, myocardial infarction, atherosclerosis, and acute respiratory distress syndrome are also known to involve a substantial increase in MMP activity [111]. Different tissues seem to have different

MMP populations. Some of the more common MMPs include MMP-1 (collagenase), MMP-3 (stromelysin), and MMP-12 (macrophage elastase).

The activity of MMP is regulated, which is accomplished by tissue inhibitors of MMPs (TIMPs). In normal conditions there should be a balance between MMPs and TIMPs [112]. Chronic oxidative stress leads to an imbalance of MMPs, which has been implicated in the pathogenesis of a variety of diseases such as cancer, osteoarthritis, and immune-mediated arthritis [113]. High levels and imbalances of TIMPs are found in fibrotic conditions such as liver fibrosis and have been found to promote the progression of fibrosis through inhibition of matrix degradation. Thus, inhibition of MMPs might be indicated in pathologic conditions. This inhibition can act as a modulator of disease and adjunct therapy for primary disease conditions. Specific biomedicines such as pharmaceuticals, antioxidants, and botanicals can modulate MMP activity. In addition, MMP expression appears to be sensitive to the redox system and oxidative stress [113]. Hence, there is good rationale for providing antioxidant therapy to modulate disruptive MMP activity, which is common in pathologic states. The biologically active components from natural products, including green tea polyphenols (GTP), resveratrol, genistein, and organosulfur compounds from garlic have been shown to inhibit MMP-2, MMP-9, and MMP-12 activities. GTP caused the strongest inhibition of these MMP enzymes [114].

Adhesion molecules

Certain protein molecules expressed on the surface of a cell mediate the adhesion of the cell to other cells onto the extracellular matrix. These molecules, called adhesion molecules, attract leukocytes and initiate the contact necessary for their attachment and transendothelial migration [115]. The cellular adhesion mechanism is complex and is a crucial step for inflammation, morphogenesis, and wound healing. This cellular process appears to be sensitive to ROS when it can initiate cell adhesions directly or indirectly. Overproduction or excessive amounts of adhesion molecules can be detrimental and are a contributing factor in the cascade of cyclic inflammation. This cyclic inflammation is perpetuated because inflammation attracts adhesion molecules and adhesion molecules promote inflammation [116]. In addition, adhesion molecules also play an essential role in the immune response by mediating the biologic interactions that are essential for immune cell trafficking and activation [117]. Integrins are one family of adhesion molecules that are used by leukocytes to interact with other cells and with components of the extracellular matrix [118]. Another type, intercellular adhesion molecule-1 (ICAM-1), is an inducible adhesion molecule of the immunoglobulin supergene family that is expressed constitutively on endothelial tissues [119]. During inflammation, expression of adhesion molecules such as ICAM and E-selectin by endothelial cells allows leukocytes to bind to the endothelium at the site of inflammation, permitting recruitment of leukocytes and platelets from blood into the extravascular tissue [120].

Adhesion molecules located along blood vessels are governed by the vascular cell adhesion molecule-1 and are involved in inflammatory conditions of the intravascular system [121]. These cell adhesion molecules act on certain specific cell adhesion receptors. These receptors function in signal transduction and have been shown to contain protein tyrosine kinase activity. These tyrosine kinases provide the pathway in which extracellular stimuli can interact with the complex network of receptor-mediated intracellular transduction molecules [122]. Tyrosine kinases have been implicated in specific signal transduction pathways that control cell growth and cellular architecture and protect cells from death. These enzymes regulate mitosis, differentiation, migration, neovascularization, and apoptosis. Excessive activity of tyrosine kinases has been implicated in the pathogenesis of cancer [123]; therefore, modulation of cell adhesion receptors that have tyrosine kinase activity would be advantageous, specifically when it relates to cause and effect of inflammation and cancer.

Certain pharmaceuticals, nutraceuticals, or antioxidants can mitigate protein tyrosine kinases signal transdution and defer inflammation or carcinogenesis. These chemicals are called protein tyrosine kinase inhibitors. One such inhibitor, α tocopherol (vitamin E) has been shown to modulate protein kinase activity by inhibiting tyrosine phosphorylation, as does N-acetylcysteine, another antioxidant [124]. The isoflavone genistein has also been demonstrated to inhibit tyrosine kinase and to modulate cancer activity. This application pertains specifically to the cellular inhibitory effects that occur because of oxidative metabolism byproducts, which account for its selective inhibition of growth in certain cancer cell lines [125]. The activity of cell adhesion molecules represents a cellular process that is sensitive to ROS. Some natural supplements can mitigate cell adhesion activity by oxidant-dependent pathways. Antioxidants appear to reduce cellular inflammation in part by decreasing genetic expression of endothelial cells containing proinflammatory cytokines and adhesion molecules [126]. In one study, tocotrienol, a certain type of vitamin E, was the most effective form for reducing endothelial expression of adhesion molecules [127]. Under the influence of antioxidants such as NAC, vascular molecule expression is downregulated, as is TNF-α–induced activation of NF-κB [128]. The use of antioxidant or botanical therapies to modulate adhesion molecules is warranted, especially when there is oxidative damage and imbalance of the cellular redox. Clinicians should strive to learn the precise molecular mechanisms that regulate tissue-specific and cytokine-specific genetic expression. That information will give clinicians a better understanding of the cellular reaction to localized inflammation. This realization might lead to the development of specific anti-inflammatory therapeutic strategies, perhaps involving antioxidants and botanical therapies.

Necrosis

Cell death is a complex cellular activity. Depending on the nature of the stimulus, there are pro-death receptors and survival receptors at odds in each cell. Certain signaling molecules act at these receptors, and when activated they stimulate other receptors. There is a significant redundancy of cellular activities, and each stimulation has numerous multiple actions besides its immediate action [129]. Cells die by necrosis or apoptosis. Necrosis is the result of cellular damage that cannot be repaired and is the result of internal or external forces or chemical or physical events that destroy cells. The progression of events as a result of necrosis is that cells swell, rupture the outer cell membrane, and eventually die and release biochemical mediators of inflammation [130], which is an energy-driven process. There is also a novel type of death of tumor cell called autoschizis, which is less energy-driven and characterized by exaggerated membrane damage and progressive loss of organelle-free cytoplasm through a series of self-excisions. During this process the nucleus becomes smaller, the cell size decreases to one half to one third its size, and most organelles surround an intact nucleus in a narrow rim of cytoplasm. Even though mitochondria are condensed, cell death does not result from ATP depletion [131].

Programmed cell death (apoptosis)

Programmed cell death (apoptosis) is different from necrosis in that it is a restrained death that is often genetically programmed and can be a normal physiological mechanism. It is a complicated physiological function that has numerous avenues of application. "Physiological cell death may be as important as cell life in a wide range of normal processes such as fetal development, aging, defense against viruses, cell homeostasis, as well as immune system processing" [132]. The activation of apoptosis in an individual cell is based on its environment, internal metabolism, genetic information, or other various external or internal forces. During this process, cell shrinkage, nuclear condensation, and DNA fragmentation occur without the release of cytokines that are involved in cellular inflammation [132], which is in contrast to necrosis, in which the outer cellular membrane is disrupted and inflammatory chemicals are released. Although apoptosis and necrosis were thought to be entirely distinct mechanisms of cell death, new evidence indicates that the processes are regulated by many of the same biochemical intermediates such as cellular ATP, Ca^{2+} influx, ROS, and thiol antioxidants (GSH inducers). Beyond a certain threshold it appears that stress-induced changes in these biologic modulators can switch the cell death mechanism from apoptosis to necrosis [133].

Accelerated apoptosis occurs during exposure to high levels of ROS, toxins, or other primary injurious events; however, drastic changes in cellular death can also occur from dysfunction of the apoptosis mechanism. Dysfunction of apoptosis occurs with cancer, immune and inflammatory disease, viral infection, and degenerative diseases [134]. The attempt to correct this dysfunction and influence apoptosis is widely appealing. The fact that it apoptosis reduced in cancer and autoimmune diseases and increased in viral and degenerative diseases suggests potential benefits in being able to modulate it. Supplements that might modulate or modify apoptosis are likely to be useful therapeutic agents. These chemicals might also act as anti-inflammatory, antiviral, antiaging, and anticancer compounds.

Research has revealed that mitochondria's integrity might be the determining factor in inducing apoptosis in individual cells depending on the death stimulus. Scientific information indicates that the mitochondria undergo major changes in membrane integrity before classical signs of apoptosis become apparent. These changes involve the inner and outer mitochondrial membrane, which leads to a disruption of the membrane and a release of activated proteins such as cytochrome C into the cytoplasm [135]. This process relies heavily on the activation of a cysteine family of proteins called caspases. Caspases are indispensable as initiators and effectors of apoptotic cell death and are directly involved in many of the biochemical and morphologic features of apoptosis. They are sensitive to the redox status of the cell, and certain levels of oxidative stress can block their activity. Thus, alterations of intracellular redox status might trigger or block the apoptotic death program depending on the severity of the oxidative stress [136]. Caspases are activated through two principal pathways, the "extrinsic pathway," such as the Fas-caspase-8–induced pathway, and the "intrinsic" or mitochondrial pathway, often involving cytochrome c release and caspase-9 as an initiator caspase. Of the many identified caspases, caspase-3 appears to be the major instigator of apoptosis and central to apoptosis induced by a variety of stimuli. The cascade of caspase activation is the mechanism responsible for nuclear degradation or fragmentation and cellular morphological changes typical of apoptotic cells [137].

Presently, there is no compelling evidence that apoptosis can occur in the absence of caspases. Although cell death can occur through caspase-independent nonapoptotic mechanisms as mentioned previously, the morphologic characteristics that define the process of apoptosis depend on the activity of caspases [138]. Additionally, not all caspases are involved primarily in apoptosis. Caspase-1 activates proinflammatory cytokines, which modulate the effects of inflammation. This inflammation often acerbates tissue injury, resulting in an elaboration of antiapoptosis-inducing proteins [139]. Several families of proteins such as Bcl-2 and BAX contain proapoptotic (Bcl-2, Bid) and antiapoptotic (BAX) members, some of which are implicated in cancer and degenerative neuronal diseases [140]. The entire life and death machinery is controlled through a complicated regulatory system heavily influenced by oxidative stress (Fig. 2).

Apoptosis-based therapies

Scientific estimates judge that too much or too little cell death contributes to much of the medical diseases for which adequate therapy or preventative measures are lacking. Great interest has emerged in devising therapeutic strategies for modulating these molecules that make life or death decisions. These efforts in finding certain biologic constituents that modulate apoptosis and modify cell death would be excellent targets for therapeutic intervention. For example, thiol antioxidants (NAC, α lipoic acid, S-adenosylmethionine [SAMe]) that increase GSH levels are ideal agents because they appear to modulate mitochondrial respiration and apoptosis. Additional biologic agents that target caspases are also logical choices for control of apoptosis. For example, caspase-modulating drugs offer a variety of choices that could be anything from specific inhibitors to broad inhibitors found in nature. Among the issues to be answered include (1) whether cell death associated with a particular disease is caspase-dependent or -independent, (2) whether or not the caspases have other physiologic functions beyond apoptosis, and (3) whether or not preservation of the cell equates with preservation of cellular function. These questions and more will be answered with future applications of these biologic agents.

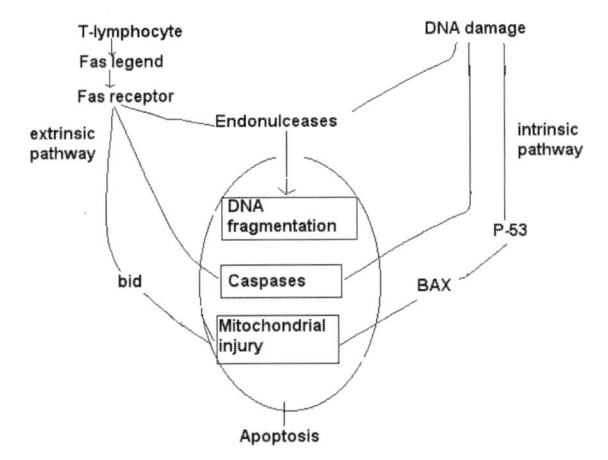

Fig. 2. Cell death process (apoptosis). It is a morphological phenomenon characterized by an intrinsic and extrinsic pathways. The cascade of caspase activation depicts the mechanism for DNA degradation or fragmentation and cellular morphological changes typical of apoptotic cells. (*Modified from* Rubin E, Farber J. Pathology. 3rd edition. Philadelphia: Lippincott-Raven; 1999; p. 27; with permission.)

Summary

There have been remarkable advances in molecular and cell biology that define the mechanisms of how various supplements function in and around cells. Current evidence strongly supports the probability that cellular functions and cellular responses that pertain to inflammation, disease, and life and death activity can be modulated with supplementation; however, the complexity of each individual's reaction and the vast differences in physiologic influences makes clinical research difficult in regard to clinical studies using antioxidant and biologic therapies. Not enough is known specifically about each supplement and its interactions with cells, nor is enough understood about how the body compensates or reacts to such applications. What works well in one individual or species might work differently in another. In addition, not all antioxidants are created equally, and discrepancies in purity and absorption can occur. It must also be determined whether or not less than optimum levels or infrequent usage will produce the same physiological effects. Not everyone—nor every species of animal—responds in the same manner to supplements, which might account for the variations in clinical research.

The cellular effects of antioxidants and other supplements are well defined and meaningful, and their clinical application looks promising despite individual variations. Combinations of antioxidants are synergistic and support cellular functions, effects that are often not apparent with individual agents. Such combinations offer a variety of mechanisms for reducing oxygen metabolites in tissues, altering signaling pathways, and modulating transcription factors, and they might play key roles in reducing the damage afforded by ROS. It is the author's opinion that combinations of antioxidants are best suited for clinical application in modulating disease and reducing premature aging when caused by excessive free radical accumulation. Clinicians should approach clinical application of these supplements based on the best available scientific research and species-specific information available.

Acknowledgment

The author thanks Kimm J. Hamann, PhD, Associate Professor, Department of Medicine, University of Chicago, for reviewing and editing this manuscript.

References

[1] Zhu C, Bao G, Wang N. Cell mechanics: mechanical response, cell adhesion, and molecular deformation. Annu Rev Biomed Eng 2000;2:189–226.
[2] Melov S. Mitochondrial oxidative stress. Physiological consequences and potential for a role in aging. Ann N Y Acad Sci 2000;908:219–25.

[3] Laupacis A. The future of evidence based medicine. Can J Clin Pharmacol 2001;8(Suppl A): 6A–9A; 908:219–25.
[4] Jewell DE, Toll PW, Wedekind KJ, Zicker SC. Effect of increasing alkenals in serum of dogs and cats. Veterinary Therapeutics 2000;1:264–72.
[5] Southorn PA, Powis G. Free radicals in medicine. I. Chemical nature and biologic reactions. Mayo Clin Proc 1988;63(4):381–9.
[6] Droge W. Free radicals in the physiological control of cell function. Physiol Rev 2002; 82(1):47–95.
[7] Sun Y, Oberly LW. Redox regulation of transcriptional activators. Free Radic Biol Med 1996;21(3):335–48.
[8] Gate L, Paul J, Tew KD, Tapiero H. Oxidative stress induced in pathologies: the role of antioxidants. Biomed Pharmacotherapy 1999;53(4):169–80.
[9] van de Vusse GJ, van Bilsen M, Glatz JF, et al. The critical steps in cellular fatty acid uptake and utilization physiololgy. Mol Cell Biochem 2002;239:9–15.
[10] Hajri T, Abumrad NA. Fatty acid transport across membranes: relevance to nutrition and metabolic pathology. Annu Rev Nutr 2002;22:383–415.
[11] Van der Vusse GJ, van Bilsen M, Glatz JF, Hasselbaink DM, Luiken JJ. Critical steps in cellular fatty acid uptake and utilization. Biochem 2002;239(1–2):9–15.
[12] Dobrescu G. Intercellular communication. Rev Med Chir Soc Med Nat Iasi 1998;102(3–4): 17–24.
[13] Kile BT, Nicola NA, Alexander WS. Negative regulators of cytokine signaling. Int J Hematol 2001;73(3):292–8.
[14] Li X, Stark GR. NFkappaB-dependent signaling pathways. Exp Hematol 2002;30(4): 285–96.
[15] Heldin CH. Protein tyrosine kinase receptors. Cancer Surv 1996;27:7–24.
[16] Horvath CM. STAT proteins and transcriptional responses to extracellular signals. Trends Biochem Sci 2000;25(10):496–502.
[17] Bromberg J, Darnell JE Jr. The role of STATs in transcriptional control and their impact on cellular function. Oncogene 2000;19(21):2468–73.
[18] Anthony CP, Thibodeau GA. Textbook of anatomy and physiology. 11th edition. Mosby; 1983.
[19] Kapit W, Macey R. The physiology book. Menlo Park (CA): Addison Wesley Longman; 1987.
[20] Orrenius S, McCabe MJ Jr, Nicotera P. $Ca(2^+)$-dependent mechanisms of cytotoxicity and programmed cell death. Toxicol Lett 1992;64–5. Spec No:357–64.
[21] Fawthrop DJ, Boobis AR, Davies DS. Mechanisms of cell death. Arch Toxicol 1991; 65(6):437–44.
[22] Allan VJ, Thompson HM, McNiven MA. Motoring around the Golgi. Nat Cell Biol 2002;10:E236–42.
[23] Marsh BJ, Howell KE. The mammalian Golgi. Nat Rev Mol Cell Biol 2002;3(10):789–95.
[24] Rutishauser M. Spiess: endoplasmic reticulum storage diseases. Swiss Med Wldy 2002; 132(17–18):211–22.
[25] Lippincott-Schwartz J. Membrane cycling between the ER and Golgi apparatus and its role in biosynthetic transport. Subcell Biochem 1993;21:95–119.
[26] Cudna RE, Dickson AJ. Endoplasmic reticulum signaling as a determinant of recombinant protein expression. Biotechnol Bioeng 2003;81(1):56–65.
[27] Shepherd VL. Intracellular pathways and mechanisms of sorting in receptor-mediated endocytosis. Trends Pharmacol Sci 1989;10(11):458–62.
[28] Winchester B, Vellodi A, Young E. The molecular basis of lysosomal storage diseases and their treatment. Biochem Soc Trans 2000;28(2):150–4.
[29] Nieminen AL. Apoptosis and necrosis in health and disease: role of mitochondria. Int Rev Cytol 2003;224:29–55.
[30] Halestrap AP, Doran E, Gillespie JP, O'Toole A. Mitochondria and cell death. Biochem Soc Trans 2000;28(2):170–7.

[31] Paumard P, Vaillier J, Coulary B, et al. The ATP synthase is involved in generating mitochondrial cristae morphology. EMBO J 2002;21(3):221–30.
[32] Balaban RS. Regulation of oxidative phosphylation in the mammalian cell. Am J Physiol 1990;258(3 Pt 1):C377–89.
[33] Roth E. Oxygen free radicals and their clinical implications. Acta Chir Hung 1997;36(1–4): 302–5.
[34] Haddad JJ. Glutathione depletion is associated with augmenting a proinflammatory signal: evidence for an antioxidant/pro-oxidant mechanism regulating cytokines in the alveolar epithelium. Cytokines Cell Mol Ther 2000;6(4):177–87.
[35] Parke DV, Sapota A. Chemical toxicity and reactive oxygen species. Int J Occup Med Environ Health 1996;9(4):331–40.
[36] Fanz YZ, Yang S, Wu G. Free radicals, antioxidants and nutrition. Nutrition 2002; 18(10):872–9.
[37] Carmody RJ, Cotter TG. Signalling apoptosis: a radical approach. Redox Rep 2001;6(2): 77–90.
[38] Exner R, Wessner B, Manhart N, Roth E. Therapeutic potential of glutathione. Wien Klin Wochenschr 2000;112(14):610–6.
[39] Wallace DC. A mitochondrial paradigm for degenerative diseases and aging. Novaritis Found Sympos 2001;235:247–63.
[40] Xu D, Finkel T. A role for mitochondria as potential regulators of cellular life span. Biochem Biophys Res Commun 2002;294(2):245–8.
[41] Mongan PD, Capacchione J, West S, Karaian J, Dubois D, Keneally R, Sharma P. Pyruvate improves redox status and decreases indicators of hepatic apoptosis during hemorrhagic shock in swine. Am J Physiol Heart Circ Physiol 2002;283(4):H1634–44.
[42] Vieira HL, Kroemer G. Pathophysiology of mitochondrial cell death control. Cell Mol Life Sci 1999;56(11–12):971–6.
[43] Yin XM. Signal transduction mediated by Bid, a pro-death Bcl-2 family proteins, connects the death receptor and mitochondria apoptosis pathways. Cell Res 2000;10(3): 161–7.
[44] Jurgensmeier JM, Xie Z, Deveraux Q, Ellerby L, Bredesen D, Reed JC. Bax directly induces release of cytochrome c from isolated mitochondria. Proc Natl Acad Sci USA 1998;95(9):4997–5002.
[45] Harris MH, Thompson CB. The role of the Bcl-2 family in the regulation of outer mitochondrial membrane permeability. Cell Death Differ 2000;7(12):1182–91.
[46] Bowser DN, Petrou S, Panchal RG, Smart ML, Williams DA. Release of mitochondrial $Ca2^+$ via the permeability transition activates endoplasmic reticulum $Ca2^+$ uptake. FASEB J 2002;16(9):1105–7.
[47] Kajimoto S, Takanashi N, Kajimoto T, et al. Sophoranone, extracted from a traditional Chinese medicine. Shan Dou Gen induces apoptosis in human leukemia cells via formation of reactive oxygen species and opening of mitochondrial transition pores. Int J Cancer 2002;99(6):879–90.
[48] Hakim J. Pharmacologic control of intracellular signaling pathways: from research to therapy. J Cardiovasc Pharmacol 1995;25(Suppl 2):S106–13.
[49] Chen F, Castranova V, Shi X. New insights into the role of nuclear factor-kappaB in cell growth regulation. Am J Pathol 2001;159(2):387–97.
[50] Blackwell TS, Christman JW. The role of nuclear factor-kappa B in cytokine gene regulation. Am J Respir Cell Mol Biol 1997;17(1):3–9.
[51] Kretz-Remy C, Mehlen P, Mirault ME, Arrigo AP. Inhibition of I kappa B-alpha phosphorylation and degradation and subsequent NF-kB activation by glutathione peroxidase overexpression. J Cell Biol 1996;133(5):1083–93.
[52] Breithaupt TB, Vazquez A, Baez I, Eylar EH. The suppression of T cell function and NF(kappa)B expression by serine protease inhibitors is blocked by N-acetylcysteine. Cell Immunol 1996;173(1):124–30.

[53] Maalouf S, El-Sabban M, Darwiche N, Gali-Muhtasib H. Protective effects of vitamin E on ultra violet light-induced damage in keratinocytes. Mol Carcinog 2002;34(3):121–30.
[54] Kretz-Remy C, Arrigo AP. Selenium: a key element that controls NF-kB activation and I kappa B alpha half life. Biofactors 2001;14(1–4):117–25.
[55] Aragno M, Mastrocola R, Brignardello E, Catalano M, Robino G, Manti R, et al. Dehydroepiandrosterone modulates nuclear factor-kappa B activation in hippocampus of diabetic rats. Endocrinology 2002;143(9):3250–8.
[56] Almawi WY, Melemedjian OK. Molecular mechanisms of glucocorticoid antiproliferative effects: antagonism of transcription factor activity by glucocorticoids receptor. J Leukoc Biol 2002;71(1):9–15.
[57] Yin MJ, Yamamoto Y, Gaynor RB. The anti-inflammatory agents aspirin and salicylate inhibit the activity of I(kappa)B kinase-beta. Nature 1998;396(6706):15–7.
[58] Sethi S, Eastman AY, Eaton JW. Inhibition of phagocyte-endothelium interactions by oxidized fatty acids: a natural anti-inflammatory mechanism?. J Lab Clin Med 1996; 128(1):27–38.
[59] Conner EM, Grisham MB. Inflammation, free radicals, and antioxidants. Nutrition 1996; 12(4):274–7.
[60] Bharti AC, Aggarwal BB. Nuclear factor-kappa B and cancer: its role in prevention and therapy. Biochem Pharmacol 2002;64(5–6):883–8.
[61] Qin Y, Camoretti-Mercado B, Blokh L, Long CG, Ko FD, Hamann KJ. Fas resistance of leukemic eosinophils is due to activation of NF-k B by Fas ligation. J Immunol 2002; 169(7):3536–44.
[62] Chung HY, Kim HJ, Kim KW, Choi JS, Yu BP. Molecular inflammation hypothesis of aging based on the anti-aging mechanism of calorie restriction. Microsc Res Tech 2002; 59(4):264–72.
[63] Davis JN, Kucuk O, Djuric Z, Sarkar FH. Soy isoflavone supplementation in healthy men prevents NF-kB activation by TNF-alpha in blood lymphocytes. Free Radic Biol Med 2001;30(11):1293–302.
[64] Unwin PN. Gap junction structure and the control of cell-to-cell communication. Ciba Found Symp 1987;125:78–91.
[65] Yamasaki H, Krutovshikh V, Mesnil M, et al. Role of connexin (gap junction) genes in cell growth and carcinogenesis. C R Acad Sci III 1999;322(2–3):151–9.
[66] Alves LA, Nihei OK, Fonseca PC, Carvalho AC, Savino W. Gap junction modulation by extracellular signaling molecules: the thymus model. Braz J Med Biol Res 2000;33(4): 457–65.
[67] Lo CW. Genes, gene knockouts, and mutations in the analysis of gap junctions. Dev Genet 1999;24(1–2):1–4.
[68] Bertram JS. Carotenoids and gene regulation. Nutr Rev 1999;57(6):182–91.
[69] Yoshizawa T, Watanabe S, Hirose M, Miyazaki A, Sato N. Dimethylsulfoxide maintains intercellular communication by preserving the gap junctional protein connexin32 in primary cultured hepatocyte doublets from rats. J Gastroenterol Hepatol 1997;12(4): 325–30.
[70] Kojima T, Mochizuki C, Mitaka T, Mochizuki Y. Effects of melatonin on proliferation, oxidative stress and Cx32 gap junction protein expression in primary cultures of adult rat hepatocytes. Cell Struct Funct 1997;22(3):347–56.
[71] Fukuda T, Ikejima K, Hirose M, Takei Y, Watanabe S, Sato N. Taurine preserves gap junctional intercellular communication in rat hepatocytes under oxidative stress. J Gastroenterol 2000;35(5):361–8.
[72] Upham BL, Kang KS, Cho HY, Trosko JE. Hydrogen peroxide inhibits gap junctional intercellular communication in glutathione sufficient but not glutathione deficient cells. Carcinogenesis 1997;18(1):37–42.
[73] Stahl W, Sies H. The role of cartenoids and retinoids in gap junctional communication. Int J Vitam Nutr Res 1998;68(6):354–9.

[74] Trosko JE, Ruch RJ. Gap junctions as targets for cancer chemoprevention and chemotherapy. Curr Drug Targets 2002;3(6):465–82.
[75] Trosko JE, Chang CC. Mechanism of up-regulated gap junctional intercellular communication during chemoprevention and chemotherapy of cancer. Mutat Res 2001; 480–481:219–29.
[76] Trosko JE, Ruch R. Cell–cell communication in carcinogenesis. Front Biosci 1998;3: D208–36.
[77] Trosko JE, Chang CC. Mechanism of up-regulated gap junctional intercellular communication during chemoprevention and chemotherapy of cancer. Mutat Res 2001; 480–481:219–29.
[78] Trump BF, Berezesky IK, Chang SH, Phelps PC. The pathways of cell death: oncosis, apoptosis, and necrosis. Toxicol Pathol 1997;25(1):82–8.
[79] Galan A, Garcia-Bermejo L, Vilaboa NE, et al. The role of intracellular oxidation in death induction (apoptosis and necrosis) in human promonocytic cells treated with stress inducers. Eur J Cell Biol 2001;80(4):312–20.
[80] Heller A, Koch T, Schmeck J, van Ackern K. Lipid mediators in inflammatory disorders. Drugs 1998;55(4):487–96.
[81] Tsudo M. Cytokines and disease. Rinsho Byori 1994;42(8):821–4.
[82] Homaidan FR, Chakroun I, Haidar HA, El-Sabban ME. Protein regulators of eicosanoid synthesis: role in inflammation. Curr Protein Pept Sci 2002;3(4):467–84.
[83] Tapiero H, Ba GN, Couvreur P, Tew KD. Polyunsaturated fatty acids (PUFA) and eicosanoids in human health and pathologies. Biomed Pharmacother 2002;56(5): 215–22.
[84] Lim JW, Kim H, Kim KH. Expression of Ku70 and Ku80 mediated by NF-kappa B and cyclooxygenase-2 is related to proliferation of human gastric cancer cells. J Biol Chem 2002;277(48):46093–100.
[85] Beharka AA, Wu D, Serafini M, Meydani SN. Mechanism of vitamin E inhibition of cyclooxygenase activity in macrophages from old mice: role of peroxynitrite. Free Radic Biol Med 2002;32(6):503–11.
[86] Simopoulos AP. Omega-3 fatty acids in inflammation and autoimmune diseases. J Am Coll Nutr 2002;21(6):495–505.
[87] Kim JW, Baek BS, Kim YK, Herlihy JT, Ikeno Y, Yu BP, et al. Gene expression of cyclooxygenase in the aging heart. J Gerontol A Biol Sci Med Sci 2001;56(8):B350–5.
[88] Lu J, Ho CT, Ghai G, Chen KY. Differential effects of theaflavin monogallates on cell growth, apoptosis, and Cox-2 gene expression in cancerous versus normal cells. Cancer Res 2000;60(22):6465–71.
[89] Mendoza Rodriguez CA, Cerbon MA. Tumor suppressor gene p53: mechanisms of action in cell proliferation and death. Clin 2001;53(3):266–73.
[90] Lof S, Poulsen HE. Antioxidant intervention studies related to DNA damage, DNA repair and gene expression. Free Radic Res 2000;33(Suppl):S67–83.
[91] Wang XD, Russell RM. Procarcinogenic and anticarcinogenic effects of beta-carotene. Nutr Rev 1999;57(9 Pt 1):263–72.
[92] Siems W, Sommerburg O, Schild L, Augustin W, Langhans CD, Wiswedel I. Beta-carotene cleavage products induce oxidative stress in vitro by impairing mitochondrial respiration. FASEB J 2002;16(10):1289–91.
[93] Hamilton KK. Antioxidant supplements during cancer treatments: where do we stand? Clin J Oncol Nurs 2001;5(4):181–2.
[94] Spector S. Leukotriene inhibitors and antagonists in asthma. Ann Allergy Asthma Immunol 1995;75:463–70.
[95] Christmas P, Weber BM, McKee M, Brown D, Soberman RJ. Membrane localization and topology of leukotriene C4 synthase. J Biol Chem 2002;277(32):28902–8.
[96] Bautz F, Denzlinger C, Kanz L, Mohle R. Chemotaxis and transendothelial migration of CD34(+) hematopoietic progenitor cells induced by the inflammatory mediator

leukotriene D4 are mediated by the 7-transmembrane receptor CysLT1. Blood 2001; 97(11):3433–40.
[97] Agrawal R, Daniel EE. Control of gap junction formation in canine trachea by arachidonic acid metabolites. Am J Physiol 1986;250(3 Pt 1):C495–505.
[98] Ohd JF, Wikstrom K, Sjolander A. Leukotrienes induce cell-survival signaling in intestinal epithelial cells. Gastroenterology 2000;119(4):1007–18.
[99] Schewe T, Kuhn H, Sies H. Flavonoids of cocoa inhibit recombinant human 5-lipoxygenase. Nutr J 2002;132(7):1825–9.
[100] Kimmatkar N, Thawani V, Hingorani L, Khiyani R. Efficacy and tolerability of Boswellia serrata extract in treatment of osteoarthritis of the knee—a randomized double blind placebo controlled trial. Phytomedicine 2003;10(1):3–7.
[101] Rath PC, Aggarwal BB. TNF-induced signaling in apoptosis. J Clin Immunol 1999;19(6): 350–64.
[102] Antwerp Van DJ, Martin SJ, Kafri T, Green DR, Verma M. Suppression of TNF-alpha induced apoptosis by NF Kappa B. Science 1996;274(5288):787–9.
[103] Habtemarian S. Natural inhibitors of tumor necrosis factor-alpha production, secretion and function. Planta Med 2000;66(4):303–13.
[104] Cairns CB, Panacek EA, Harken AH, Banerjee A. Bench to bedside: tumor necrosis factor-alpha: from inflammation to resuscitation. Acad Emerg Med 2000;7(8):930–41.
[105] Dijkstra G, Moshage H, Jansen PL. Blockade of NF-kappaB activation and donation of nitric oxide: new treatment options in inflammatory bowel disease? Scand J Gastroenterol Suppl2002;7(236):37–41.
[106] Baines M, Shenkin A. Use of antioxidants in surgery: a measure to reduce postoperative complications. Curr Opinion Clin Nutr Metab Care 2002;6:665–70.
[107] Cammer W. Protection of cultured oligodendrocytes against tumor necrosis factor-alpha by the antioxidants coenzyme Q(10) and N-acetyl cysteine. Brain Res Bull 2002;58(6):587–92.
[108] Raza SL, Cornelius LA. Matrix metalloproteinases pro- and anti-angiogenic activities. J Investing Dermatol Symp Proc 2000;5(1):47–54.
[109] Bergers G, Cousens LM. Matrix metalloproteinase product information. Curr Opin Genet Dev 2002;10:20.
[110] Galis ZS, Khatri JJ. Matrix metalloproteinases in vascular remodeling and atherogenesis: the good, the bad, and the ugly. Circ Res 2002;90(3):251–62.
[111] Nagase H. Activation mechanisms of matrix metalloproteinases. Biol Chem 1997;378(3–4): 151–60.
[112] Bee A, Barnes A, Jones MD, Robertson DH, et al. Canine TIMP-2 purification, characterization and molecular detection. Vet J 2000;160(2):126–34.
[113] Kelly EA, Jarjour NN. Role of matrix metalloproteinases in asthma. Curr Opin Pulm Med 2003;9(1):28–33.
[114] Demeule M, Brossard M, Page M, Gingras D, Beliveau R. Matrix metalloproteinase inhibition by green tea catechins. Biochem Biophys Acta 2000;1478(1):51–60.
[115] Krieglstein CF, Granger DN. Adhesion molecules and their role in vascular disease. Am J Hypertens 2001;14(6 Pt 2):44S–54S.
[116] Roebuck KA. Oxidant stress regulation of IL-8 and ICAM-1 gene expression: differential activation and binding of the transcription factors AP-1 and NF-kappaB. Int J Mol Med 1999;4(3):223–30.
[117] Tailor A, Granger DN. Role of adhesion molecules in vascular regulation and damage. Curr Hypertens Rep 2000;2(1):78–83.
[118] Tanaka Y. T cell integrin activation by chemokines in inflammation. Arch Immunol Ther Exp [Warsz] 2000;48(6):443–50.
[119] Hubbard AK, Rothlein R. Intercellular adhesion molecule-1 (ICAM-1) expression and cell signaling cascades. Free Radic Biol Med 2000;28(9):1379–86.
[120] Sahnoun Z, Jamoussi K, Zeghal KM. Free radicals and antioxidants: physiology, human pathology and therapeutic aspects. Therapie 1998;53(4):315–39.

[121] Peter K, Weirich U, Nordt TK, Ruef J, Bode C. Soluble vascular cell adhesion molecule-1 (VCAM-1) as potential marker of atherosclerosis. Thromb Haemost 1999;82(Suppl 1): 38–43.
[122] Green PJ, Walsh FS, Doherty P. Signal transduction mechanisms underlying axonal growth responses stimulated by cell adhesion molecules. Rev Neurol [Paris] 1997;153(8–9): 509–14.
[123] Roussidis AE, Karamanos NK. Inhibition of receptor tyrosine kinase-based signal transduction as specific target for cancer treatment. In Vivo 2002;16(6):459–69.
[124] Sylvester PW, McIntyre BS, Gapor A, Briski KP. Vitamin E inhibition of normal mammary epithelial cell growth is associated with a reduction in protein kinase C (alpha) activation. Cell Prolif 2001;34(6):347–57.
[125] Barnes S, Boersma B, Patel R, Kirk M, Darley-Usmar VM, Kim H, et al. Isoflavonoids and chronic disease: mechanisms of action. Biofactors 2000;12(1–4):209–15.
[126] Nathens AB, Bitar R, Marshall JC, Watson RW, Dackiw AP, Fan J, et al. Antioxidants increase lipopolysaccharide-stimulated TNF alpha release in murine macrophages: role for altered TNF alpha mRNA stability. Shock 2001;16(5):361–7.
[127] Theriault A, Chao JT, Gapor A, Chao JT, Gapor A. Tocotrienol is the most effective vitamin E for reducing endothelial expression of adhesion molecules and adhesion to monocytes. Atherosclerosis 2002;160(1):21–30.
[128] Schubert SY, Neeman I, Resnick N. A novel mechanism for the inhibition of NF-kappaB activation in vascular endothelial cells by natural antioxidants. FASEB J 2002;16(14): 1931–3.
[129] Nicola NA. Cytokine pleiotropy and redundancy: a view from the receptor. Stem Cells 1994;12(Suppl 1):3–12 [discussion 12].
[130] Zimmermann KC, Green DR. How cells die: apoptosis pathways. J Allergy Clin Immunol 2001;108(4 Suppl):S99–103.
[131] Jamison JM, Gilloteaux J, Taper HS, Calderon PB, Summers JL. Autoschizis: a novel cell death. Biochem Pharmacol 2002;63(10):1773–83.
[132] Lovschall H, Mosekilde L. Apoptosis: cellular and clinical aspects. Nord Med 1997; 112(4):133–7.
[133] Susin SA, Zamzami N, Kroemer G. Mitochondria as regulators of apoptosis: doubt no more. Biochim Biophys Acta 1998;1366(1–2):151–65.
[134] McConkey DL. Biochemical determinants of apoptosis and necrosis. Toxicoll Lett 1998; 99(3):157–68.
[135] Reed JC. Mechanisms of apoptosis. Am J Pathol 2000;157(5):1415–30.
[136] Hampton MB, Orrenius S. Redox regulation of apoptotic cell death. Biofactors 1998; 8(1–2):1–5.
[137] Ueda S, Masutani H, Nakamura H, Tanaka T, Ueno M, Yodoi J. Redox control of cell death. Antioxid Redox Signal 2002;4(3):405–14.
[138] Depraetere V, Golstein P. Dismantling in cell death: molecular mechanisms and relationship to caspase activation. Scand J Immunol 1998;47(6):523–31.
[139] Zeuner A, Eramo A, Peschle C, De Maria R. Caspase activation without death. Cell Death Differ 1999;6(11):1075–80.
[140] Tsujimoto Y. Role of Bcl-2 family proteins in apoptosis: apoptosomes or mitochondria? Genes Cells 1998;3(11):697–707.

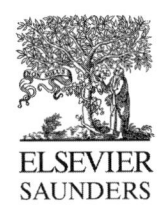

// Metabolic, antioxidant, nutraceutical, probiotic, and herbal therapies relating to the management of hepatobiliary disorders

Sharon A. Center, DVM

College of Veterinary Medicine, Cornell University, Ithaca, NY 14853, USA

Conventional education in the medical sciences is based on facts evolved from organized experiments or observations involving bench laboratory methods, animal models of disease, and clinical patients; however, for many medicinal, nutraceutical, and herbal substances, benefit and hazard odds for particular applications are derived from uncontrolled anecdotal observations. With the popularity of so-called evidence-based medicine, an expression used by clinician–scientists looking for proof that treatment surpasses the placebo effect (causing no harm), many clinicians are searching for data that justify the use of novel products. Evidence-based data are complicated; recently even the use of a placebo control group was called into question [1]. Many nutraceutical, conditionally essential nutrients and botanical extracts have been proposed as useful in the management of liver disease. The most studied of these are addressed in terms of proposed mechanisms of action, benefits, hazards, and safe dosing recommendations allowed by current information. While this is an area of soft science, it is important to keep an open and tolerant mind, considering that many major treatment discoveries were in fact serendipitous accidents. Consider, for example, the realization by Western medicine that the ancient Asian custom of using bear bile in the treatment of liver disease provides ursodeoxycholic acid (UDCA), now known to provide a number of diverse and important therapeutic benefits in cholestatic and necroinflammatory liver disease.

Hepatocellular death: apoptosis and cytolytic cell death (necrosis)

Hepatocellular injury and death can be initiated by a variety of insults derived from the extra- or intrahepatic environment. Cell death can occur as

E-mail address: sac6@cornell.edu

a result of biologic pathways culminating in apoptosis (non-necrolytic programmed cell death, an energy-requiring process) or cell (cytolytic) necrosis. While these responses are often described as being separate and unique, recent evidence suggests that the distinction is not always clear [2].

An important mechanism of *cytolytic hepatocyte death* is cytochrome P_{450}-dependent formation of reactive metabolites. Covalent binding of reactive metabolites to hepatic proteins can trigger direct cell injury or an immune response. Reactive metabolites can damage DNA directly, cause overexpression of proapoptotic proteins (eg, p 53), deplete essential antioxidants, damage mitochondria, or increase cytosolic calcium. Cytotoxic T lymphocytes can kill hepatocytes through (1) binding to hepatocyte surface receptors (eg, Fas–ligand binding to the hepatocyte Fas receptor), (2) production of death-signaling cytokines (eg, tumor necrosis factor-α [TNF-α]), or (3) release of cytotoxic mediators (eg, granzyme B) [3]. Necrosis classically involves cell swelling, loss of plasma membrane integrity, and subsequent cell lysis and secondary inflammation, and it typically produces zonal injury except in the rare circumstance of fulminant hepatic necrosis.

Apoptosis, or programmed cell death, eliminates inessential or pathologically altered cells, and in most circumstances it is presumed to be beneficial; however, in some hepatobiliary disorders premature apoptosis eliminates a critical number of hepatocytes, leading to impaired liver function. Apoptosis is characterized morphologically on the basis of microscopic or ultrastructural changes in cells and organelles, or it is characterized mechanistically on the basis of mediator activation and release. Microscopically, it is characterized by cell shrinkage and cytoplasmic and nuclear condensation and fragmentation without loss of plasma membrane integrity (eg, the classic Councilman or acidophilic bodies historically described in diseased liver) [2]. Mechanistically it is a controlled, usually focal or spotty process that unobtrusively eliminates cells [2]. While apoptotic cells classically are phagocytosed rapidly by neighboring macrophages without induction of an inflammatory response, the response also can initiate or modulate hepatic inflammation [4]. Hepatocyte apoptosis interrupts mitochondrial electron transport promoting secondary oxidative stress that can damage adjacent cells. Oxidant injury and loss of cytosolic ATP disables normal cell processes, causing abnormal canalicular bile formation (canalicular bile stasis), reduced synthesis of constituitively expressed proteins (albumin, fibrinogen, acute phase proteins), impaired transport and exportation processes involving cytoskeletal elements (eg, canalicular bile stasis, hepatocellular copper [Cu] retention), and impaired membrane pumps (eg, cell swelling, cytosolic granular appearance, hydropic degeneration on microscopic examination).

Mitochondria and hepatic oxidative injury

All cells generate reactive oxygen species (ROS), primarily from normal mitochondrial function, which in the highly metabolic hepatocyte accounts for approximately 2% to 5% of the oxygen consumed in conducting oxidative phosphorylation [2]. Because mitochondria are an important source of ROS, they have pivotal importance in disease processes in which oxidative stress or altered cell redox status play a pathophysiologic role. Many intracellular processes invoking apoptosis and necrosis target mitochondria directly or indirectly [2,5]. Enhanced mitochondrial ROS production can result from exposure to a number of biologic mediators, drugs, toxins, and conditions (eg, tumor necrosis factor-α [TNF-α], bile acids, ischemia–reperfusion injury). Impaired electron transport leads to release of reduced mitochondrial intermediates that can autoxidize, yielding free radicals and lipid peroxides, which can induce mitochondrial permeability transition (MPT), a process that precedes organelle/cell suicide. A number of drugs, biomolecules, and factors are recognized that can induce hepatocyte MPT, such as ROS, thiol crosslinkers, bile acids (direct effect), salicylic acid and valproic acid (which can disrupt cell calcium management), and certain chemotherapeutic agents (eg, induce Fas-receptor/Fas-ligand [Fas-L]–initiated MPT) [5–7]. Cell redox balance influences normal cell function through effects on gene expression and transcription factors. Oxidative stress is known to (1) upregulate production of inflammatory cytokines, chemokines, and adhesion molecules; (2) increase expression and binding of Fas-L; (3) induce survival genes (ie, NF-κβ) that can block TNF-α–initiated apoptosis; and (4) induce MPT directly. Depending on the extent and nature of oxidative stress, cell death can result from apoptosis or necrosis. The latter is favored by high-level oxidant exposure.

Kupffer cells: resident hepatic macrophages

A common source of oxidant stress in liver disease emanates from activated hepatic phagocytes (Kupffer cells). These resident cells represent 80% to 90% of the fixed macrophages in the body, unique because of their proximity to the site of acute phase protein synthesis and chronic priming exposure to endotoxins derived from the portal circulation. Kupffer cells are implicated as a cause of liver injury in systemic sepsis, endotoxemia, and ischemia–reperfusion injury, and they participate in all forms of chronic inflammatory liver disease [8–10]. Activated Kupffer cells produce a complex and highly interactive repertoire of inflammatory mediators and cytokines. Signaling from these cells is pivotal to host response in necroinflammatory processes, in which they crosstalk with and activate Stellate cells, resulting in enhanced deposition of extracellular matrix (ECM). Further, Kupffer cells provide a critical storage site for transition metals, particularly iron. Transition metals are those that fluctuate between benign and reactive forms. Iron housed in this capacity contributes to oxidative injury in acute or chronic necroinflammatory liver disease.

Activated Kupffer cells amplify and augment tissue inflammatory responses damaging "innocent bystanders," for example (1) directly from oxidative burst activity, (2) secondarily from chemikines and cytokines, (3) through attraction and adhesion of neutrophils and mast cells, and (4) by elaboration of mediators that attract and aggregate platelets that obstruct local microcirculation causing an ischemic–reperfusion challenge. Their involvement in liver disease can represent their recruitment as a tissue response to oxidative stress or can lead the way as a primary pathologic process. Kupffer cells contribute to hepatocellular dysfunction associated with the proinflammatory cytokines released in early sepsis before circulatory dysfunction becomes apparent [11]. Antioxidants can modulate Kupffer cell activation during early sepsis, producing beneficial effects extending beyond the liver [12]. Pretreatment with N-acetylcysteine (NAC) or vitamin E before endotoxin exposure suppresses lipopolysaccharide (LPS)-mediated production of TNF-α in Kupffer cells and disease responses signaled by Kupffer cells, including tissue neutrophil migration, prostaglandin release, and increased procoagulant activity typical of the sepsis syndrome [13,14].

Stellate cells (Ito cell, hepatic myofibroblast)

The hepatic Stellate cells, also known as Ito cells or retinoid storage cells, reside in the space of Disse in close contact with sinusoidal endothelial cells, hepatocytes, and Kupffer cells. These cells normally represent about 15% of the total liver cell population [15]. Stellate cells have long branching cytoplasmic processes that extend to the intersinusoidal, perisinusoidal (subendothelial position), and interhepatocellular spaces. Encircling the sinusoids allows them to influence sinusoidal blood flow (pericapillary constriction). Normal resting Stellate cells are rich in retinoic acid (vitamin A storage, Ito cell capacity), have minimal ECM, few receptors, and show little proliferative response; however, upon activation, phenotypic transformation occurs whereby they acquire myofibroblast-like features (ie, they lose retinoid stores, express smooth muscle proteins [actin], develop the ability to produce collagen, express numerous surface receptors, behave in a proinflammatory capacity, and demonstrate remarkable proliferative responses) [15]. Activated Stellate cells produce interstitial collagens I and III and are the source of pathologic fibroplasia. Along with Kupffer cells, activated Stellate cells also function as a source of metalloproteinases (collagenases), which can degrade ECM collagen; however, their dual production of metalloproteinase inhibitors typically permits a net accumulation of ECM collagen, promoting hepatic fibrogenesis. The major mediator of the Stellate cell population and recovery from the dynamic process of fibrosis is apoptosis.

Kupffer cells mediate hepatic Stellate cell responses through cytokine elaboration. The immediacy of their communication is exemplified by changes in acute-phase responses following bacteremia or endotoxemia. Kupffer cell secretion of interleukin (IL)-1, IL-6, and TNF is followed within 48 hours by altered gene expression in Stellate cells, increasing ECM proteins and reducing metalloproteinases. With more constant injury (eg, exposure to a necrotizing toxin), induction of transforming growth factor-β (TGF-β) protects against Stellate cell apoptosis. Differences in initiated Kupffer cell cytokine responses in different forms of injury send different urgency regarding Stellate cell response.

Numerous therapeutic agents including certain dietary supplements and herbal derivatives are considered to be antioxidants or are touted as providing anti-inflammatory effects because they influence the accumulation or activity of Stellate cells [14], which might include an ability to inhibit cell activation or proliferation, to control signaling from neighboring cells (elaboration of cytokines or vasoactive mediators from Kupffer cells), quench ROS, or inhibit ROS production. Some agents appear to suppress Stellate cell collagen synthesis directly or enhance metalloproteinase production. Antioxidants are of special interest in controlling adverse Stellate cell behavior because they modulate Kupffer cells and consequently Stellate cell activation, collagen production, and progression into apoptosis [15–18]. Hepatic fibrogenesis depends on signals that maintain Stellate cell activation or prohibit their apoptotic removal. While these cells tend to undergo spontaneous apoptosis, this is diverted by certain inflammatory cytokines (TNF and TGF-β) that typically induce apoptosis in other cell lines.

Hepatic fibrosis

Hepatic fibrogenesis is a dynamic process involving an imbalance between the synthesis of ECM and its dissolution by metalloproteinases. Basic fibrogenesis is a nonspecific mechanism that continues as long as injury or inflammatory signaling persists. The process initiates with the intent of limiting extension of inflammation and tissue damage and becomes pathologic as the balance between ECM deposition, remodeling, and removal favors its net accumulation. The ECM is a complex mixture of glycoproteins (collagen, elastin, fibronectin, laminin) and proteoglycans organized in a tridimensional network [19]. Excessive deposition of ECM changes liver architecture disturbing normal perfusion. The final stage culminates as cirrhosis, denoted by extensive fibrosis linking acinar zones (representing the areas of chronic injury), nodular regeneration (regenerated hepatic tissue lacking normal architectural landmarks, encircled by connective tissue), and impaired sinusoidal perfusion (loss of dynamic fenestrae in sinusoidal endothelium, deposition of ECM in the space of Disse or focal zonal regions, and intrahepatic formation of arteriovenous and venovenous shunts). Implicit in the development of hepatic fibrosis is the limited exposure of hepatocytes to sinusoidal blood, perturbing exchange of substances between the liver and splanchnic and systemic circulations. The process defined as *sinusoidal capillarization* describes loss of the normally dynamic fenestrae present in the sinusoidal endothelial barrier. The process described by *collagenization* defines the deposition of ECM in zonal or perisinusoidal locations. Zonal fibrosis is most prominent in companion animals that have chronic necroinflammatory liver disease, which is primarily periportal. Perisinusoidal fibrosis describes the deposition of excessive ECM in the space of Disse (the area beneath the endothelium where ultrafiltrate bathes the hepatocyte surface) and sinusoidal capillarization. Accumulated ECM can function as a storage site for inflammatory mediators and cytokines, promoting and prolonging tissue injury. While certain therapeutic applications might describe increased collagenase activity as a beneficial effect, there are many different metalloproteinases, each of which acts on a specific ECM component. Furthermore, collagenases are collagen type-specific. Thus, increased collagenase activity as a therapeutic claim has importance only if proven in a hepatobiliary disease model or clinical scenario. While it was long thought that hepatic fibrosis was a progressive one-way pathologic process inevitably leading to cirrhosis, recent work proves that it can resolve if underlying inflammatory processes are controlled and eliminated [16–20].

The crosstalk between cells driving inflammation and fibrosis is complex, and the blend of stimuli determining the net balance of ECM deposition is changing constantly. Exactly where and what in this myriad of responses and communications can be manipulated therapeutically remains unclear; however, it is unlikely that single-agent therapy can change the process pivotally. Rather, a complementary, adjunctive, or synergistic approach is more likely to provide better clinical responses.

Cholestatic liver disease: special considerations

Cholestatic liver disease encompasses a heterogeneous group of abnormalities associated with compromised bile formation or flow. Causes include structural, genetic, immunologic, and inflammatory processes and complex metabolic abnormalities (eg, associated with sepsis). Proven treatments, besides mechanical decompression of an obstructed biliary tree, are largely inadequate and unproven except for administration of UDCA in selected disorders and antimicrobial treatment in sepsis. Recognizing the complexities of cellular and molecular mechanisms leading to liver injury and fibrosis in cholestasis is critical to selecting interventional strategies. Free radicals contribute importantly to the pathogenesis of cholestatic liver injury. Although the initial insult might be mechanical or immunologic, cell injury is worsened by direct damage from hydrophobic bile acids. Polymorphonuclear leukocytes are also involved as an initial response.

Hepatic copper (Cu) retention, secondary to reduced biliary Cu egress, contributes to injury by promoting ROS generation through its transition metal status (Haber-Weiss reaction).

Much evidence substantiates that hydrophobic bile acids contribute to cholestatic liver injury. The hepatotoxic potential of bile acids, in decreasing order, includes (1) lithocholic acid, (2) deoxycholic acid, (3) chenodeoxycholic acid, (4) cholic acid, and (5) UDCA [21]. Chenodeoxycholic acid, which was once prescribed for gallstone dissolution in humans, produces morphologic and clinical hepatotoxicity. Lithocholic acid is used for in vivo and in vitro disease modeling, where it provokes severe hepatocellular injury reliably. Sulfation and conjugation of bile acids attenuates their hepatotoxicity. In order of least to greatest toxic potential, they are (1) sulfation, (2) taurine conjugation, (3) glycine conjugation, and (4) unconjugated. Despite the amphipathic characteristic of bile acids, their hepatotoxicity is more complex than a simple detergent effect on lipid membranes. Rather, bile acid hepatotoxicity is associated with induction of apoptosis or necrosis (associated with lipid peroxidation) and depends upon the concentration achieved (higher concentrations favor necrosis). Bile acid-induced apoptosis is mediated through the Fas death receptor, protein kinase C, activation of cathepsin B, or by direct mitochondrial toxicity. Much experimental and clinical evidence supports a role of ROS as a mechanism of hepatocellular injury in cholestasis (eg, increased plasma and red blood cell [RBC] lipid peroxides, reduced liver antioxidant enzyme activity and glutathione (GSH) values, and improvement derived from correction of antioxidant insufficiencies) [22–27]. Lipid peroxidation involving mitochondria is proven in chronic bile duct obstruction, in which tissue injury is enhanced by feeding a high-lipid, vitamin E insufficient diet while injury is attenuated by vitamin E supplementation [22,23]. Hydrophobic bile acids have an inhibitory effect on egress of triglycerides from the liver as very-low-density lipoproteins (VLDL) [28,29]. Human and rat hepatocytes exposed to physiologic concentrations of taurocholic acid (10–200 umol/L, similar to zone 1 hepatocyte bile acid exposure) demonstrated a dose-dependent suppression of triglyceride exportation. Hydrophobic bile acids also inhibit mitochondrial respiration, generating ROS that overwhelm in situ mitochondrial antioxidants (eg, GSH, superoxide dismutate [SOD], coenzyme Q_{10}), culminating in oxidative injury [23]. Increased ROS oxidize critical thiol sites in membranes, enhancing MPT and activating proapoptotic proteases that amplify initial injury. Depleting cell GSH before exposure to bile acids increases their sensitivity to necrosis but not apoptosis [27]. Because attempted rescue after bile acid exposure by increasing cell GSH does not protect against either mode of cell death, the importance of a preemptive therapeutic approach for avoiding antioxidant depletion in cholestasis is obvious. A number of antioxidants and UDCA have been shown to modulate cholestatic liver injury, albeit through different mechanisms. For example, merely improving the efficiency of mitochondrial electron transport with a coenzyme Q_{10} analog (idebenone) limits production of free radicals [24]. UDCA combined with antioxidants as polymodal therapy seems logical as an interventional strategy because hepatoprotection afforded by UDCA relates to effects that are mechanistically distinct from direct mediation of redox status [24–27].

Therapeutic agents: functional interaction and product claims

In Fig. 1, important aspects in the pathobiology of liver injury are emphasized. Cytoprotective agents work, in part, by inhibiting inflammation and fibrosis, initiation of apoptosis, and by preemptively protecting against oxidant injury to ensure full ability to maintain an appropriate redox balance. Effects might be highly influenced by unique species-specific responses or disease mechanisms, and it is these factors that complicate interpretation of treatment and response. For example, γ-interferon inhibits proliferation/activation of Stellate cells and reduces expression of ECM components in liver disease models inconsistently. Pentoxyphillin (pentoxyphylline), which theoretically inhibits platelet-derived growth factor (PDGF), making it theoretically attractive for reducing Stellate cell collagen formation where PDGF is a potent agonist, provides no antifibrotic benefit in vivo. The list of contradictory and confusing findings and testimonials is long and difficult to decipher; however, an indisputable area of therapeutic benefit involves attenuation of oxidant injury. Thus, antioxidant activity has become a buzzword in the world of alternative therapies involving the liver.

All liver injury involves collateral oxidative/peroxidative organelle or cell membrane injury

While pathomechanisms of liver injury and fibrosis are multifactorial, nearly all involve collateral oxidative/peroxidative damage of cell and organelle membranes, proteins, and enzymes [30]. As a prototype antioxidant, and as the most important systemic and intracellular antioxidant mechanism, thiol management has been studied most intensively. Hepatobiliary thiol status is importantly influenced in inflammatory, necrotizing, cholestatic, and fibrosing disorders and by pathologic hepatocellular triglyceride accumulation. Altered thiol status has protean effects on hepatocytes and other resident and transient cells within the liver.

While administration of antioxidants for liver disorders has generated much interest, mixed results of administration of various products can be found. Data are still accumulating relevant to vitamin E, nicotinamide adenosine dinucleotide (NADH), SOD, ubiquinone (coenzyme Q_{10}), s-adenosylmethionine (SAMe), NAC, milk thistle (Silibinin), polyunsaturated phosphatidylcholine, and many herbal products. While in vitro work

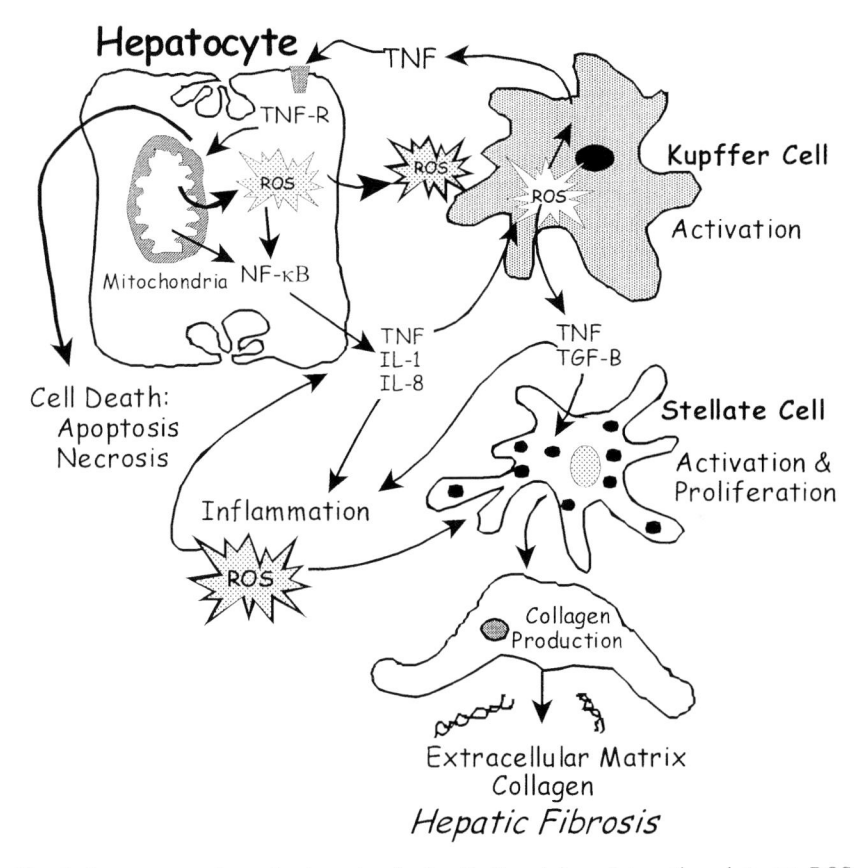

Fig. 1. Important pathomechanisms involved with liver injury. Interactions between ROS initially derived from mitochondria (toxins, endotoxins, infectious organisms, and so forth) activate hepatic Kupffer cells, initiating a chain of biologic responses leading to hepatocyte NF-κβ activation as one mechanism. Production of tumor necrosis factor (TNF) can directly or indirectly provoke hepatocyte cell death. Expression of the TNF-receptor (TNF-R) on the hepatocyte surface is shown. TNF and other mediators (transforming growth factor-β [TGF-β] shown) stimulate hepatic Stellate cells (activation and proliferation), augmenting inflammatory responses. Mediators and cytokines contributed from neighboring and transient cells can be stored within the ECM fostering the inflammatory response. When activated, Stellate cells phenotypically resemble myofibroblasts, lose their retinal stores, express surface receptors, and produce ECM collagen leading to hepatic fibrosis.

provides compelling data supporting specific nutraceuticals, studies in human patients have been less consistent and less convincing. Complicating factors include (1) incomplete understanding of the role of oxidative mechanisms in particular disorders, (2) inconsistent associations between serum antioxidant concentrations and peripheral markers of tissue injury and actual tissue circumstances, (3) different antioxidants or signals measured between studies, and (4) inconsistent analytic methods for measuring products and case outcome. Because most oxidants and antioxidants are labile, rapidly transitioning molecules, their quantitative measurement in spontaneous disease is difficult. Furthermore, tissue antioxidant status is not reflected reliably by measuring circulating antioxidants or their biologic markers [31–33]. Consequently, a peripherally collected blood or urine sample does not generally reflect the propriety of antioxidant therapy and cannot be used for monitoring treatment response—this problem greatly compromises documentation of an evidence-based response.

While most clinical studies have focused on single-agent therapy, this approach is unlikely to succeed considering the complex biochemical and cell interactions associated with liver disease. Initial studies using a polypharmacy approach support this point of view [25,26,34,35]. Free radical association with hepatobiliary disease is the foundation around which a majority of nutraceutical recommendations are formulated. The remainder are involved in different ways in intermediary metabolism unique to the liver, having extraordinary prominence in the system, or having an ability to modify apoptosis.

Metals and liver disease

Considering the involvement of oxidative injury in most forms of hepatobiliary disease, the role of metals has considerable importance. Metals importantly contribute to catalytic processes generating free radicals important to their detoxification [36–41]. Cu and iron (Fe) play a critical role in formation of ROS, and selenium and zinc contribute to ROS detoxification. Because the liver is the first organ perfused by portal blood containing absorbed minerals, it can serve as a reservoir for excessive quantities of potentially toxic metals. The biliary system serves as a major route of mineral excretion and there is an enterohepatic circulation of some of these.

Copper

Copper has pro-oxidant and antioxidant functions. As a constituent of Cu–zinc superoxide dismutase (Cu–Zn SOD), it contributes to an important antioxidant enzyme that detoxifies the superoxide radical, converting it to a nonradical product. Hepatocellular Cu overload has been well described in dogs as a genetic defect, as a random defect in individual dogs, rarely in cats, and as a complicating feature of cholestatic liver disease. While the mechanism of hepatocellular Cu retention is variable, the effect of pathologic quantities of accumulated hepatic Cu is well defined, with the mitochondria being a major target [37–40]. Excessive hepatic Cu initiates mitochondrial membrane peroxidation and morphologic abnormalities long before tissue histologic features are apparent. Mitochondrial changes are associated with diminished organelle GSH and α-tocopherol concentrations and correlate with serum alanine aminotransferase (ALT) activity, impaired mitochondrial respiration, and cytolytic necrosis. Most dogs that have an inborne error causing pathologic hepatic Cu retention develop high liver Cu concentrations within the first 5 years of life.

Normally, absorbed Cu circulates bound to transport proteins to the liver and other systemic organs. In the liver, Cu is bound to cytosolic transport proteins, used in some enzyme pathways, and ultimately is stored associated with metallothionein. In health, egress into bile maintains a neutral Cu balance. Tissue Cu concentrations are increased in patients that have cholestatic disorders as a consequence of impaired biliary elimination. Cu accumulating in the hepatocyte bound to binding proteins is identified as red-pink granules with routine hematoxylin and eosin staining. Special stains for Cu confirm the nature of the red granules. Finding Cu-positive granules in patients that have severe hepatitis or cholestasis might lead to an erroneous deduction that pathologic Cu retention is the primary disease pathomechanism rather than an epiphenomenon of cholestasis. Quantitative tissue Cu measurement helps determine the seriousness of the Cu storage and the need for chelation therapy (Fig. 2) [42,43]. Generally, tissue Cu values of 1800 ppm or more (ug/g dry liver) that coordinate with biopsy findings are considered to be pathologically increased and deserving of medical chelation. While the approach to these cases remains controversial, dogs that have Cu values greater than 1800 ppm (ug/g) dry liver tissue are usually chelated using d-penicillamine (with supplemental pyridoxine) or trientine. Chelation is continued for 6 months or longer, and optimally a second liver biopsy is obtained to judge the success of hepatic Cu removal. If Cu concentrations are reduced to less than 1000 ppm (ug/g), chronic oral zinc therapy is initiated (for Cu storage disease 5-10 mg/kg elemental zinc per day in two divided doses 30-60 minutes before meals; for chronic hepatic disease 1-5 mg/kg elemental zinc per day in two divided doses); consult the later section on zinc therapy. Chelation therapy and zinc are not used together because of the chelators' avidity for heavy metals. Caution is necessary when interpreting tissue Cu concentrations because small liver biopsy specimens, as obtained with needle sampling techniques, might retrieve nonrepresentative tissue (regenerative nodule only, fibrotic scar only). Consideration of the extent of Cu retention should be judged based on histologic appearance and quantitative determinations.

Cu-affiliated liver injury leads to reduced circulating antioxidant concentrations, reduced hepatic α-tocopherol and GSH concentrations, and compromised production of hepatic cytosolic Cu-Zn SOD [39,40]. Because in vivo work substantiates that vitamin E deficiency potentiates Cu hepatotoxicosis, all patients that have pathologic Cu retention should receive supplemental α-tocopherol, a thiol donor, therapy targeting the process provoking pathologic Cu retention, and control of enteric Cu uptake, which might involve nutritional adjustments and restriction of Cu ingestion in contaminated water.

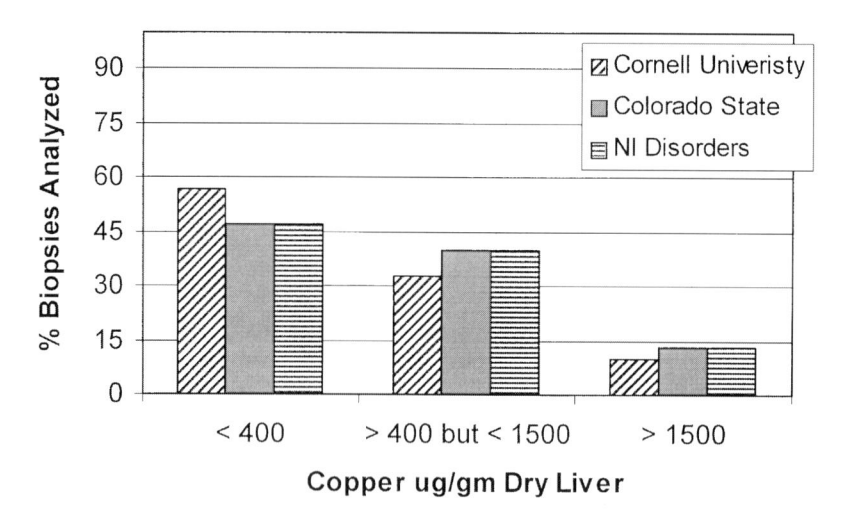

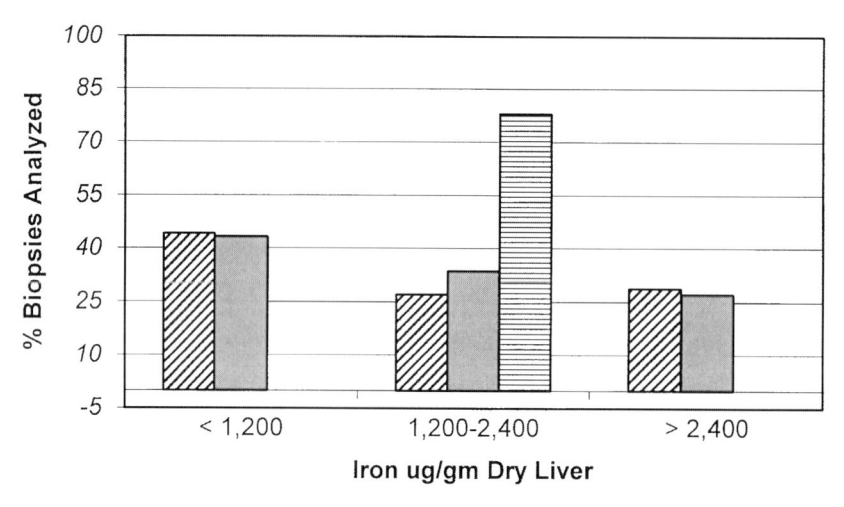

Fig. 2. Hepatic tissue transition metal status in dogs that have spontaneous liver disease showing number of patients (% of submitted specimens) with copper and iron concentrations exceeding normal limits [42,43]. Tissue metal determinations completed by atomic absorption spectroscopy with values expressed on a dry weight basis. Normal copper tissue concentrations ≤400 ug/g; normal iron tissue concentrations < 1200 ug/g dry liver tissue. NI = necro-inflammatory liver disease.

Iron

Iron (Fe) plays an essential role in biology, where its transition property permits it to fluctuate between the ferrous ion (Fe^{2+}) and ferric ion (Fe^{3+}) state important for energy production in mitochondria and transport of oxygen in hemoglobin. Fe is the most efficient transition metal catalyzing the formation of ROS from oxygen by way of the Fenton-driven Haber-Weiss reaction; nonchelated and chelated Fe^{2+} or Cu^{2+} can catalyze the reaction ($H_2O_2 + Fe^{2+} \rightarrow OH\cdot + OH^- + Fe^{3+}$). This capacity to drive single electron transfers makes iron a major player in production and metabolism of free radicals in biological systems (Fe^{2+} can reduce O_2 to $O_2^{\cdot-}$ in cellular and extracellular compartments) [41,44–48]. It is widely recognized that Fe contributes to liver injury in many forms of hepatobiliary disease because under pathologic conditions, accumulation of even small amounts generates free radicals. Like humans, animals that have chronic necroinflammatory liver disease usually develop tissue Fe concentrations (within Kupffer cells) that exceed the normal limits (Fig. 2) [41–48]. This state is described morphologically as hemosiderosis or siderosis or as golden brown particulate granules in Kupffer cells.

Kupffer cells ordinarily recycle a large amount of Fe derived from senescent erythrocytes and preferentially accumulate Fe in the circumstance of hepatocellular injury. Because the Kupffer cell serves as a major source of ROS in inflammatory liver disease, it is not surprising that Fe augments tissue damage. It has long been dogma that Fe and other transition metals sequestered in macrophages are unable to catalyze free radical reactions; however, apparent sequestration does not segregate Fe into an innocuous form [44–48]. Fe remains constantly in flux within and between cells with even the minute pool of intracellular free Fe being available for free radical reactions [44,45].

The profibrogenic influence of Fe on Kupffer cells is widely recognized. Priming or activation of Kupffer cells, such as what occurs following challenge by injurious or hepatotoxic events (eg, toxins, infectious agents, gut-derived endotoxin, xenobiotics, ischemia, phagocytosis of necrotic debris, or exposure to ROS or other oxidative products) amplifies their pro-oxidant activity and Fe-associated fibrogenesis [44,49–52]. Iron might also mediate collagen gene activation in the hepatic Stellate cell or otherwise trigger signals promoting Stellate cell activation [44]. The relationship between circulating Fe indices, hepatic Fe status, and liver lesions has been repeatedly shown to be poor in experimental disease models, humans (even those who have hemochromatosis), and dogs and cats that have acquired and congenital liver disease. Serum Fe indices provide limited information regarding Fe balance because of interference from acute phase responses, hemolysis, and hepatic synthetic failure. Consequently, peripheral sampling cannot be used to assess the extent of hepatic Fe storage nor to recommend antioxidant therapy. Because Fe imposes significant and potent fibrogenic and cytotoxic potential, whether it is in Kupffer cells or hepatocytes, tissue concentrations of Fe should be measured routinely. This information is used to guide the propriety of antioxidant administration [49–52]. A summary of hepatic Fe concentrations in two populations of canine liver patients is shown in Fig. 2, where more than 50% of total biopsies and approximately 80% of dogs that had necroinflammatory liver disease demonstrated increased tissue Fe concentrations [42,43].

Therapeutic modulation of Fe-related liver injury has been investigated using Fe loading disease models (enteral or parenteral) and humans who have hematochromatosis (a genetic defect causing pathologic Fe loading in the liver). Increased hepatic Fe depletes tissue SOD activity and vitamin E stores, alters the tissue GSH/glutathione disulfide (GSSG) ratio, and leads to low circulating α-tocopherol concentrations [52]. Abnormal cell redox status is associated with low GSH reductase activity (enzyme recycling GSSG to GSH) and Fe interference with selenium incorporation in selenium-dependent GSH peroxidase. These enzymes are essential for GSH detoxification reactions and redox cycling [53,54]. Hepatocytes depleted of reduced GSH are known to be more susceptible to Fe-induced lipid peroxidation. Because antioxidants can inhibit Fe-induced lipid peroxidation in vitro and in vivo, confirming high tissue Fe concentrations sanctions thiol donor and α-tocopherol supplemenation [55–59]. While single treatment with GSH, NAC, or α-tocopherol reduces cell damage and death experimentally, the best in vivo responses have been achieved using combinations [41,58]. Flavonoids also might impart a beneficial influence on tissue injury affiliated with Fe. Flavonoid polyphenols derived from plants (eg, green tea, red wine, purple grape juice, coca products, apples, milk thistle, and certain nuts) can participate in Fe chelation and free radical trapping, protecting lipids from Fe-mediated oxidation [59,60]. Flavonoids can impart diverse influences on disease, many occurring subsequent to modulation of NF-κβ [59].

Mechanisms of defense involving cell redox status

Oxidative stress is a well-known inducer of gene transcription involving complex mechanisms such as NF-κβ, activator proteins, and mediators conferring inducible gene expression [61,62]. A good example is the tumor suppressor gene p53, which plays a role in cell response to circumstances damaging DNA, where it activates transcription of genes, controlling cell cycle arrest or apoptosis. Binding of p53 to DNA and its subsequent transcriptional activities are controlled by a cell's thiol redox status. Four of nine cysteine groups in thiol-bearing amino acids in the p53 DNA-binding domain are essential for its expression. Oxidation of thiol groups effects structural change in p53, abolishing its ability to interact with its DNA target sequence. Glutathionylation (when GSH conserves thiol groups) in proteases and caspases explains the regulatory effect of intracellular GSH in a multitude of pathologic conditions and its influence on apoptosis. A reduced cysteine site is requisite for proper activity of many enzymes. Cytosolic oxidative stress activates NF-κβ by degrading its Iκβ-binding anchor, allowing NF-κβ to translocate to the nucleus, where it interacts with DNA. Certain antioxidants can therefore inhibit NF-κβ activation and its proinflammatory consequences (eg, NAC, α-tocopherol, GSH) [14,63–65].

Corticosteroids and lipoxygenase inhibitors also influence cell redox status by inhibiting NF-κβ activation [66]. TNF-α, a pleiotropic cytokine produced by biliary epithelia, sinusoidal endothelium, and activated Kupffer cells, can induce proliferative, apoptotic, or cytotoxic responses through NF-κβ activation [62,66]. A number of antioxidants are thought to modulate NF-κβ by inhibiting induction of TNF-α in hepatic Kupffer and other resident nonparenchymal hepatic cells.

The link between oxidative stress and hepatic fibrosis has been proven in a number of models of chronic liver disease and in spontaneous liver disorders, in which it plays an important role in activating the Stellate cell. While a direct link between GSH concentrations and an ability to modulate behavior of activated Stellate cells has not been proven, a number of antioxidants influencing GSH redox status discourage Stellate cell transformation into its myofibroblast phenotype. Antifibrotic and anti-inflammatory effects can be derived from antioxidant supplementation. A good example is α-tocopherol proven to inhibit collagen gene expression and collagen deposition, but also to influence complexly intercellular signaling, resulting in beneficial immunomodulatory, anti-inflammatory, antiproliferative, and antifibrotic effects.

Hepatic antioxidant systems

Owing to its pivotal location interfacing between the splanchnic and central circulatory beds, its central role in intermediary metabolism and detoxification, and its large resident macrophage population, the liver has great risk for exposure to injurious substances, infectious agents, toxic adducts, and potentially oxidizing substrates. It therefore comes as no surprise that the liver is richly endowed with a diverse repertoire of antioxidant/detoxification mechanisms (Fig. 3). Despite the fact that exposure to oxidative challenge is an ongoing process in the liver, in health little significant tissue injury results because of the highly complex, multifactorial, interactive, and complementary antioxidant network. It is convenient to discuss hepatoprotectant antioxidants in terms of whether they are enzymatic or nonenzymatic.

Enzymatic antioxidants

Antioxidative enzymes are assumed to constitute the first line of defense. Enzymatic antioxidants include enzymes in specific subcellular compartments routinely trafficked by radicals (mitochondria, peroxisome, cell cytosol) or in the systemic circulation. SOD catalyzes the dismutation of $O_2^{\cdot -}$ to H_2O_2 with specific forms existing in cytosolic, mitochondrial, and extracellular locations (Cu–Zn–SOD being cytosolic, Mn–SOD being primarily mitochondrial). Catalase, located predominantly in peroxisomes,

Nonenzymatic

Zinc
Metallothionein
Ascorbate
α-Tocopherol
CoEnzyme-Q₁₀
Thiol Donors:
  SAMe, Lipoic Acid
  N-acetylcysteine
Polunsaturated
  Phosphatidylcholine
Silibinin
Plasma Proteins:
  albumin, ceruloplasmin,
  transferrin
Ursodeoxycholic Acid

Enzymatic

Transition Metals
Cu & Fe^{+2}

$OH\bullet$

Membrane

$O\bullet$

SOD
O_2 (CuZn-SOD)
(Mn-SOD)

H_2O_2 — Catalase

GSH
GSH — GSSG
GSSG reductase — GSH

GSH-Peroxidase

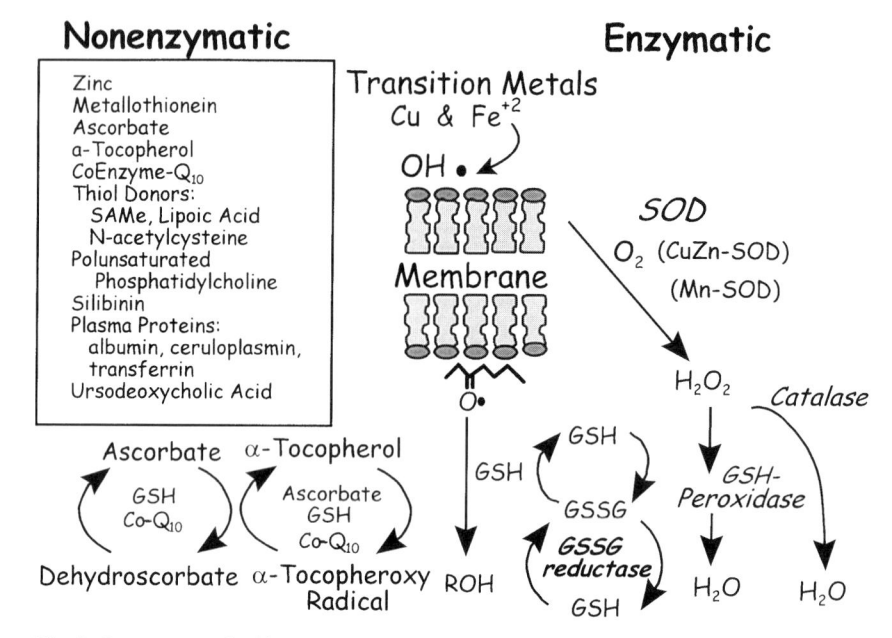

H_2O H_2O

Ascorbate   α-Tocopherol
GSH   Ascorbate
Co-Q₁₀   GSH
             Co-Q₁₀
Dehydroscorbate α-Tocopheroxy ROH
                 Radical

Fig. 3. Important antioxidant mechanisms for the liver (natural and therapeutic) depicted as nonenzymatic (molecular) antioxidants and enzymatic antioxidants (*italicized*), as discussed in the text. In the center of the diagram a cartoon depicts a biologic membrane with hydrophilic polarity indicated by the oval structures and lipid tails (paired polyunsaturated fatty acids in the hydrophobic portion). Note the reappearing and important contributions made by GSH.

catalyzes conversion of H_2O_2, produced during oxidation of very long chain fatty acids, to water. GSH–peroxidases (GSH-Px), a family of cytosolic, mitochondrial, and extracellular enzymes, converts lipid hydroperoxides and H_2O_2 to water and stable alcohols by oxidizing GSH to its oxidized disulfide form (GSSG). Several GSH-Pxs require selenium at their reactive site. An additional group of extracellular selenoproteins also provides antioxidant protection. GSH reductase, which requires riboflavin as a cofactor, regenerates reduced GSH from its oxidized GSSG form. Enzymatic antioxidants cannot be supplemented orally except for provision of cofactors that might upregulate enzyme production or activity when actual or conditional deficiencies exist.

Soluble nonenzymatic antioxidants

Protein binding of toxic adducts or transition metals (Cu or Fe) to albumin, transferrin, ferritin, ceruloplasmin, or metallothionein provides another rapid means of protection. GSH, used here to simply represent thiol status, α-tocopherol, ascorbic acid, bilirubin, ubiquinol (coenzyme Q_{10}), dihydrolipoic acid (lipoic acid), and therapeutic NAC and s-adenosylmethionine (SAMe) are members of the nonenzymatic molecular antioxidant class. An expanding group of soluble antioxidants play a role in circulating blood, interstitial fluids, and on or within extracellular cell and lipoprotein surfaces. Combinations working cooperatively provide the breadth of protection necessary within body systems. Emulating this cooperative antioxidant interaction with a combined or polymodal therapeutic approach is therefore recommended. For example, a cooperative approach in necroinflammatory liver disease could include glucocorticoids or other anti-inflammatory or immunomodulatory prescription medications combined with various antioxidants. Because glucocorticoids mediate NF-κβ inhibition, adjunctive therapy with thiol donors such as NAC or SAMe and vitamin E would theoretically provide a wider breadth of effects for controlling inflammatory mediator release and adverse cell responses [67,68].

Thiols

Thiol-containing compounds provide S–H sulfhydryl (SH) bonds supplied by cysteine residues. Cysteine residues are readily metabolized and participate in thiol–disulfide exchange reactions. The major nonprotein thiol source in intermediary metabolism is GSH, which carries a single cysteine group. The major protein thiol source is thioredoxin, a small protein containing two redox-active half-cysteine residues. GSH and thioredoxins have complementary—and to some extent overlapping—roles. In most cells GSH is the most abundant nonprotein thiol. Thioredoxin represents the smallest member of a family of proteins containing a thioredoxin fold; each family member contributes to antioxidant defense, protein folding, or signal transduction. Thioredoxin is ubiquitous as it is essential for gene expression, where it facilitates protein–nucleic acid interactions by reducing cysteine in the DNA binding loop of transcription factors. A fluctuating thiol status reflects a range of normal and abnormal cell responses that can be influenced pivotally by GSH and thioredoxins [68]. It is well established that altered cell and organelle redox balance trigger responses directing gene transcription. The earliest and best-studied cell demonstrating this interaction is the lymphocyte, where even partial thiol depletion has profound consequences on blast transformation, cell proliferation, and cytotoxic T cell generation.

Glutathione

The tripeptide L-γ-glutamyl-L cysteinyl-glycine, or GSH, is the most prevalent low molecular mass thiol donor in most cells. It achieves tissue concentrations ranging between 0.2 and 10 mM/g. In cells, tissues, and plasma, GSH exists in several forms: (1) as reduced GSH, (2) as GSSG formed upon GSH oxidation (also called oxidized GSH), and (3) as further oxidation products including sulfonates and glutathionylated or thiolated proteins [69–71]. While the term total GSH represents all free and bound GSH moieties including protein–thiols, conventional application indicates GSH plus twice the GSSG concentration (a single GSH molecule yielding two GSSG molecules). The GSH molecule is unique because its γ-glutamyl bond confers resistant to intracellular degradation. This bond can only be catabolized extracellularly near membranes that have bound γ-glutamyl transpeptidase (γGT). The product formed by reaction between GSH and γGT is a γ-glutamyl enzyme that becomes an amino acid acceptor yielding γ-glutamyl amino acids (Fig. 4) [70,71]. The γ-glutamyl amino acids are easily transported into cells, where they function as GSH substrate transporters and can be partitioned into the γ-glutamyl cycle, which generates GSH. One of the best acceptor amino acids for γGT is cystine. The presence of a more direct cystine shuttle system in the hepatocyte simplifies the process and explains the high efficacy of certain therapeutic agents functioning as thiol donors (eg, NAC).

There is a constant turnover of GSH in the body, with the liver occupying a central position in this dynamic flux; turnover of GSH in normal liver, estimated in rodents and humans, approximates 20% per hour [72]. The liver contains one of the highest organ GSH concentrations and serves as a major source of systemic GSH. The hepatocyte has the unique ability to convert methionine to cysteine for GSH production in the transsulfuration pathway and to export GSH into plasma and bile at a rate that accounts for nearly all of its de novo GSH synthesis [73,74]. GSH can undergo transport only across selected biological membranes, notably the mitochondrial membrane and hepatocellular plasma and canalicular membranes. Hepatic GSH exportation provides 90% of the plasma GSH [74]. Hepatocytes also release a substantial amount of GSH and GSSG across canalicular membranes into bile in a process involving specialized transporters. Biliary excretion of GSH metabolites (thioether s-conjugates as part of mercapturate biosynthesis) eliminates metabolic and toxic waste products. The hepatocyte cytosol supplies GSH to its mitochondria, which are unable to synthesize GSH, have limited ability to recycle GSH, and are unable to export GSSG.

Hepatocellular GSH concentration therefore reflects the balance between its synthesis, use, and exportation. Synthesis is constitutive, regulated, and occurs through several pathways (Fig. 4) [70,71]. The direct and simple synthetic pathway involves only its constituent amino acids and the sequential action of two cytosolic ATP-dependent enzymes: (1) γ-glutamylcysteine synthetase (γ-GCS, also known as glutamate–cysteine ligase), and (2) GSH synthetase (also known as GSH synthase). A more complicated pathway (the γ-glutamyl cycle) involves conversion of γ-glutamyl amino acids derived from γGT membrane activity to glutamic acid, which then combines with cysteine and enters the simple GSH pathway. An alternative or salvage pathway of GSH biosynthesis derives

Fig. 4. Overview of hepatocyte GSH synthesis, including: (1) membrane γGT and transport of γ-glutamyl amino acids, (2) amino acid γ-glutamyl cycle, (3) GSH salvage pathway permitting direct GSH synthesis, bypassing the (4) rate-controlling enzyme. The direct and simple pathway of GSH synthesis involves only its constituent amino acids and the sequential action of two cytosolic ATP-dependent enzymes: (1) γ-glutamylcysteine synthetase (γ-GCS; also known as glutamate-cysteine ligase) and (2) GSH synthetase (also known as GSH synthase). A more complicated pathway (the γ-glutamyl cycle) involves γ-glutamyl amino acids (derived from γGT membrane activity) and γ-glutamyl cyclotransferase and cysteinyl-glycine dipeptidase. These reactions yield glutamic acid, glycine and cysteine, which can then enter the direct synthetic pathway. L-γ-glutamyl-L-cysteine also can be shuttled directly to GSH synthetase bypassing the normally rate-limiting enzymatic step of GSH synthesis (γ-GCS) in the alternative or salvage pathway of GSH biosynthesis.

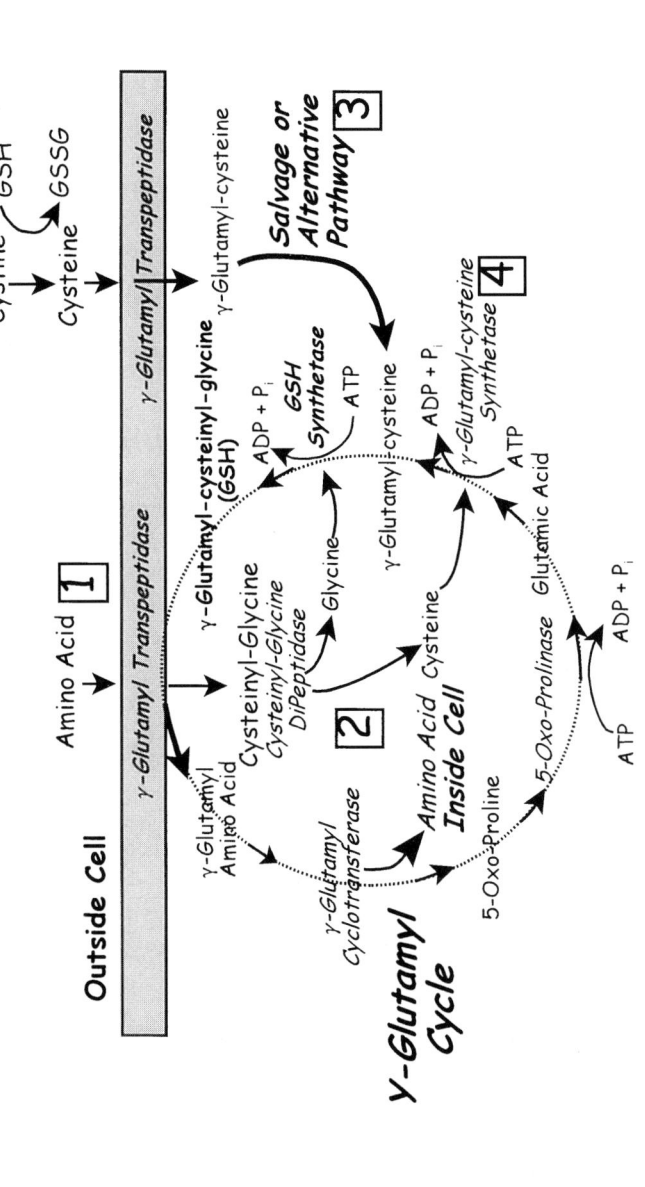

from reduction of cystine to cysteine by GSH, formation of L-γ-glutamyl-L-cysteine by interaction with γGT, and direct interaction with GSH synthetase, bypassing the rate limiting enzymatic step (γ-GCS) of the γ-glutamyl cycle [71].

De novo hepatic GSH synthesis is regulated by three factors: (1) the level of γ-GCS (the rate-limiting step), (2) availability of its substrates (L-cysteine especially), and (3) feedback inhibition of GSH on γ-GCS. Because of enzyme kinetics and the typically low levels of γ-GCS, more than than 95% of γ-GCS is converted to GSH [72]. Although intracellular concentrations of precursor amino acids vary with the species and tissues studied and the patient's nutritional status, the consistently lower concentrations of L-cysteine compared with L-glutamate and glycine impose a rate-limiting influence. Realization of this rate-limiting effect has led to the development of pharmacologic L-cysteine prodrugs.

Glutamate and glycine for GSH synthesis are derived from several metabolic pathways in the hepatocyte. Cysteine is unique because its SH form is predominantly found intracellularly. The disulfide form of cysteine (cystine) is predominant extracellularly owing to the high lability of the cysteine SH bond and its auto-oxidation in the extracellular environment. While hepatocytes do not readily transport cystine, release of GSH from the cell permits thiol–disulfide exchange with cystine at the cell interface, yielding cysteine for transcellular uptake [75]. In the hepatocyte, cysteine is protected by its affiliation with comparatively high concentrations of cytosolic GSH [76]. The hepatocellular cysteine uptake mechanism is quantitatively important to GSH synthesis and is approximated as three-fold greater than for methionine and 13-fold higher than for cystine. Sources of hepatic cysteine include portally delivered dietary protein and L-cyst(e)ine derived from biliary GSH and GSSG undergoing enterohepatic circulation, endogenous protein breakdown, and methionine catabolism in the hepatic transsulfuration pathway. The hepatic ability to convert methionine to cysteine by way of the transsulfuration pathway permits the liver to function as a major storage organ for GSH and as a reservoir for cysteine that critically influences hepatic GSH biosynthesis and systemic GSH availability [76]. Most nonhepatic tissues rely on degradation of plasma GSH and GSSG and uptake of released L-cyst(e)ine as a source of new L-cysteine for GSH and protein synthesis. Therefore, considering the dynamic flux of GSH in the hepatocyte and its importance to systemic GSH, it is implicit that impaired hepatocyte GSH concentrations have polysystemic ramifications.

It has long been recognized that metabolism of methionine is disrupted in patients that have severe liver disease in which impaired methionine clearance is known to coincide with hepatic encephalopathy (HE). Down-regulation of an enzyme (methionine adenosinetransferase, MAT1) limiting methionine conversion to SAMe in the liver is a major causal factor. This phenomenon compromises the hepatic ability to generate adequate GSH concentrations in the face of hepatic disease. Low hepatic concentrations of GSH have been substantiated in spontaneous liver disease (humans, dogs, and cats) and in a myriad of models of serious liver disease (Fig. 5) [77]. Administration of SAMe can bypass the metabolic blockade imposed by low MAT1 activity and overcome nutritional deficiencies limiting cyst(e)ine. In addition to replenishing tissue and circulating GSH, SAMe

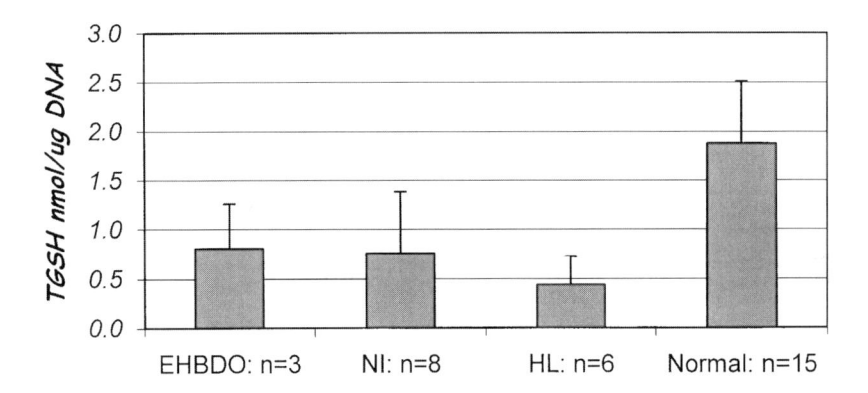

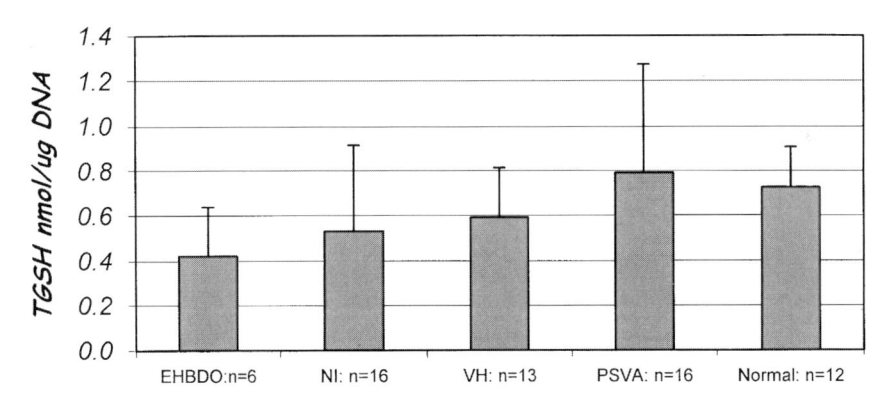

Fig. 5. Total glutathione (TGSH) nmol/ug/DNA concentrations (mean +1 SD) in liver tissue from healthy cats and dogs and clinical patients with various liver disorders. Subnormal TGSH concentrations were found irrespective of the unit of expression (tissue wet weight, protein, or DNA) in many patients. The number of animals included is shown by n; EHBDO = extrahepatic bile duct obstruction; HL = hepatic lipidosis; NI = necroinflammatory disorders; PSVA = portosystemic vascular anomaly; VH = vacuolar hepatopathy (corticosteroid associated). Cats are depicted in the upper graph, dogs in the lower graph. Significantly lower liver tissue TGSH concentrations compared with healthy animals were found in nearly 45% of dogs and 77% of cats that have necroinflammatory and cholestatic disorders. Profound reduction in tissue GSH concentrations were observed in cats that have severe hepatic lipidosis. (*Data from* Center SA, Warner KL, Erb HN. Liver glutathione concentrations in dogs and cats with naturally occurring liver disease. Am J Vet Res 2002;63:1187–97.)

supplementation can attenuate pathophysiologic effects of liver disease including tissue inflammation, cholestasis, and fibroplasia (consult the section on SAMe). Another factor potentially limiting GSH synthesis is the availability of cellular ATP, for example in cells that have limited ability to produce ATP (eg, erythrocytes) or tissues suffering from ischemic injury.

The essential role played by GSH in stabilizing cell redox status is catalyzed by GSH-Px. Thereafter, recovery of GSH is accomplished by reduction of GSSG in a reaction catalyzed by GSSG reductase with nicotinamide adenine dinucleotide phosphate (NADPH) serving as a reducing equivalent. This series of reactions is termed the GSH redox cycle (Fig. 6). The GSH redox cycle is quantitatively important because flux through it is generally high relative to de novo hepatic GSH synthesis. In health, the high efficiency of GSSG reductase can maintain the hepatocellular GSH pool in a predominately reduced state (intracellular GSH/GSSG >98%) [78,79]; however, reduction of GSSG to GSH occurs at the expense of NADPH, which in most cells is produced in the mitochondria and cell cytosol. NADPH has critical importance in the mitochondria, where it scavenges toxic free radicals and repairs biomolecule-derived radicals. It also functions as an essential coenzyme in several metabolic pathways (including glycolysis and maintenance of the lipoate cycle). In certain situations NADPH availability might be a limiting factor in GSH regeneration. GSH-Px is a selenoprotein interactive only with soluble hydroperoxides (eg, H_2O_2) and some organic hydroperoxides (eg, hydroperoxy fatty acids). Biosynthesis of selenoproteins such as GSH-Px depend on selenium availability and its incorporation as selenocysteine. Thioredoxin peroxidase also is an important redox-regulating enzyme that is dependent on selenium. Hepatic GSH-Px activity is readily diminished by selenium deficiency; it is this relationship that explains the historical perspective that selenium yields important antioxidant benefits.

A number of factors might contribute to finding subnormal hepatic GSH concentrations in patients that have serious liver disease (Box 1). In addition to diminished hepatocellular GSH synthesis, enhanced exportation for

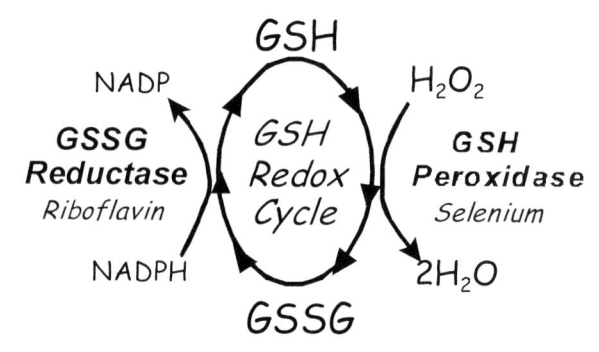

Fig. 6. GSH redox cycle reaction showing essentiality of reducing equivalents (NADPH or NADH) and cycle enzyme cofactors (*in italics*).

Box 1. Factors contributing to impaired hepatocellular glutathione

Poor nutritional status
Insufficient protein intake
Limited substrate amino acids: L-cyste(i)ine
Vitamin insufficiency: riboflavin (GSSG reductase), NADPH
Hepatic insufficiency → altered competition for shared transporters
B_{12}, folate, or other vitamin deficiencies

Impaired s-adenosylmethionine synthetic pathway enzymes or intermediates
Downregulation of hepatic MAT1 isoform
Loss of pathway enzymes from lack of GSH thiol protection
B_{12} or folate deficiency
Impaired hepatocellular ATP: mitochondrial dysfunction, NADPH depletion

Enhanced formation of peroxynitrate/hydroxyl radicals
Transition metal-associated injury
Ischemic–reperfusion insult
Vitamin E deficiency
Zinc deficiency
Imbalanced antioxidant network

Increased glutathione-S-transferase conjugation → cell glutathione exportation
Detoxification reactions: toxins, xenobiotics

Hepatotoxicity
Xenobiotics → free radical formation → GSH use
Endogenous oxidative products (mitochondrial dysfunction, membrane oxidation) → GSH use
Toxins → peroxidative membrane injury, toxic adduct or electrophile formation → GSH use
Membranocytolytic bile acids → mitochondrial injury and membrane damage → ↓ GSH/GSSG

Impaired glutathione redox cycle: impaired rejuvenation reduced glutathione
Increased GSSG formation → exportation from cell → net GSH loss
Insufficient NADPH (reducing equivalent)

Inborne errors of metabolism
Deficiency of GSH reductase
Deficiency of γ-GCS or GSH synthetase
Deficiency of other antioxidant enzymes
Excessive loss of amino acid substrates: renal tubular defects

systemic needs, increased participation in redox neutralization or detoxifying conjugation functions, heightened challenge by ROS imposed by the hepatic disease processes and poor nutritional intake of selenium, riboflavin, other essential cofactors, and protein necessary for GSH synthesis might each impose limiting influences.

Hepatocellular glutathione functions

While the thiol status of GSH is best acknowledged to mitigate oxidant injury, this molecule also is integrally involved in numerous cellular and metabolic processes, summarized in Fig. 7. Briefly, GSH is involved in the (1) metabolism and maintenance of thiol moieties (eg, proteins and low molecular weight thiols such as cysteine and coenzyme A); (2) maintenance of the reduced protective forms of ascorbic acid and α-tocopherol; (3) modulation of critical cell processes influencing the cell cycle, gene expression, signal transduction, microtubular-related processes, immune function, cell proliferation, and apoptosis; (4) metabolism of diverse substrates (eg, xenobiotics, eicosnoids, vitamin K); (5) formation of GSH conjugates essential for elimination or detoxification processes by way of enzymatic (GSH-S-transferase family of enzymes) or nonenzymatic mechanisms; (6) protection against generation of ROS simply from aerobic metabolism and mitochondrial electron leakage and from pathologic processes (enzymatic or nonenzymatic reactions); and (7) coenzyme functions involved in cell defense in addition to its role with GSH-Pxs and GSH-S-transferases. Accumulation of intracellular GSSG alters cell thiol redox status, activating oxidant-responsive transcriptional elements. GSSG accumulation might also lead to a net loss of GSH because GSSG might be exported preferentially. Extracellular GSSG is not taken up by intact cells but degraded, necessitating increased de novo GSH synthesis. In severe liver disease, when synthesis of GSH might be compromised by multiple factors (Box 1), this chain of events amplifies GSH tissue depletion [74].

While conjugation reactions involving GSH occur spontaneously with some electrophiles, most are catalyzed by an enzyme from the family of GSH-S-transferases, producing thioesters that prepare toxic adducts for elimination. Such GSH conjugation mitigates toxicity of a variety of substances (eg, free radicals, ROS, heavy metals, and cytotoxic electrophiles). Several transport mechanisms (eg, multidrug resistance-associated protein [MRP1], canalicular multispecific organic anion transporter [cMOAT/MRP2]) extrude GSH conjugates from the cell [80]. Different transporters are found on different cell populations. MRP1 transporter is found on the plasma membrane of many cells but not the liver, whereas the cMOAT/MRP2 is localized to specific transporting biliary epithelia and canalicular membranes. It is through the canalicular cMOAT mechanism

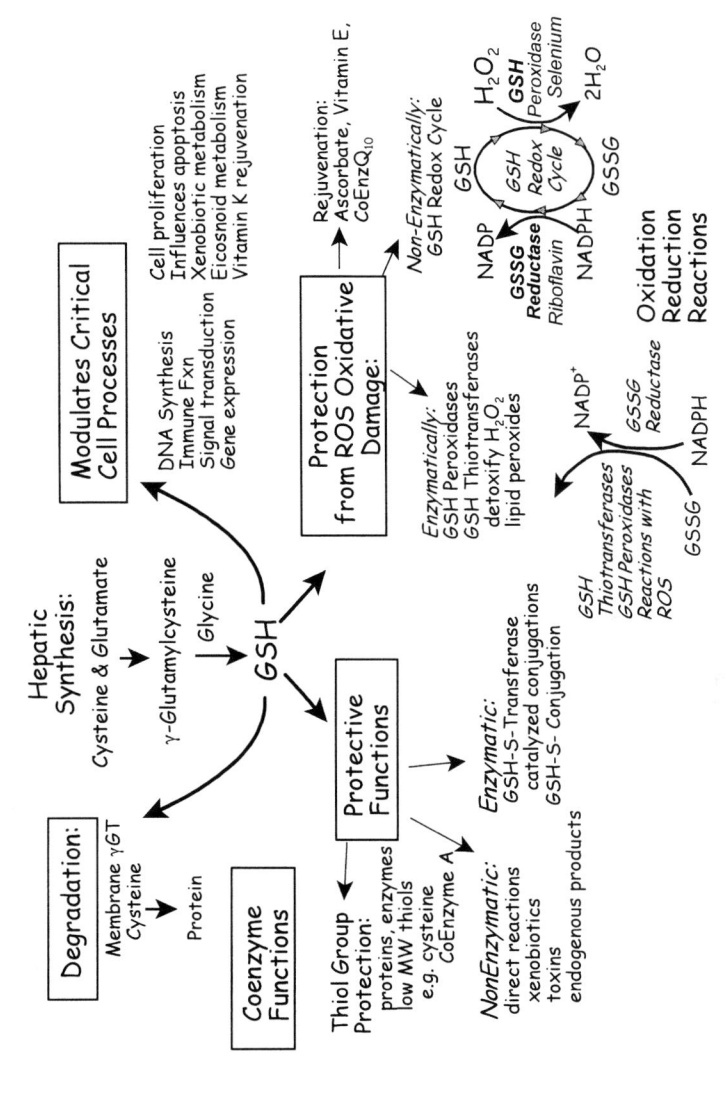

Fig. 7. Metabolic interactions of GSH in the liver, including synthesis, degradation, and major functional categories.

that hepatocyte bile acid and GSH extrusion occurs [81,82]. GSH is the most abundant organic molecule in bile, where it achieves concentrations approximating 8 to 10 mM, comparatively 2.5- to 10-fold greater than concentrations of biliary bile acids and bile pigments. High GSH concentration in canalicular bile, together with its hydrophilic nature, generates a potent osmotic driving force for bile secretion [81,82]. Because bile functions as a major elimination route for transition metals that might augment redox reactions (eg, Cu, Fe, manganese), high biliary GSH concentrations might modulate the chemical reactivity of these metals as they sojourn the biliary tree. Because thiols are important mucolytic agents, biliary GSH also influences bile composition considering that large amounts of mucin are produced by the biliary epithelium, especially within the gallbladder. The presence of biliary thiols is also believed to accelerate dissolution of choleliths and might reduce the risk for cholelith formation [83,84].

Mitochondria, unable to synthesize GSH, depend on hepatocellular cytosolic GSH. Because they can exchange reduced GSH with cytosol but cannot export GSSG, they have a predisposition for an unstable redox status. Lacking catalase, which neutralizes H_2O_2 efficiently, they rely on GSH-Px and nonenzymatic reactions involving GSH to adjust their redox status. Lacking an efficient antioxidant network that increases on demand, mitochondria have high risk for ROS-derived injury [85–87]. Experimental work confirms that mitochondrial GSH depletion and oxidant damage precede microscopic and biochemical detection of hepatocellular GSH insufficiency and oxidant injury. Mitochondrial GSH depletion influences organelle metabolism and MPT directly and indirectly, triggering onset of apoptosis and cell necrosis [87]. It is now well established that mitochondrial GSH depletion augments TNF-α cytotoxicity in several models of liver disease. Ordinarily, TNF-α targets mitochondria and a diversity of cell responses imparting cytotoxic effects that promote ROS and free radical generation and gene regulatory influences [87,88]. The ability of hepatic mitochondrial GSH to regulate organelle redox status importantly influences expression of survival genes responsive to ROS-sensitive transcription signals (eg, NF-$\kappa\beta$). Restoring mitochondrial GSH might play a key therapeutic role in a number of liver disorders, and experimental evidences shows that this can be accomplished with certain thiol donors. For instance, NAC and SAMe can attenuate hepatocellular injury associated with mitochondrial GSH depletion.

Mitochondrial GSH uptake is facilitated by a specific transporter that requires normal mitochondrial membrane fluidity for optimal function [85–87]. Certain hepatotoxins impair this transport system or diminish organelle membrane fluidity, compromising mitochondrial integrity and GSH availability, leading to cell apoptosis. UDCA can mitigate such mitochondrial toxicity and conserve organelle GSH in the face of injury imposed by ethanol, TNF-α, TGF-β, Fas ligand, and membranocytolytic hydrophobic bile acids [87,89,90]. Treatment with SAMe similarly restores the mitochondrial GSH response to a number of hepatotoxins by normalizing its transorganelle GSH transport and membrane fluidity [91–97]. Mitochondrial GSH plays an essential role in maintaining cell calcium homeostasis; low organelle GSH predisposes to hepatocellular MTP expression and permeability of the inner mitochondrial membrane to calcium. Certain hepatotoxic drugs known to dysregulate cell calcium homeostasis deplete mitochondrial GSH as their pathomechanism; examples include BCNU, adriamycin, ethacrynic acid (a drug related to furosemide), and acetaminophen. Toxicity of some of these has been attenuated by thiol supplementation.

Thioredoxin

Thioredoxin (Trx) represents a family of small redox proteins that undergo reversible oxidation to form a cysteine disulfide (Trx-S2) bond through transfer of reducing equivalents from the cysteine residue catalytic site to a disulfide substrate [98,99]. Oxidized Trx is spontaneously reduced back to the cystine form by the NADPH-dependent flavoprotein Trx reductase. A cytosolic form and mitochondrial form of Trx are recognized that perform many biological actions, including (1) supplying reducing equivalents to Trx-Px and RNA reductase, (2) regulating transcription factors, and (3) regulating activity of enzymes containing critical thiol groups. While GSH is a more important intracellular antioxidant because it is present in concentrations that are 500- to 1000-fold greater than Trx and NADPH, Trx exerts redox control over the activity of many DNA-binding transcription factors (eg, the transcription factor NF-κβ and the glucocorticoid receptor). Changes in cell thiol status can therefore affect the functions of Trx and modulate hepatocellular response in disease directly.

Supplementing hepatocellular thiols/glutathione

Therapeutic manipulation of thiols and GSH has received considerable attention; however, for thiol supplements to meet expectations, other members of the interactive antioxidant network need to be replete (Fig. 8) [100]. Most commonly, an L-cysteine precursor is administered to directly provide the limiting amino acid for GSH synthesis and to replace L-cysteine irreversibly lost with GSH-S-transferase products. Because L-cysteine autooxidizes to insoluble L-cystine and can be toxic in some in vitro circumstances, therapeutic administration is typically done using NAC, an agent that can be given orally or intravenously (IV); however, the efficacy of cysteine delivery systems on GSH synthesis are limited by feedback inhibition of γ-GCS by GSH. Therapeutic use of NAC is advantageous because this molecule can directly provide cysteine after hydrolysis, it might reduce plasma cystine to cysteine by way of thiol–disulfide exchange, or it can function directly in redox and detoxication reactions. Under normal

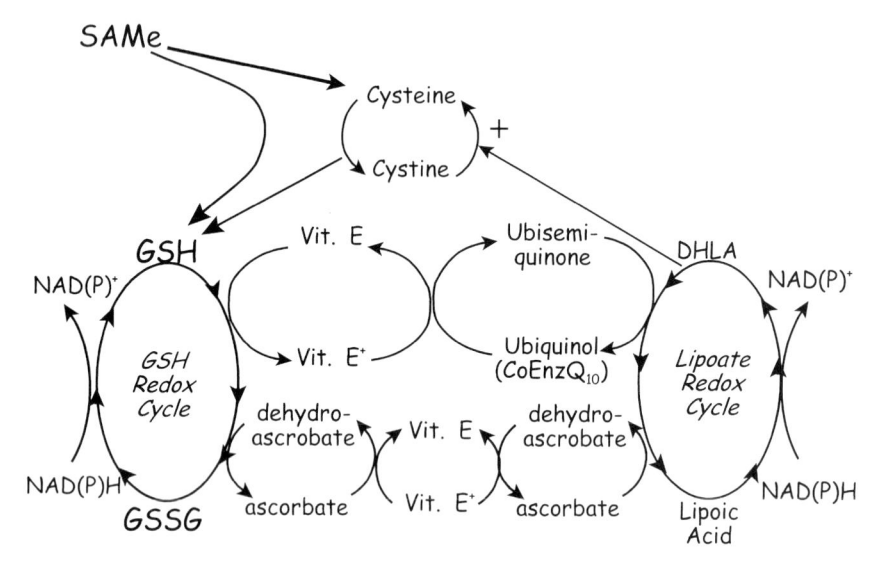

Fig. 8. Antioxidant network and interacting systems necessary for optimal response to thiol supplementation. Adequate nutrition along with vitamin and mineral intake are necessary to maintain balance in this series of interactions. (*Adapted from* Sen CK, Packer L. Thiol homeostasis and supplements in physical exercise. Am J Clin Nutr 2000;72(Suppl):653S–69S.)

conditions NAC will not increase total hepatic GSH because intracellular concentrations are closely regulated by feedback control; however, in the circumstance of hepatic GSH depletion, NAC can normalize liver and circulating GSH values.

While a wide range of L-cysteine precursors have been developed, most of these are compared therapeutically to effects provided by NAC that are considered to be the standard. Because GSH itself is poorly taken up or not at all by most cells and it is degraded rapidly in the gut and circulation, oral or IV administration of GSH mainly provides constituent amino acids [101,102]. Products labeled as providing GSH directly should realistically be considered to be good but expensive L-cysteine precursors or delivery agents, functioning in the same capacity as methionine and NAC. Use of oral or IV GSH esters has been explored and might provide a pharmacologic way to mimic physiologic release of GSH from the liver in the future. Certain GSH esters are taken up readily by cells and release GSH intracellularly. These esters will theoretically have great therapeutic potential bypassing steps regulating intracellular GSH synthesis [101–104]. Experimental work proves that such GSH esters can increase intracellular GSH significantly within hours above physiologic concentrations and protect against lethal acetaminophen hepatotoxicosis [103]; however, metabolism of GSH esters in humans differs from their metabolism in rodents, and there is no referenced work in dogs or cats. A liposomally delivered GSH prodrug is also under investigation that provides similar benefits in experimental models [102].

Alternative methods of thiol supplementation involve methionine, SAMe, parenteral administration of γ-glutamyl amino acids, and nutritional supplementation by ingestion of a specially processed whey protein. Because the utility of methionine as a cysteine precursor relies on entry into the transsulfuration pathway, this method of supplementing thiols might be inappropriate for patients that have low MAT1 activity (hepatic dysfunction), and it might increase risk for HE. Administration of SAMe permits ready access to the transsulfuration pathway and provides numerous additional metabolic/biochemical advantages discussed in detail in a later section. Parenterally infused γ-glutamyl amino acids (γ-glutamylcysteine, its disulfide and mixed disulfide forms, along with γ-glutamylcystine) are transported readily into the kidney and possibly other tissues, reduced, and generate GSH by way of GSH synthetase (see Fig. 4) [102]. Feeding a specially processed whey protein (protein isolation protecting thermolabile amino acids and oligopeptides) functioning as a cysteine/cystine delivery nutrient can increase circulating GSH concentrations in humans who have chronic hepatitis and other diseases [105,106]; however, the ability of whey protein to therapeutically improve hepatic tissue GSH concentrations has not yet been demonstrated convincingly.

N-acetylcysteine

NAC, the acetylated form of the amino acid L-cysteine, is an excellent therapeutic source of SH groups and functions as the standard to which all other thiol donors are compared. Only the L-NAC form is metabolically active; the D-NAC form is useless. In veterinary patients L-NAC is used therapeutically as a direct thiol donor when supplementation is needed urgently. It is absorbed rapidly following oral administration, undergoes extensive first-pass metabolism by enterocytes and the liver, and is readily deacetylated intracellularly. Usually, it is administered intravenously. Metabolic incorporation into other molecules occurs extensively in the intestines (lumen and mucosa). Cysteine and inorganic sulfites constitute major metabolites reaching the liver and provide the majority of its therapeutic effect (Fig. 9). Bioavailability and pharmacokinetics of NAC have been studied in humans and animals (mostly rodents). Because of extensive enteric metabolism, oral bioavailability of intact NAC is estimated to be between 4% and 10%. Less than 3% of an oral dose is eliminated directly in feces, and between 13% and 38% is recovered in urine within 1 day. In humans, the free NAC plasma half-life is approximately 2 hours with virtually no NAC detectable 10 to 12 hours after administration [107,108]. As a thiol source, beneficial effects of NAC derived from its ability to stimulate GSH

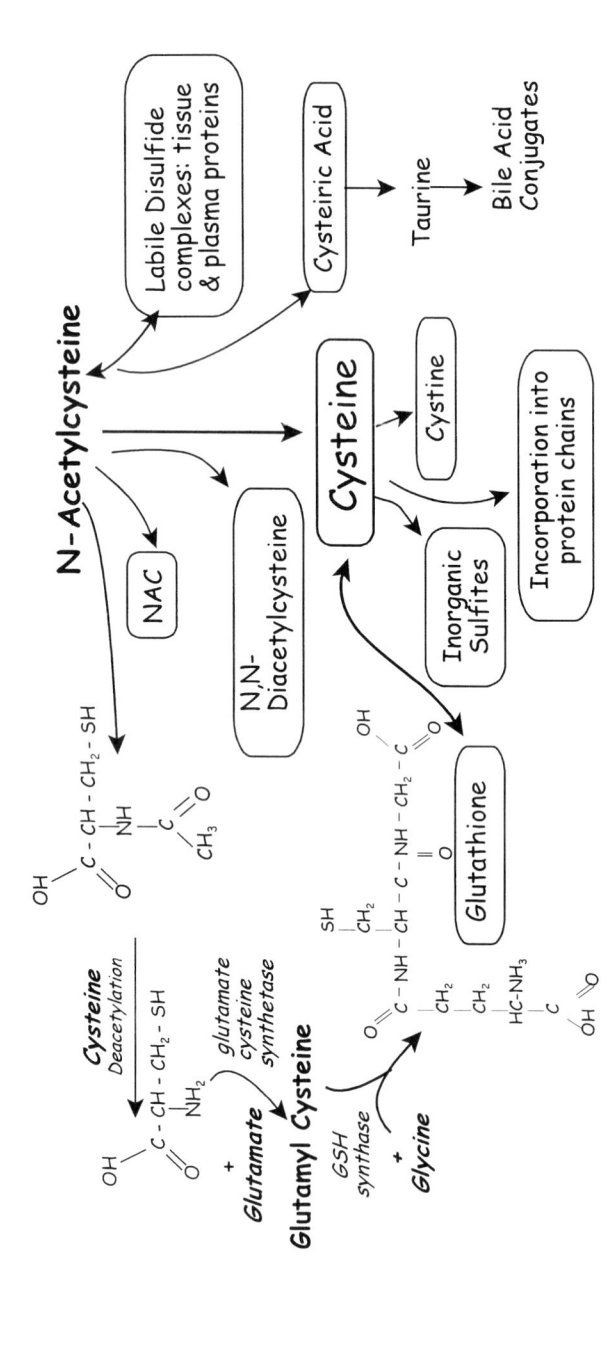

Fig. 9. Metabolic fate of NAC after intravenous administration. While NAC undergoes deacetylation to cysteine, the amino acid limiting the rate of GSH synthesis, it also provides systemic protection against oxidants and toxins even before GSH formation. Products/metabolites derived from NAC cysteine donation are shown. As a thiol delivery agent NAC is considered the standard to which others are compared.

synthesis, enhance glutathione-S-transferase activity, promote detoxification of certain hepatotoxins, and act directly quenching oxidant radicals (specifically, $HOCl$, $O_2^{\bullet-}$, $OH\cdot$, and H_2O_2). To derive GSH, NAC must be deacetylated to cysteine, and both enzymes necessary for GSH synthesis are required (Figs. 4, 9) [101,102].

Proven medical applications of NAC are numerous and varied. It can enhance RBC GSH in hypoxic patients and can improve/preserve hepatocyte membrane fluidity and antioxidant enzyme activities in the cytosol and mitochondria in complete biliary tree occlusion [109]. It can enhance hepatic detoxification of a number of toxins through effects on GSH synthesis/metabolism and by restricting toxic adduct production. Although it does not influence cytochrome p450 oxidases directly, it can stimulate cytosolic enzymes, augmenting NADP and GSH reduction and reductive detoxification of xenobiotics. It has proven benefit in treatment of a number of hepatotoxins including, but not limited to, organic solvents, heavy metals, and acetaminophen (in which it has undergone the largest scrutiny as a therapeutic agent and serves as the standard of care) [110,111]. NAC has a protective effect in hepatic ischemia–reperfusion injury, perhaps by inhibiting Kupffer cell activation and in altering (improving) regional blood flow [112–114]. Its inhibitory influence on NF-κβ activation under a variety of conditions is linked to its thiol status [115]. It can prevent Kupffer cell NF-κβ activation induced by physiologically relevant concentrations of LPS [115]. Its ability to attenuate expression of endothelial adhesion molecules mitigates pathologic effects of oxidative stress beyond its capacity as a thiol donor. It can alter response in various vascular beds (peripheral, cardiac, sinusoidal) and improves oxygenation/perfusion in fulminant hepatic failure [112,116–118].

The role of NAC in treatment of sepsis and septic complications remains controversial [13,14]. Hepatocellular dysfunction is an early event in sepsis associated with proinflammatory cytokines before circulatory dysfunction becomes apparent [11]. A number of antioxidants including NAC modulate Kupffer cell activation in sepsis and are thought to yield benefit extending beyond the liver [12]. In conjunction with α-tocopherol, NAC reverses the inflammatory response in activated Kupffer cells in vitro, an effect mediated by suppression of cytokine mRNA, reduced production of TNF-α, and NF-κβ activation [14,65]. Pretreatment before endotoxin exposure with NAC or vitamin E suppresses many LPS-mediated changes independent of GSH. Cell redox balance influencing thiol groups, rather than specific ROS, govern key signaling events that trigger release of NF-κβ from its cytosolic anchor and expression of its dependent proinflammatory genes [115]. Activation of NF-κβ is inhibited by several thiol donors including NAC (in pharmacologic concentrations). However, there is some evidence that NAC might impair the neutrophil-killing capability irrespective of its augmenting effect on phagocytosis, an undesirable influence in sepsis [119,120].

In animals that have Heinz body hemolysis or when severe toxin-related liver injury is suspected, treatment with IV NAC is recommended. NAC is delivered through a nonpyrogenic filter (0.25 μm) using a 10% solution diluted 1:2 or more with saline and administered over 20 to 30 minutes. Dose recommendations follow therapeutic guidelines for humans who have acetaminophen toxicity: 140 mg/kg IV is given initially, thereafter followed by 70 mg/kg IV or orally for multiple treatments as frequently as every 4 hours but usually at 8- to 12-hour intervals for animals that have liver disease and are in crisis. Frequency of administration has not been evaluated. Higher doses of NAC have been used in humans for metal-associated systemic toxicity [121]. Treatment is tailored to the urgency of situation; for chronic treatment, oral NAC is usually replaced by SAMe for reasons detailed in the next section [121]. NAC might be particularly suited for animals that have fulminant hepatic failure caused by suspected hepatotoxicosis (eg, diazepam hepatotoxicity in cats, carprofen or tri-methoprim sulfa hepatotoxicity in dogs) and in cats that have the severe hepatic lipidosis (HL) syndrome associated with Heinz body anemia, hemolysis, or that demonstrate overt signs of hepatic failure. Whole blood and hepatic GSH concentrations measured in a small number of cats that have severe HL has verified profound depletions.

Despite the fact that the pharmacokinetics of NAC are altered significantly in humans who have hepatic dysfunction, using conventional dosing recommendations in dogs and cats that have severe liver disease has not produced toxic effects. Nevertheless, prolonged administration as a constant rate infusion of NAC must be avoided in hepatic insufficiency because this can result in excessive cysteine catabolism, yielding an overabundance of protons that block urea formation, favoring glutamine synthesis rather than ammonia detoxification in the urea cycle [122,123]. For this reason, parenteral NAC administration is given in 20- to 30-minute bolus doses.

Some work suggests that NAC behaves as a pro-oxidant when administered chronically in small doses. In healthy humans, doses as low as 1.2 g of NAC daily significantly reduce the GSH:GSSG ratio. In vitro work similarly confirms a pro-oxidant potential under certain circumstances (eg, NAC promoting oxidative DNA damage in the presence of Cu^{2+}) [124,125]. This finding argues against the prophylactic administration of low-dose NAC to patients that have liver disease as a means of achieving low-level thiol supplementation.

In humans, side effects after IV bolus administration of NAC might include hemodynamic changes (increased or decreased blood pressure) thought to reflect cysteine interaction with endothelial nitrates (an enhanced nitrate effect or elimination of nitrate tolerance through sulfhydryl group donation). Intracranial vasodilation also is considered to be a potential risk because it could theoretically compromise a patient that had cerebral edema associated with HE. Infrequent allergic reactions have been described in humans but have not been witnessed in animals by the author [125–128]. Large oral doses in humans (usually for acetaminophen overdose) have rarely been associated with nausea, rash, pruritus, angioedema, bronchospasm, tachycardia, or hypo- or hypertensive responses. The median lethal dose (LD_{50}) of oral NAC is 7888 mg/kg in mice and greater than 6000 mg/kg in rats.

S-adenosylmethionine

Dietary methionine is converted to SAMe under the influence of MAT1 (the hapatic SAMe synthetase isoform; E.c. 2.5.1.6) and ATP [129–131]. This is the only reaction that catabolizes methionine in mammals because this essential amino acid does not normally undergo transamination. Because 85% of transmethylation reactions and as much as 48% of methionine metabolism occurs in the liver, it is no surprise that hepatic SAMe adequacy is integrally important to many liver functions and to intermediary metabolism (Fig. 10) [130–135]. More than a half a century ago, abnormal metabolism of methionine was confirmed as a metabolic feature of cirrhosis and linked with HE [136–138]. In health, the amount of methionine necessary to generate enough SAMe for normal physiologic purposes is derived by de novo synthesis through (1) a salvage pathway involving methyltetrahydrofolate and vitamin B_{12} or trimethylglycine (betaine derived from choline), each combining with homocysteine; (2) dietary methionine intake; or (3) protein catabolism (a major mechanism) [129]. SAMe has important impact on intermediary metabolism through its function as a methyl group donor (transmethylation pathway), as a precursor of sulfur-containing compounds (transsulfuration pathway), and in production of polyamines (polyamine pathway) [130–132].

SAMe influences more than 100 reactions catalyzed by methyltransferases. Among these are biosynthesis of phospholipids (ie, phosphatidylcholine, essential for normal cell and organelle membrane integrity, fluidity, receptor expression, and signaling); biosynthesis of l-carnitine (a conditionally essential nutrient facilitating fatty acid oxidation); biosynthesis of creatine (essential for energy in muscles); formation of neurotransmitters and certain neuroreceptors; and reactions involving DNA, RNA, proteins, and many other endogenous metabolites (eg, steroid hormones). A number of products and reactions have special importance for normal hepatobiliary function and structure, gene transcription, and cell replication.

The transsulfuration pathway functions primarily in the liver, where it provides endogenous sulfur compounds including GSH and taurine (except that sufficient taurine is not derived from the transsulfuration pathway in cats) and sulfates. Hepatic SAMe thus serves as the major source of hepatic GSH and systemic thiol availability. Through this pathway SAMe plays a major role in hepatic and systemic redox status, resistance to oxidative

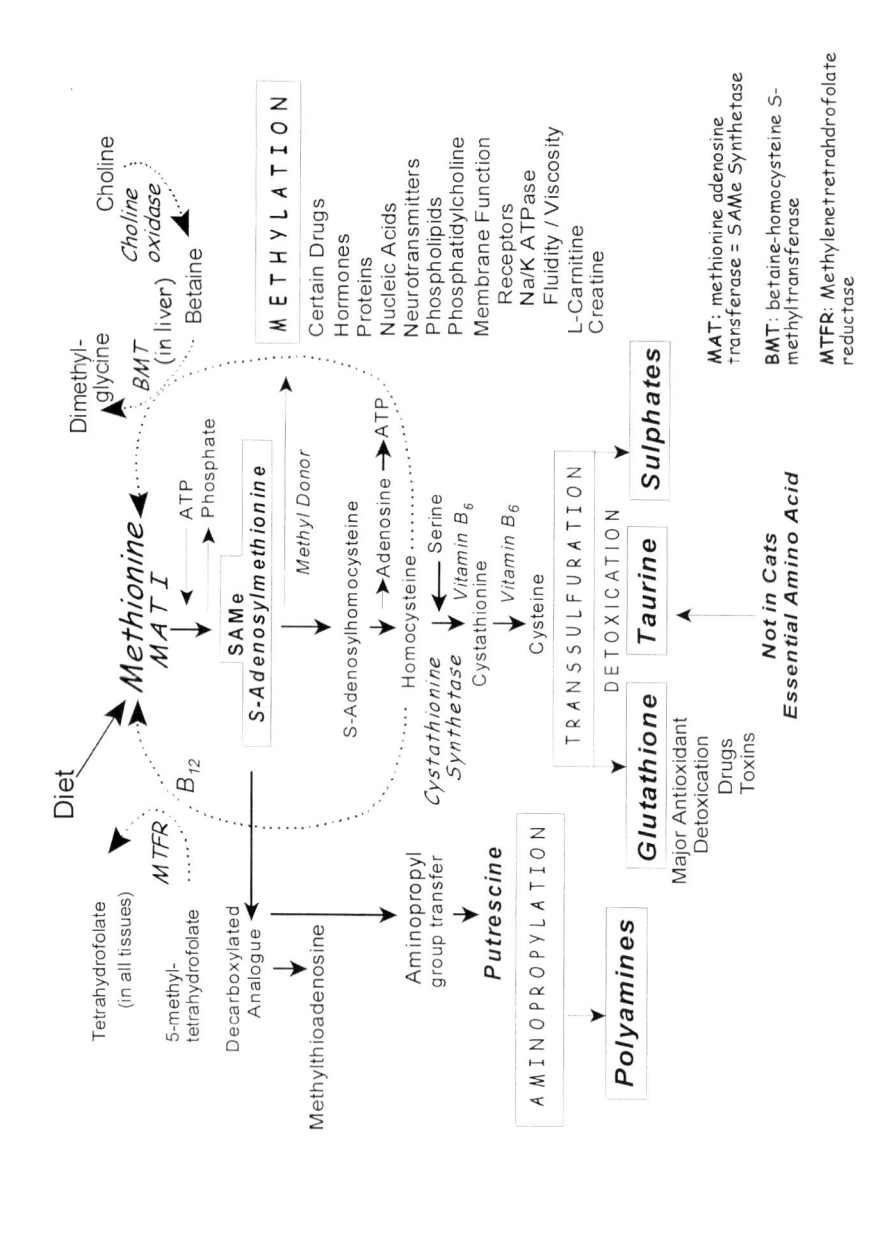

Fig. 10. Metabolic pathways and products of SAMe. Consult text for discussion of rate controlling enzymes and importance of its metabolic products.

injury, protection from toxic electrophiles or adducts, and xenobiotic metabolism.

The polyamine pathway influences cell replication, tissue regeneration and growth, DNA synthesis, and cell response to apoptotic signals. This pathway also generates methylthioadenosine (MTA), a decarboxylation product of SAMe recently implicated as a key hepatocyte signaling molecule that can also be used to resynthesize methionine [133].

While adequacy of hepatocellular GSH can be limited by nutritional status (protein, vitamins, micronutrients), excessive ROS exposure, or overwhelming toxic adduct formation, it also is importantly restricted by downregulation of the hepatic MAT1 isoform that governs methionine catabolism to SAMe in the liver (Fig. 10). In normal liver, most SAMe is used for methylation reactions, with decarboxylation yielding MTA accounting for approximately 5% of its use [132]. This designation can be increased when conditions require increased polyamine synthesis (eg, during liver regeneration). The predominant importance of SAMe for methylation reactions is shown by the shift in designated function in the face of dietary methyl group restriction. Normally, the fraction of available homocysteine converted to cystathionine (a precursor for GSH, taurine, and sulfate synthesis) during each transsulfuration cycle approximates 50% in humans. This rate declines to approximately 20% in the circumstance of dietary methyl group restriction [134,135]. Thus, a major factor governing SAMe use is methionine conservation to ensure its repletion for transmethylations. With appropriate cues, homocysteine can deviate precursors to salvage pathways to generate and conserve methionine. Coexistent folate, vitamin B_{12}, or choline deficiencies can impair sufficient SAMe resynthesis through the salvage pathways. In addition to the inability to catabolize methionine to SAMe, humans who have hepatic insufficiency might develop an acquired folate or B_{12} deficiency (nutritional, reduced enteric uptake, reduced hepatic storage) that can further compromise methionine availability. B_{12} deficiency has been amply documented in cats that have liver disease (cholangiohepatitis, HL) coexistent with severe small bowel malassimilation. This might importantly contribute to the confirmed whole blood and hepatic GSH depletion in individual cases.

The SAMe molecule imposes self-limiting feedback through direct influence on activity of cystathione β synthase (SAMe activates this enzyme; EC 4.2.1.22), betaine–homocysteine S-methyltransferase (SAMe inhibits this enzyme; EC 4.2.1.1.5), and methylenetetrahydrofolate reductase (SAMe inhibits this enzyme; EC 1.7.99.5; Fig. 10). SAMe thereby designates fractional use of homocysteine for methylation processes (generating and conserving methionine) or for the post-homocysteine transsulfuration pathway (GSH, sulfate generation).

While SAMe is the first product of methionine metabolism in all cells, it has greatest importance in the liver, where it can enter biochemical pathways not fully functional in other organs. In the liver there is a dynamic flux between its synthesis, use, and exportation. Initial medical attention focused on SAMe regarded it as a potential safe and universally effective thiol donor because of its pivotal role at the metabolic crossroads between methylation, transulphuration, and aminopropylation pathways, but a number of other important functions have been clarified since. In combination with its decarboxylation derivative, MTA, SAMe has been shown to influence gene expression, the apoptotic cascade, cell response to cytokines, membrane integrity (cell and mitochondrial), mitochondrial function, and hepatocellular and mitochondrial redox status under a variety of in vitro and in vivo circumstances [132,134–140]. Exactly whether SAMe or MTA is responsible for specific biologic responses is difficult to determine because most studies have not measured MTA. Discerning the role of MTA is further complicated by the fact that it resynthesizes methionine and SAMe [135,136].

Studies indicate that SAMe administration can beneficially alter the rate of liver disease progression, clinicopathologic markers, hepatic GSH stores, mitochondrial function, and detrimental cytokine effects [25,26,91,93–97,130,131,139–152]; however, because the amount of SAMe entering the liver after oral administration is small and has an extremely rapid half-life (~5 minutes), mechanisms other than those directly mediated by GSH status are likely involved [133,136]. An amplification effect driven by control of MAT genes has been postulated [133].

Methylation reactions facilitated by SAMe are indispensable in intermediary metabolism. Methylation of DNA cystine residues (c-5 position) affects their interaction with proteins, inhibits transcription, and gene expression. Hypomethylation of DNA can lead to chromosomal instability and mutations. Abnormal methylation at transcription sites can influence expression of tumor suppressor genes, leading to neoplastic transformation. In the context of liver disease, one particularly important methylation process converts phosphatidylethanolamine to phosphatidylcholine (PPC), an essential membrane component. SAMe orchestrates the addition of three methyl groups to the amino moiety of phosphatidylethanolamine. During methylation, phosphatidylethanolamine translocates from the cytoplasmic to the extracellular surface of the cell membrane, where PPC plays an integral role maintaining membrane function and binding domains. External localization maintains the appropriate ratio of phosphatidylethanolamine:PPC, determining membrane fluidity or viscosity. Increased phospholipid methylation reduces membrane viscosity, creating a more fluid interface that facilitates transmembrane movement of proteins through the lipid bilayer (important for membrane receptor expression), cell signaling, and metabolite exchange [129,151]. Influence on PPC might have an important effect in chronic necroinflammatory liver disease, limiting fibrosis (see section regarding PPC).

There is much evidence implicating age, injury, or disease associated SAMe deficiency as an enabling factor in liver disorders. SAMe provides hepatoprotection against a wide variety of hepatotoxins, including therapeutic agents. Case reports described successful responses in humans who had idiosyncratic drug hepatotoxicity in which SAMe mitigated drug toxicity [130,131]. Xenobiotic toxicity attenuated by SAMe administration in humans (idiosyncratic reactions) and toxins in animal models include acetaminophen, ethanol, CCl_4, galactosamine, α-nathpylisothiocyanate (ANIT), estrogen therapy (in women), anticonvulsants (including primidone and phenobarbital), chemotherapeutic agents (including methotrexate, prednisone, azathioprine, and cyclosporine), and certain antidepressants. The extent of therapeutic benefit achieved in case reports describing individual patients is difficult to discern; however, there is a large database documenting its benefit in acetaminophen and alcohol hepatotoxicity in humans and animals, and other toxins studied in vivo [130,153–155]. Attenuation of xenobiotic toxicity is attributed to increased availability of GSH and sulfates, implementing conjugation and detoxification reactions, the enabling of methylation reactions, or altering enzyme pathways (preserving thiol bonds) associated with toxic adduct formation or elimination. Protection against acetaminophen toxicosis is believed to largely reflect thiol donation. Extensive work using animal models (hepatotoxicity secondary to bile acids, extrahepatic bile duct obstruction, ischemia–reperfusion injury, ethanol, CCl_4) shows that SAMe prohibits hepatocellular SAMe depletion, conserves hepatocyte and mitochondrial GSH, and mitigates deleterious mitochondrial effects including MPT, transition to the apoptotic or necrotic death pathways, and development of organ fibrosis [25,26,93–95,132,142,150,156–161]. One of the most analyzed outcomes is its influence on hepatic and mitochondrial GSH and restoration of GSH in face of oxidative injury. Oral SAMe replenishes hepatic GSH in humans who have cirrhosis and improves tolerance to free radical, cholestatic, and ischemic–reperfusion liver injury [161,162].

Inadequate antioxidant protection permissively augments progression of liver disease and its systemic complications. Because mitochondrial GSH depletion precedes measurable tissue GSH depletion, demonstrating low hepatic tissue GSH concentrations is thought to reflect severely altered cell thiol and redox status and to represent patient vulnerability to oxidant injury [3,5,16,163]. Low hepatic tissue GSH concentrations have been proven in companion animals that have spontaneous liver disease, analogous to the situation in humans and numerous animal models of liver disease (see Fig. 5) [77]. The proportion of cats that have spontaneous liver disease that develop subnormal hepatic GSH values exceeds the proportion of dogs, suggesting that cats might have greater risk. Whether this relates to comparatively lower γGT activity in the cat, greater methionine turnover, or different disease processes compared with dogs has not been determined. Preventing tissue SAMe deficiency should be considered as a rational therapeutic intervention for animals, as it is now proposed for humans who have necroinflammatory and cholestatic liver disorders. A number of clinical studies in humans with liver disease support the claim that orally administered SAMe provides benefit. A double blind, placebo-controlled, multicenter clinical trial involving humans (n = 220) who had chronic liver disease (chronic active hepatitis, cirrhosis) showed that SAMe improved clinicopathologic features and, subjectively, cholestatic symptoms [145]. Similar results have been shown in a variety of large and small blind and open studies with meta-analysis confirming clinical benefit in patients with chronic liver disease. SAMe improved survival in chronic alcohol hepatotoxicosis (SAMe 1.2 g daily for 6 months), and delayed liver transplantation in patients with cirrhosis when treatment was initiated early in the disease process and improved clinical status in women who had severe cholestasis of pregnancy [97,143–149,161,162,164].

Considering the broad range of metabolism influenced by SAMe, and that the liver serves as the largest source of SAMe and GSH precursors for the body, impaired hepatic availability of either substance has wide systemic permutations. Because SAMe is essential for maintaining DNA methylation, a broad range of potential adverse effects becomes possible. The influence of SAMe on cytokines has been detailed clearly, and it includes modulation of TNF-α, a pivotal signal for mitochondrial death pathways and production of a broad repertoire of inflammatory and fibrogenic cytokines. The ability of SAMe to attenuate LPS-stimulated transcription of the gene for TNF-α provides an important anti-inflammatory and antifibrotic effect in the liver, considering that the liver is continuously exposed to LPS derived from the alimentary canal [165]. Treatment with SAMe is therefore thought to suppress hepatic injury and reactive fibrosis in response to this signaling pathway [96,140,165]. In view of this response, SAMe might prove to be useful in attenuating reactive hepatic injury commonly found in dogs and cats that have inflammatory bowel disease that is thought to reflect an ''innocent bystander'' injury related to inflammatory mediator and endotoxin delivery through the portal circulation. Because TNF-α cytotoxicity is mediated in part through its effects on mitochondria and by promoting oxidative stress, it is possible that SAMe might also attenuate TNF-α cytotoxicity by mitigating its mitochondrial influence and rectifying altered cell and mitochondrial redox status. SAMe and its decarboxylation product MTA are known to protect hepatocytes from toxin-induced apoptosis mediated at the level of the mitochondria [166,167]. The protective effect of SAMe on hepatic mitochondria in alcohol toxicity is but one example of this action. For many years SAMe has been known to function as an hepatoprotectant against development of dysplastic and neoplastic hepatocellular foci in hepatotoxic (but not infectious) models of hepatocarcinogenesis. While the exact mechanism has yet to be elucidated, an influence on growth-regulating genes is suspected (DNA methylation) and through production of its catabolite MTA, which has an inhibitory influence on cell growth [141,168].

There is sparse information regarding SAMe adequacy in extrahepatic tissues or in primary disease in other organ systems. Studies in humans, relevant animal models, and in vitro investigations suggest that SAMe can rectify RBC membrane abnormalities associated with liver disease [148,151,169]. There is increasing evidence that SAMe also can attenuate cytokine-mediated injury in other tissues based on preliminary work in pancreatitis and gastric ulceration [170,171]. SAMe has also been evaluated in humans as a treatment for depression and for its analgesic and anti-inflammatory properties for osteoarthritic pain and inflammation; in each case it was shown to provide clinical benefit [130,172].

Pharmacologic applications of s-adenosylmethionine

When provided exogenously as a supernutrient, SAMe can impart a variety of benefits without noxious effects. Since March 1999 SAMe has been available in the United States under the Dietary Supplement and Health Education Act as an over-the-counter supplement. While a relatively new product in the North America, SAMe has been available in Europe since 1979 as a prescription medication. In its native form, SAMe is labile and degrades rapidly. Patented stable salts, toluenedisulfonate and 1,4-butanedisulfonate forms, are used for pharmaceutical purposes. SAMe is absorbed enterically in the small bowel; however, enteric coated tablets are necessary to achieve pharmacologically relevant dosing. Because there is minimal protein binding, orally administered SAMe can gain access to the central nervous system (CNS) crossing the blood–brain barrier [129,130]. Several studies have proven that parenteral and oral SAMe can achieve CSF concentrations; dogs given 8 mg/kg followed by 12 mg/kg CRI for 6 hours had a steady hourly increase in CSF SAMe concentrations, achieving 20- to 40-fold basal values at 6 hours [172]. Experimental studies and clinical trials in humans, dogs, and cats have shown that parenteral and oral SAMe can increase GSH in RBCs and hepatic tissue, but how SAMe accesses hepatocytes remains controversial. Treatment of humans who have liver disease, dogs that have glucocorticoid-induced vacuolar hepatopathy, and healthy cats has proven that oral SAMe can increase hepatic GSH concentrations significantly [130,144,148,149,173,174]. Uptake into mitochondria occurs by way of a carrier-mediated transport system; approximately one third of total hepatic SAMe concentrations reside within this organelle known to be deficient in the MAT1 enzyme [175]. Oral administration of SAMe also increases SAMe concentrations in synovial fluid.

SAMe has a favorable side effect profile comparable with placebo controls in numerous clinical studies in human patients. Overall it has a low incidence of side effects and excellent tolerability. In humans, gastrointestinal distress, flatulence, mania/agitation, and headache are described occasionally. A "serotonin syndrome" has occurred in humans when SAMe was coadministered with a monoamine oxidase inhibitor. Enteric coating of tablets is reported to minimize occasional adverse gastrointestinal effects in humans. Starting a small dose and gradually scaling up to the intended therapeutic dose has been used to ameliorate minor gastrointestinal upset. Single-dose oral toxicity studies in rodents derived an LD_{50} of greater than 4650 mg/kg for SAMe; chronic administration in rats given 200 mg/kg body weight per day for 104 weeks failed to produce toxicity, as has administration for greater than 100 days at 40 to 65 mg/kg in healthy cats and 20 mg/kg for 6 months in healthy dogs. Companion animals treated with SAMe rarely show intolerance. Occasionally an owner might note nausea or food refusal coordinating with the immediate postpill interval (within hours). In several animals these effects have self resolved over time. Rarely, anxiety has been observed, necessitating treatment discontinuation. In a few cats, persistent postdosing emesis has necessitated treatment discontinuation. Loading for 3 to 6 weeks with a daily dose of 20 mg/kg followed by a smaller twice weekly maintenance dose has been recommended in some human treatment protocols. This regimen has not been studied in animals and remains a speculative practice.

A dose of approximately 20 mg/kg of SAMe (stabilized salt) per day in dogs of approximately 53 mg/kg using an enteric coated tablet on an empty stomach increases plasma SAMe concentrations significantly in dogs and cats [173,174]. Maximal plasma concentrations are individually quite variable but are generally achieved between 1 to 4 hours in dogs and 2 to 8 hours in cats. Plasma SAMe concentrations are detectable after an overnight fast in animals chronically treated for 3 weeks or longer. Significantly increased hepatic total GSH concentrations were achieved after 118 days of SAMe administration in healthy cats (mean dose 53 mg/kg) [173]. Dogs given oral SAMe at a dose of approximately 20 mg/kg in a double-blind placebo-controlled crossover trial with prednisolone modeled vacuolar hepatopathy also developed significantly increased hepatic total GSH concentrations [173]. Exactly what minimum dose of SAMe is efficacious in management of spontaneous liver disease has yet to be determined in humans or animals. Prospective clinical studies of SAMe might be complicated by the over-the-counter purchase of products lacking bioavailability. Oral administration of enteric coated, stabilized SAMe to dogs and cats that have necroinflammatory and cholestatic liver disease has been supervised by the author for more than 4 years without any signs of toxicity.

Despite the underlying cause, the pathologic effects of liver disease are fairly predictable, involving common mechanisms that damage cell structure and function while impairing avenues of cellular protection, toxin neutralization/excretion, and cell repair and regeneration. Measures restoring hepatocellular function that can simultaneously stimulate cell repair, attenuate free radical production/accumulation and cytokine-induced injury, suppress inflammation, and improve detoxication mechanisms and toxin elimination and membrane function are desirable in a large spectrum of disorders. It is in this regard that SAMe is relevant as a therapeutic agent in the diverse forms of liver damage encountered in veterinary patients. Because membrane damage by free radicals and oxidation is a basic pathomechanism of cell injury in diseases of the liver and biliary tree, supplementation with SAMe might protect the liver and provide thiol substrates to the systemic circulation.

In severe liver disease, reduced hepatic mass, impaired hepatic perfusion, and nutritional deficiencies might impair hepatic synthesis of SAMe directly. Acquired SAMe deficiency impairs availability of transsulfuration products used in conjugation reactions. While this impairment limits taurine only in dogs, it might limit sulfation reactions in cats. It has recently been shown that bile acid sulfation plays a role in detoxifying bile acids in cats that have liver disease, enabling their urinary elimination [176]. Studies show that SAMe can attenuate bile acid-induced hepatotoxicity, leading to apoptosis and with this effect has been verified in humans with cholestatic liver disease. An adjunctive benefit might be derived when SAMe and ursodeoxycholic acid are coadministered [25,26]. A beneficial influence of SAMe on hepatocellular regeneration/cell division, hepatic mass replacement, and protein synthesis has also been shown, which validates its use in the context of acute hepatocellular necrosis or following extensive hepatic mass resection. Products derived from transmethylation have pivotal importance in liver disease, especially production of PPC, which is essential for optimal membrane structure, integrity, and function. As membrane function deteriorates in liver disease, so does the repertoire of an individual hepatocyte limiting its ability to accommodate to declining organ function. Part of this cell debilitation derives from impaired signaling imposed by deleterious membrane changes. Normalizing membrane PPC not only improves intercellular communication and cell health but also provides an antifibrotic effect, described in detail later in this article. Normalizing membrane structure might also improve GSH-motivated canalicular bile flow and membrane Na^+/K^+ ATPase initiated bile formation, which might explain the attenuation of cholestasis observed in disease models. Anti-inflammatory effects have been shown in vitro and in humans concordant with an influence of SAMe on GSH concentrations and other antioxidant processes that might relate to improved thiol and redox status, diminished signaling by TNF-α, membrane methylation (production of PPC), or in response to enhanced MTA availability.

Oral treatment with SAMe appears to be warranted in dogs and cats that have necroinflammatory and cholestatic liver injury because (1) SAMe is absorbed, (2) it can influence hepatic GSH concentrations, (3) it is nontoxic in healthy and ill animals, and (4) each species undergoes liver tissue GSH depletion in spontaneous disease. SAMe administration to cats that have HL syndrome might be important based on the many metabolic abnormalities that have been documented in this disorder that might reflect SAMe and GSH depletion. Many chronically inappetent cats that have HL present with subnormal vitamin B_{12} concentrations. Deficiency of this vitamin compromises conversion of homocysteine to methionine in the salvage pathway. Because inappetent cats are known to develop low plasma methionine concentrations (~50% of normal) [177], they seemingly have high risk for low hepatocellular SAMe and its direct metabolic products. The extraordinarily high serum bile acids in HL have a fractionation pattern that is nearly identical to that of major bile duct occlusion, suggesting impaired enterohepatic bile acid circulation [178]. Finding low GSH in whole blood and liver tissue in representative cases, observing the tendency for the HL cat to develop Heinz body hemolysis and fat-soluble vitamin deficiency (vitamin K responsive coagulopathies), provides strong circumstantial evidence of critical oxidant challenge and insufficient antioxidant protection. Compromised ability to perform methylation reactions might also limit synthesis of L-carnitine in amounts sufficient to resolve hepatic triglyceride accumulation (consult section on L-carnitine). Clinical work in humans, experimental work in rodents, and in vitro work with hepatocytes substantiates that low tissue GSH concentrations and high bile acid concentrations impair egress of fat from hepatocytes, that an impaired antioxidant defense correlates with fatty liver, that starvation amplifies tissue GSH depletion, and that antioxidants contribute to syndrome regression [25,26,179–184]. Thus, SAMe and vitamin E are used in HL in an adjunctive capacity with supportive care apropos for this syndrome, with nutritional support being the key to recovery. Because no parenteral form of SAMe is currently available, enterically coated tablets are crushed and given with feedings. A doubled dose of SAMe is empirically used because bioavailability is markedly reduced in the presence of food. Fasting the HL cat to administer medication is unacceptable because many of these cats require a constant rate of food delivery during early recovery.

As publication of studies involving SAMe continue to increase in human medicine it is becoming more apparent that a polypharmacy approach likely offers the most reasonable treatment and best response. There is evidence that SAMe has a sparing effect on vitamin E and a synergistic effect with vitamin E and UDCA. The important modulatory influence of SAMe against cytokine-mediated injury, disease progression, and cell commitment to death pathways suggests that it might attenuate hepatic disease phenomenon in ways that differ from other therapeutic agents. There is ample evidence to firmly recommend prescription SAMe as an antioxidant in companion animals that have liver disease, yet like most drugs in veterinary medicine there are no controlled studies that have evaluated its efficacy in animals other than the cited pilot investigations.

α-lipoic acid (thioctic acid)

While the metabolic role of lipoic acid has been realized for decades, little information has been included in the veterinary literature. Lipoic acid was initially classified as a vitamin until it was proven to be synthesized by mammals. Known by a variety of names, α-lipoic acid also is referred to as α-lipoate, thioctic acid, 1,2-dithiolane-3 pentanoic acid, and 1,2-dithiolane-3 valeric acid. At physiologic pH, lipoic acid is anionic and referred to as lipoate [185]. Octanoate serves as the immediate precursor for its carbon fatty acid chain and cysteine, its sulfur donor. α-lipoic acid is readily absorbed from the diet or from supplements (oral bioavailability in humans is ~30%, and free lipoic acid distributes widely throughout the body with a mean plasma half-life of ~30 minutes in humans) [185]. Thereafter it is taken into cells and reduced to dihydrolipoate (DHLA) by several enzymes (GSH reductase, Txn reductase, mitochondrial DHLA-dehydrogenase [also known as lipoyl or lipoamide dehydrogenase]) with NADH serving as a reducing equivalent. DHLA dehydrogenase, a membrane-bound protein containing a flavin adenine α-keto acid dehydrogenase complex, is located in mitochondrial and cell plasma membranes, where it catalyzes reversible redox cycling of disulfide bonds within the enzyme, transferring electrons to protein adducts and from NADH or NADPH using lipoic acid or coenzyme Q_{10} as a cofactor [185,186]. Together DHLA and lipoic acid form a redox couple, each being exchanged across cell membranes, where they function as antioxidants in the extra- and intracellular compartments.

α-lipoic acid also is metabolized to lipoamide, an essential cofactor in various multienzyme systems, mostly within the mitochondria, that are involved with oxidation of pyruvate (pyruvate dehydrogenase enzyme complex) and of α-ketoglutarate (α-ketoglutarate dehydrogenase enzyme complex). It is also functions as a cofactor for the oxidation of branched-chain amino acids (branched-chain α-keto acid dehydrogenase enzyme complex) [187,188]. Free α-lipoic acid influences different biochemical pathways at various levels, interacting with protein systems functioning as a substrate, an inhibitor, or an effector [188]. It provides antioxidant effects in aqueous and lipid phases and also chelates transition metals, especially iron. Acting synergistically with other antioxidants, DHLA assists in regeneration of the reduced (functional) forms for vitamin E, GSH, ascorbate, ubiquinol (coenzyme Q_{10}), and NADPH (see Fig. 8). It also might influence regulatory proteins and genes involved in normal growth and metabolism and promote apoptosis in cancer cells [189].

Interacting with transition metals, DHLA can limit their oxidant potential; it can remove Fe from ferritin in the Fe^{2+} and Fe^{3+} state. Affiliation with transition metals, however, might impose a pro-oxidant challenge that might occur during rejuvenation of reduced ascorbate, which is not surprising considering the oxidant effects of vitamin C in biologic systems [189]. While DHLA also manifests other pro-oxidant effects in liver test systems in vitro, in general it should be considered to be a powerful reducing agent because it quantitatively enhances GSH availability in several ways. After synthesis it is released from the cell, where it can reduce cystine to cysteine facilitating GSH formation. By increasing intracellular cysteine, it is quantitatively important for increasing intracellular GSH [190]. It also can reduce GSSG to GSH and increases the sulfhydryl content of bile by increasing biliary GSH exportation [188]. In addition to its powerful antioxidant properties, lipoate can also increase the efficiency of glucose uptake into skeletal muscle cells (in vitro) to a magnitude comparable to insulin. Lipoate supplementation has consequently been of interest to athletes and patients who have diabetes mellitus.

As a treatment for liver disease, a number of studies in rodent models and humans have been undertaken, but none in the dog or cat. There are no compelling data to recommend its specific use in liver disease. The LD_{50} of lipoic acid approximates 400 to 500 mg/kg after oral dosing in dogs but it appears to be 10 times more toxic in cats [189,191,502]. Caution is warranted in supplementing lipoic acid especially in ill, anorectic cats subject to thiamine deficiency because fatal complications have occurred in thiamine deficient rats with doses as low as 20 mg/kg [192]. Side effects in humans include allergic skin reactions and hypoglycemia in diabetic patients as a consequence of enhanced glucose uptake [189]. There is limited information regarding dose recommendations for humans or animals. Metabolic studies in dogs show that they uniquely metabolize lipoic acid compared with rodents and humans [497]. Metabolism in the cat remains uncharacterized. Chronic feeding of α-lipoic acid in dogs by incorporation of 150, 1500, 3000, and 4500 ppm (dry matter diet) in a basal diet increased the whole blood GSH:GSSG ratio (improved redox status), did not induce adverse hematologic or biochemical effects, but did induce weight loss at the highest intake level (whether this represented a metabolic effect or inappetence was unclear) [191]. The lowest intake level produced the largest numeric improvement in GSH:GSSG. Studies in cats describing their unique susceptibility to the toxic effects of lipoic acid are in press.

Vitamin E

Vitamin E represents a family of highly lipophilic compounds found in all cell membranes, considered to be the most important lipid-soluble antioxidant. It is an essential nutrient derived from food and nutritional supplements because mammalian cells are unable to synthesize it [193–195]. Eight vitamin E isomers are widely distributed in nature; while the γ forms are found predominately in plants and are the primary form ingested, α-tocopherol is most bioavailable, and nutritional recommendations for vitamin E should be based on this form. Commercially available vitamin E consists of an isomer mixture or naturally occurring tocopherols and tocotrienols; d-α-tocopherol is a synthetic form comprised of the eight possible stereoisomers in equal amounts (all rac-α-tocopherol, formerly called dl-α-tocopherol) or their esters. Different bioavailability and bioequivalence of the various forms of vitamin E is proven, natural vitamin E (RRR-α-tocopherol) having greater bioavailability than synthetic vitamin E in humans

(2:1 bioavailability) [196]. Because of high lipid solubility and hydrophobicity, vitamin E requires adaptations to facilitate transport and uptake into the aqueous phase of plasma, body fluids, and cells. Ingested vitamin E is taken up in the proximal intestine depending on the amount of co-ingested lipid, released bile, and digestive esterases. Lipolysis and emulsification lead to its incorporation into mixed micelles, passive absorption, and incorporation into chylomicrons for lymphatic dispersal. Upon hepatic delivery, Vitamin E is extracted, sorted, and distributed to lysosomes. Thereafter, a specific α-tocopherol transfer protein (α-TPP) segregates desired forms and mediates transfer to lipoproteins. Excluded isomers are eliminated in bile or urine or they are metabolized. Vitamin E functions in the midst of an interactive group of redox antioxidant cycles called the antioxidant network (see Fig. 8).

Vitamin E is a potent defender against propagation of peroxidation membrane damage. After catalytically terminating membrane peroxidation reactions, the oxidized tochopheroxy radical is transformed to the reduced functional state through interactions with water- and lipid-soluble molecular and enzymatic antioxidants. Nearby companion reactants (vitamin C directly and indirectly through thiol antioxidants) conserve functional vitamin E, thereby protecting tissues from tocopheroxy radical oxidation.

Vitamin E also imparts a number of nonantioxidant functions, many of which reflect its influence inhibiting protein kinase C (PKC), are anti-inflammatory, and have potential to impart a dampening effect on necroinflammatory liver disease [197,198]. Nonantioxidant functions include an antiproliferative effect on vascular smooth muscle, an inhibitory influence on platelet aggregation/adhesion, suppressive influence on inflammatory cells (circulating and tissue macrophages, neutrophils, fibroblasts, and other cells in areas of PKC-primed oxidant injury), inhibitory influence on NF-κβ activation, suppressive influence on injurious immune responses, reduction of free radical production, ability to alter gene expression, inhibitory influence on thrombin-induced PKC activation, suppression of endothelin secretion, and inhibition of 5-lipoxygenase and cyclooxygenase (possibly by integration into cell and organelle membranes) [198–201]. The mechanism whereby vitamin E inhibits PKC might involve attenuated generation of membrane-derived diacylglycerol, a lipid known to facilitate PKC translocation and activity, or through membrane integration, which interferes directly with PKC [197,198]. It also is known to suppress hepatic collagen gene expression in the inflamed or injured liver [199–201].

Hepatic concentrations of α-tocopherol in humans who have cirrhosis are subnormal (3-fold below normal control values) despite normal serum concentrations [202]. Many studies substantiate that tissue concentrations of α-tocopherol are not reliably reflected by measuring plasma α-tocopherol concentrations collected during the same diagnostic interval; therefore, measuring circulating vitamin E concentrations in dogs or cats to predict tissue α-tocopherol concentrations or to guide therapeutic recommendations cannot be endorsed.

Vitamin E should be used for management of hepatobiliary disorders likely to involve oxidative membrane injury based on a plethora of data accumulated from many in vitro and in vivo studies [14, 22,23,32,40,64,196,202,203]. Hepatic injury derived from specific toxins (including CCl_4, phenobarbital, ethanol, and others), major bile duct obstruction, membranocytolytic bile acids, ischemia–reperfusion injury, and transition-metal–associated injury (Cu and Fe) has been shown to be attenuated by supplementary vitamin E. Studies show clearly that vitamin E-depleted hepatocytes have enhanced susceptibility to a variety of hepatotoxins, provoking lipid peroxidation-dependent and -independent cytotoxicity. The importance of a healthy antioxidant network for conservation of vitamin E has been shown in which SAMe administration conserves hepatic vitamin E while diminishing oxidant tissue injury from toxin (CCl_4) exposure [204]. Co-administration of vitamin E with other therapeutic agents in humans who have chronic viral hepatitis has improved response, reduced plasma markers of oxidative stress, and diminished fibrogenesis—even without significant change in circulating vitamin E status [64].

Studies of vitamin E supplementation in dogs and cats are sparse. The influence of a total dietary vitamin E intake ranging from a 153 to 598 IU/kg diet in dogs and from a 98 to 540 IU/kg diet in cats on parameters reflecting oxidant stress (total serum alkenal concentrations representing combined concentrations of malonaldehyde equivalents and 4-hydroxynonenal [4HNE]) and serum vitamin E concentrations have been reported [205]. All supplemented dogs developed significant increases in serum vitamin E concentrations. Only dogs receiving more than a 400 IU/kg diet and cats receiving a 540 IU/kg diet had significantly reduced serum alkenal concentrations reflecting improved systemic antioxidant status. In abstract presentation, dietary vitamin E (fed to provide 0.58 IU or 7 IU α-tocopherol acetate per kg body weight) given over 3 months to dogs that had histologically confirmed chronic inflammatory liver disease demonstrated that a 7 IU/kg vitamin E dose significantly reduced serum ALT activity, increased serum and hepatic vitamin E concentrations, and improved hepatic GSH:GSSG status, without increasing total GSH concentration or changing hepatic histology or metal content [206]. This study suggests that vitamin E can improve hepatic redox status in dogs that have necroinflammatory liver disease as early as 3 months.

Currently, use of vitamin E (synthetic α-tocopherol product) is recommended for dogs and cats that have necroinflammatory and cholestatic liver disorders using a dose of 10 IU/kg per day. High doses (50–100 IU/kg) might be indicated in animals that have chronic severe cholestatic liver disease compromising the enterohepatic circulation of bile acids and fat-soluble substances. Such cases will typically demonstrate sequential response to parenteral vitamin K administration (ie, correction of prolonged proteins invoked by vitamin K absence or antagonism [PIVKA] or optimized prothrombin clotting times). Vitamin E insufficiency is subsequently inferred.

Oral supplementation with α-tocopherol does not increase plasma concentrations greater than 2- to 3-fold irrespective of the amount or duration of vitamin supplementation in healthy humans; however, this represents a considerable functional increase because only approximately one molecule of vitamin E per 1000 to 2000 membrane phospholipid molecules protects the typical biologic membrane [207]. Large interindividual differences in uptake and pharmacokinetics have been shown in healthy humans, thus adequate or optimal vitamin E intake can differ widely between individuals. Increased consumption of polyunsaturated fatty acids (PUFA) increases the dietary requirement for vitamin E, with a number of studies suggesting that n-3 PUFA imposes a greater demand compared with n-6 PUFA [208–210]; however, there is great complexity in this relationship involving the PUFA source, the amount of dietary fat, the dietary ratio of n-3:n-6 PUFA, the form of vitamin E consumed, and the tissues examined.

Vitamin E is has relatively low toxicity in animals and humans. Supplemental doses ranging from 200 to 2400 IU/day (about 13- to 160-fold current normal dietary human allowances) given for up to 4.5 years are safe in humans [211,212,498]. Acute oral LD_{50} for synthetic vitamin E in rats, mice, and rabbits is greater than 2 g/kg body weight [213]; however, high doses of vitamin E ($\geq$5000 IU/d) given to humans can antagonize other fat-soluble vitamins, impairing bone mineralization, reducing hepatic vitamin A stores, and producing coagulopathies caused by vitamin K insufficiency [213,214]. Because tocopherol and some of its metabolites can inhibit platelet aggregation, it is recommended that supplementation be suspended if anticoagulants are administered or vitamin K deficiency is suspected [215]. Further, because vitamin E is metabolized extensively before excretion by cytochrome oxidases (p450 system), certain drugs that induce these enzymes might potentiate formation of the tocopheroxy radical, especially if supranutritional amounts are administered. Irrespective of cytochrome induction, supranutritional dosing of tocopherol promotes tocopheroxy radical accumulation if other protective cofactors facilitating its rejuvenation are imbalanced or relatively deficient.

Vitamin C

Ascorbic acid, a hydrophilic vitamin, acts in an antioxidant and pro-oxidant capacity [216]. In normal circumstances it functions as a cooperative member of the well-balanced antioxidant network. Excess vitamin C might be pro-oxidant in the presence of metals, especially Fe and Cu, by generating cofactors of activated oxygen radicals collateral to lipid peroxidation [217,218]. Vitamin C has important metabolic roles as a cofactor of at least eight specific enzymes involved in collagen, hormone, amino acid, and carnitine synthesis or metabolism, and it is involved in the synthesis or modulation of some components of the nervous system, the microsomal drug metabolizing system, synthesis of corticosteroids, catecholamines, metabolism of tryptophan, tyrosine, histamine, and conversion of cholesterol into bile acids [216–218]. Some of its enzyme-related functions are coordinate with Fe- or Cu-dependent enzymes in pathways where it functions as a cofactor. Vitamin C also participates in detoxification of many pharmacologic agents and toxins, and plays a role in immune function. Although some of its interactive mechanisms remain elusive, many are thought to involve its antioxidant abilities, a direct antimicrobial effect, or its influence as an immunomodulator [216].

As an antioxidant, vitamin C reduces a number of ROS, exerts a sparing effect on vitamin E and selenium, can regenerate vitamin E directly, and in cooperation with thiol antioxidants indirectly protects against GSH depletion and facilitates GSH regeneration. In some disease models, ascorbate actually promotes collagen synthesis; whether or not this occurs in the chronically inflamed liver has not been resolved. What is most concerning about use of vitamin C in liver disease is its potential to facilitate enteric Fe uptake, to promote release of Fe from ferritin, to promote Fe storage, and augment transition metal-mediated tissue injury [217–219]. The biologic importance of interactions between vitamin C and transition metals remains controversial. In vitro work might reflect test system peculiarities not achieved in biological systems; however, because hepatic Fe commonly exceeds the normal range in animals that have necroinflammatory liver disorders [42,43], it is recommended that supplementation be avoided in animals that have high tissue metal concentrations or lack quantitative metal analyses.

Milk thistle

Milk thistle, also referred to as *Carduus marianus*, Mariendistel, *Silybum marianum*, Silymarin, and silibinin is currently the most well researched plant extract used in the treatment of liver disease [220,499]. *Silybum marianum*, a member of the daisy family (Compositae), is a thistle growing 1 to 3 meters tall in sunny locations but tolerating a variety of soils and climates worldwide. Mature plants have characteristic spiked leaves with distinct white milky veins, bright purple flowers, and strong spines. The derivative of milk thistle is a complex of flavonolignans including silibinin, isosilibinin, silidianin, and silicristin, collectively referred to as Silymarin. While the active derivatives are found in the entire plant, they are concentrated in the fruit and seeds. The seeds also contain betaine (trimethylglycine) and essential fatty acids. Silymarin is extracted with 95% ethyl alcohol yielding a bright yellow fluid standard extract containing a 60% to 80% Silymarin. Despite labeling claims, there are significant variations between commercially available products and no assurance of extract purity [220,221]. Proportions of extract depend on the cultivar seed source, the cultivation conditions, and the processing techniques [222]. Most advertisements for Silymarin cite its value for enhancing liver regeneration and as a hepatoprotectant.

A considerable number of in vitro studies (and fewer in vivo studies) of Silymarin confirm that it provides antioxidant effects against relevant biological ROS and lipid peroxidation [59,60,223–227]. Studies investigating microangiopathies confirm antioxidant benefit equivalent to ubiquinol (coenzyme Q_{10}) and vitamin E [228]. Antioxidant effects mitigate hepatocellular and mitochondrial membrane oxidation and GSH depletion in hepatic iron overload, in which it significantly improves mitochondrial function, and reduces hepatic fibrogenesis and tissue iron [60,229,230]. Silymarin, and specifically purified silibinin and silicristin, accelerate hepatocellular regeneration as a result of increased gene transcription/translation and enhanced DNA biosynthesis [231–236]. This response serves for its recommendation during recovery from fulminant hepatic injury or large hepatic mass resections.

Silymarin also has been shown to mitigate the severity of hepatic fibrosis in several forms of liver injury with effects comparable to colchicine in some models [237–240]. Antifibrotic effects derive from it ability to inhibit Stellate cell activation and proliferation, signaling for type 1 collagen synthesis, and production of metalloproteinase-1 tissue inhibitor. The latter effect allows metalloproteinase ECM remodeling and ECM dissolution [241,242]. Studies substantiate that Silymarin inhibits reactive collagen formation in live animal models of hepatotoxic and obstructive cholestatic liver injury. A dose of 50 mg/kg/day successfully inhibited collagen deposition to approximately 12% of untreated controls with major bile duct occlusion. Early and advanced stages of liver injury were inhibited whether Silymarin was given during the entire 6 weeks of study or only during the last 2 weeks. It also induced a choleretic response associated with expansion of the endogenous pool of bile salts (by increased bile acid synthesis), including the hepatoprotective bile acid ursodeoxycholic acid [243].

Silymarin modulates cytosolic Ca^{2+} flux induced by oxidant injury, consistent with events triggering MPT and caspase activation [244]. In vitro work has confirmed strong inhibition of the 5-lipoxygenase pathway in Kupffer cells with pharmacologic concentrations relevant to conventional dosing, providing hepatoprotective and antifibrotic properties [245]. Silymarin also potently suppresses NF-κβ nuclear DNA binding and acute phase gene expression, consistent with clinical anti-inflammatory, antifibrotic, and antioxidant effects [246]. It also blocks TNF-α–induced activation of NF-κβ in a dose-dependent manner through several mechanisms [247]. Antioxidant properties of Silymarin have been characterized in a multitude of studies addressing specific hepatotoxins or their mechanisms. Protection against lipid peroxidation and ROS production is fairly universal. Direct and indirect antioxidant effects are recognized, impeding formation of specific oxidant toxins (eg, suppressed adduct formation, accelerated adduct degradation or disposal, or direct blocking of toxin binding sites or receptors) [248–251]. In some studies it has increased activity of antioxidant enzymes considered to offer tissue protection.

A large number of in vivo studies in animals have investigated the influence of Silymarin on ischemic liver injury and xenobiotic-induced hepatotoxicity leading to oxidative stress or direct hepatocellular damage (eg, aflatoxin B_1 lipid peroxidation, acetaminophen, ethanol, CCl_4, D-galactosamine, phallodin and α-amanitin [toxins of the "death cap" mushroom *Amanita phalloides*], thioacetamide, microcystin [small hepatotoxic peptides produced by a number of cyanobacteria], phenylhydrazine, methotrexate, cisplatin, cyclosporin and iron) and radiation-induced injury. Demonstrated hepatoprotective influences include (1) anti-inflammatory effects, (2) cell and mitochondrial membrane protection, (3) blockade of cell membrane transporters or receptors, (4) altered xenobiotic metabolism, or (5) augmented toxic adduct elimination [252–262]. Silymarin imposes a dose-dependent inhibition if certain on p450 cytochrome and might modulate phase I detoxification pathways, reducing toxic adduct formation in certain cases [263–265]. Concentrations required to achieve this effect are high compared with therapeutic doses. Its hepatotrophic influences promote recovery from xenobiotic toxicity by boosting the rate and extent of hepatic regenerative response, which might be most useful in the circumstance of diffuse injury following single exposure injury.

The greatest notoriety attributed to Silymarin is as a treatment for "death cap" mushroom (*A phalloides*) hepatotoxicity. Amanitins (primarily α-amanitin) are responsible for severe liver injury that can lead to fulminant and fatal hepatic necrosis. α-Amanitin is readily absorbed across the small bowel. It binds weakly to serum proteins and penetrates cells rapidly. In the liver it is transported into the hepatocyte by a shared organic anion transporter (phalloidine transporting system), and approximately 60% of the toxin is excreted in bile and undergoes enterohepatic circulation. Cytotoxicity results subsequent to inhibition of RNA polymerase II that impairs the ability to produce vital structural proteins, leading to cytolytic cell death. Recovery of poisoned humans, rats, and dogs has been accomplished following treatment with Silymarin combined with thioctic acid (lipoic acid), cytochrome C, and penicillin G (penicillin G is purported to block amanitin cell membrane binding sites) along with standard supportive care. Meta-analyses of treatment outcome in humans who have amanitin hepatotoxicity (individual cases and case series, n = 452) confirm a highly significant treatment response to Silymarin [223–225]. Mechanistic studies describe synergism between amanitin and TNF-α whereby the toxin enhances the cytokines oxidative and cytotoxic injury and might induce its production [220,253]. The efficacy of silibinin in mitigating amanita hepatotoxicity complements this proposal considering that it strongly blocks signals/effects attributed to TNF-α. While much is known about silymarin in experimentally modeled circumstances, its ability to attenuate the cytotoxicity of many other toxins and xenobiotics remains uncharacterized. Thus, a general use recommendation for Silymarin administration in suspected hepatotoxicity cannot be given confidently; however, it is not known whether or not such use is inappropriate, has no benefit, or is dangerous.

A number of clinical trials challenging Silymarin efficacy have been conducted in humans who had hepatobiliary disorders [220,223,225–227]. Doses including 420, 600, and 800 mg/day given orally are divided into three treatments given just before meals. Meta-analysis of the best clinical placebo-controlled studies (n = 433 patients; only four trials reported outcomes for mortality and only three assessed tissue histology) found no significant changes except a greater reduction in ALT activity among treated patients who had chronic liver disease. Frequency of adverse effects was low and indistinguishable from placebo. While there was no reduction in mortality, a trend toward improved histology in necroinflammatory liver disease was suggested. There were no features substantiating unequivocal treatment effect in patients with chronic liver disease. While data were too limited to exclude a benefit on mortality, a conclusion could not be made to recommend Silymarin for routine prescription. However, critical evaluation of Silymarin meta-analyses discloses numerous factors that complicate and invalidate study comparisons. Individual review of clinical studies usually demonstrates one or more improved treatment outcome criteria, suggesting that Silymarin has therapeutic value.

Silymarin contains four structural flavonolignan isomers: silibinin ($\sim$50–60%), isosilibinin ($\sim$5%), silicristin ($\sim$20%), and silidianin ($\sim$10%), along with other less important components (eg, taxifolin, $\sim$5%). Silibinin is the most active biologic ingredient. Pharmacokinetic parameters of Silymarin and active principles of its pharmacokinetic behavior reflect a standardized 60% extract from dried seeds [223].

Silymarin is water-insoluble and is administered as an encapsulated standardized extract. Pharmacologic study has been done extensively in humans and rodents. Although enteral absorption appears to be low, there is adequate bioavailability to allow an oral dose-related concentration in the liver and high concentrations in bile [223,266]. Compounding efforts to increase intestinal bioavailability with solubilizing substances have involved complexing silibinin with phosphatidylcholine [34,35,267–271]. Pharmacokinetic studies detail rapid uptake of silibinin after oral administration with peak plasma concentrations within 2 to 9 hours (animals and humans), an elimination T1/2 of total silibinin of 6 to 8 hours, peak plasma concentrations (a single therapeutic dose in humans) ranging from 1.5 to 6.0 mg/L of Silymarin (equivalent to 3–12 umol/L), and peak intrahepatic concentrations ranging up to 300 umol/L (relevant to achieving a therapeutic response) [223,269–272]. Because plasma protein binding of Silymarin ranges between 90% and 95%; only 3% to 8% of an oral dose is excreted in urine [269,273]. Silymarin is cleared predominantly in bile, with biliary excretion continuing for more than 24 hours after a single oral dose. Approximately 20% to 40% of Silymarin can be recovered from bile as a glucuronide or sulfate conjugate in rats and humans; the 10% to 15% of plasma total silibinin that is unconjugated has a T1/2 less than 1 hour [267,269,272–278]. Concentrations in bile exceed serum concentrations by approximately 100-fold, with peak values occurring within 2 to 9 hours of dosing. A choleretic response is associated with biliary excretion and is associated with enhanced bile acid elimination, which might be therapeutically useful in attenuating liver injury associated with membranocytolytic bile acids [223,243,270,271]. Achieved plasma silibinin concentrations linearly correlate with administered oral dose in humans with a standardized extract. A less consistent dose to plasma concentration relationship was shown with the silybinin–phosphatidylcholine complexed product (silipide) [223]. There is no tissue accumulation in humans after chronic dosing [278]. Humans with cirrhosis achieve a lower and delayed peak drug concentration compared to healthy volunteers [34,35], which suggests that dosing in patients who have hepatic insufficiency and portosystemic shunting might require modification (increased dosing).

While there are no available pharmacokinetic studies in dogs or cats, early research establishing the efficacy of Silymarin for rescue from *A phalloides* hepatotoxicosis used 50 to 150 mg/kg successfully in dogs. Given 5 and 24 hours after *A phalloides* intoxication, this dose range provided remarkable protection against lethal toxicity [254]. A 15 mg/kg Silymarin dose protected dogs, rabbits, and rodents from *A phalloides* toxicity when given 10 minutes following toxin administration; a 100 mg/kg dose provided total protection [255]. A dose comparable to that used chronically in humans with hepatitis would approximate 7–15 mg/kg/day. A dose comparable to that controlling fibrosis in rats with bile duct occlusion would approximate 40–50 mg/kg/day. However, there are no specific studies in dogs or cats with these conditions. The lack of a standard product further complicates therapeutic recommendations.

While encouraging findings have been derived from in vitro and in vivo investigations of Silymarin, there still are no well controlled trials in humans who have spontaneous necroinflammatory or cholestatic liver disease with a single form of liver disease and large enough case numbers to satisfy evidence-based criteria. There is broad indication that Silymarin has hepatoprotective, anti-inflammatory, antifibrotic, and antioxidant effects overlapping with several other vitamins and nutraceuticals (specifically vitamin E, SAMe, NAC, and PPC). Mechanistic investigations for each of these agents describe modulatory influences on central signaling pathways and cytokine responses. Silymarin has undergone a considerable repertoire of live animal disease modeling, which is clinically relevant despite the fact that little of it includes companion animals. While there is ample experience in dogs that a dose of 50 to 150 mg/kg is safe, there is limited experience in cats. A role for Silymarin in treatment of a variety of xenobiotic hepatoxicoses and other scenarios causing acute necrosis (ischemic–reperfusion injury) seems appropriate. Specifically, its role in treatment of amanitin toxicity cannot be denied. Work in the bile duct obstruction model provides compelling evidence for a potent antifibrotic response rivaling colchicine, suggesting that Silymarin should have a considered role in patients who have obstructive cholestasis that is not amenable to surgical bypass or decompression. It is possible that cholestatic disorders associated with high bile acid concentrations might also benefit from Silymarin. Because there is evidence that Silymarin can suppress activity of certain p450 cytochrome oxidases, the possibility of drug interactions must be considered in polymedicated patients [263–265]. In humans, a mild laxative effect and allergic reactions (pruritis, urticaria) have been the most commonly reported adverse effects, found in 1% of patients or less. There are no reports of hepatotoxicity from products limited to Silymarin extract; however, products containing multiple nutraceutical agents in addition to Silymarin have sometimes contained toxic contaminants.

Polyenylphosphatidylcholine or polyunsaturated phosphatidylcholine lecithin

While PPC is a mixture of seven phospholipid species, current evidence suggests that dilinoleoylphaphatidyl choline (DLPC), accounting for approximately 50% (w/w) of PPC, is the biologically active moiety. PPC derived from the diet or bile is hydrolyzed in the proximal small intestine by pancreatic phospholipases and absorbed in the distal small bowel and upper colon, whereupon it is re-esterified in the enterocyte and enters the portal circulation as PPC [279,280]. Plasma kinetics of DLPC in humans shows a residence time of 60 days and stable (high) concentrations over a 12-hour interval. The metabolic products choline and triglycerides are incorporated into high-density lipoproteins (HDL) and VLDL, respectively. DLPC accumulates in RBC lipids that seemingly serve as a long-term reservoir. Its presence in lipoproteins (especially low density lipoproteins [LDL]) provides significant protection against oxidation, exceeding that of α-tocopherol as a chain terminator [280,281]. Consequently, PPC is currently being considered to have a potential role in control of atherosclerosis in humans [282–285].

PPC and DLCP have been repeatedly shown in various models of liver disease to prevent fibrogenesis, to diminish oxidative mitochondrial and hepatocellular membrane injury and accumulation of ROS, and to conserve hepatocyte and mitochondrial GSH [286–293]. While it is generally believed that polyunsaturation of fatty acids favors their lipoperoxidation because double bonds are more vulnerable than saturated or monounsaturated bonds to free radical attack, PPC in vivo and in vitro performs consistently as an antioxidant. Using rodent and primate disease models, prophylactic treatment with DLPC protectively enriches hepatocellular membranes with PPC and phosphatidylethanolamine, conferring resistance against oxidative injury [292,293]. Each of these moieties is essential for normal cell structure and signaling; PPC enrichment involves 16:0 to 20:4 and 18:0 to 20:4 species. When DLPC and SAMe were administered prophylactically, similar lipid membrane enrichment occurred with each; however, DLPC only minimally attenuated increased liver enzyme activity and cholestasis imparted by ethanol exposure compared with impressive improvements achieved with SAMe [293]. DLPC did not, but SAMe did, restore total hepatocellular and mitochondrial GSH and improved cell oxygen use. This model suggests that SAMe might duplicate beneficial effects shown for PPC or DLPC because it enhances their synthesis (methylations). Hepatic fibrogenesis in models of liver disease in which injury is not derived from direct ROS or membrane oxidation is also attenuated with PPC, DLPC, and SAMe.

A series of mechanistic in vitro investigations clarified that PPC and DLPC reduce signaling and activation of hepatic Stellate and Kupffer cells derived from oxidant stresses imposed by inflammatory reactants and cytokines [294–299]. Responses in vitro and in vivo provide compelling evidence that each substance inhibits hepatic fibrogenesis significantly [287,290,298–300]. The only form of liver injury not significantly attenuated by DLPC administration is Fe toxicity, in which DLPC rectifies hepatic GSH without controlling oxidative injury [301].

Exactly how PPC and DLPC impose their antifibrotic influences remains unresolved. This property is unique and not shared by phospholipids containing saturated fatty acids of the same chain length as linoleate, in positions 1 and 2, or a single linoleate bound to position 1 or 2 of the glycerol backbone. The presence of two linoleate acid chains on the PPC backbone (18:2–18:2) appears to be critical for the biologic effect because substitutions of either one of the fatty acid chains results in loss of beneficial effects.

Most work with PPC has occurred in alcohol hepatotoxicosis disease models or affected humans. Studies confirm that PPC attenuates induction of the ethanol-specific cytochrome p450 (CYP2E1) and reduces hepatocyte apoptosis by approximately 50% in this form of injury [296,302]. Clinical trials in humans who had chronic necroinflammatory liver disease and acute severe hepatopathies showed clinical and histological improvement. Reduction in hepatic fibrogenesis was specifically documented in humans who had chronic hepatitis virus B (HBV)-associated cirrhosis and chronic active hepatitis, whereas PPC was used in polypharmacy combination with immunosuppressive therapy [303–308]. A sparing effect on glucocorticoid requirements was shown in patients who had immune-mediated liver disease. In a randomized, double-blind, placebo-controlled multicenter trial (n = 176; 92 patients received PPC and 84 an identical appearing placebo) PPC improved response to conventional therapy and delayed disease relapse in humans who had hepatitis C, resulting in a recommendation for adjunctive use during and after interferon-α treatment [308]. Collective findings solidly suggest that PPC/DLPC should provide therapeutic benefit in many forms of necroinflammatory liver disease.

Clinical trials with PPC in humans have shown that it has a high safety profile with no reported side effects with doses ranging between 350 mg orally every 8 hours up to a total maximal dose of 3 g per day (which equates to an approximate dosing range of 25–60 mg/kg/d). There have been no side effects observed in studies in rats or primates used to model alcohol hepatotoxicosis (3 mg PPC per kcal alcohol, or in baboons fed 3 to 4 g/d of essential phospholipid [0.4 mg choline/kcal] for up to 8 years). Dosing for dogs and cats has been extrapolated from experimental work and human studies; a range of 25 to 50 mg/kg/day is used (not exceeding the maximum human 3 g dose for large breed dogs). No side effects have been observed in more than 10 years of use in clinical patients in whom PPC has been used as a component of polymodal therapy. Dosing in cats is achieved with the supplement mixed in food. No evaluations have been conducted in dogs or cats that have spontaneous liver disease to assess treatment response. There are no pharmacokinetic studies in dogs or cats.

Ubiquinol (coenzyme Q_{10})

Ubiquinol (coenzyme Q_{10}) is the only lipid-soluble antioxidant that animal cells can synthesize de novo and regenerate with a committed enzyme system (a cytosolic ubiquinol reductase; ubiquinol is the reduced state and ubiquinone the oxidized state) [309,310]. Rejuvenation of ubiquinol from ubiquinone is dependently linked with dihydrolipoic acid (DHLP) but not with vitamin E [311,312]. Because it is synthesized in all animal tissues, ubiquinol it is not regarded as a vitamin. Its physiological role is to protect against lipid peroxidation and in this capacity, ubiquinol functions as an antioxidant in multiple systems, including liposomes, LDL, membranes of mitochondria, and peroxisomes. It also functions as a coenzyme in the mitochondrial respiratory chain, where it mediates electron transport. Tissue distributions vary greatly, with largest amounts in the myocardium, kidney, and liver. In health most hepatic ubiquinol (95%) is maintained in its reduced state. Because mitochondrial dysfunction impairs ubiquinol availability, it is presumed to be limited in hepatic disease accompanied by oxidative injury. The plasma ubiquinone:ubiquinol ratio, used to indicate systemic oxidant stress, is significantly higher in humans who have necroinflammatory liver disease or cirrhosis compared with healthy individuals [313,314]. While it is known that drugs interfering with cholesterol synthesis (eg, mevalonate synthesis inhibition) impair ubiquinol synthesis, it is unknown if hepatic disease leading to impaired cholesterol concentrations influences this pathway [310].

Ubiquinol supplementation significantly increases its circulating blood concentrations, where important functions relating to vascular disease and atherosclerosis are proposed [315–317]. However, effects on endothelial cells might influence systemic disease more broadly through influence on microvasculature. This may be pertinent to hepatobiliary disease considering the liver's expansive endothelial network and especially in the context of ischemic–reperfusion or oxidant injury.

There is some evidence that ubiquinols provided in an oil suspension have the highest bioavailability [315–318]. Currently, there is no dose recommendation that can be made with confidence for dogs and cats that have liver disease. Extrapolation from human studies suggests that a dose range of 1 to 2 mg/kg/day is safe and might provide beneficial effects. A dose of 90 mg/day has been used in large dogs that had cardiomyopathy without side effects.

Ursodeoxycholic acid

UDCA is a nontoxic hydrophilic dihydroxylated bile acid (3α, 7β-dihydroxy-5β-cholanoic acid) that was first identified in bile of the Chinese black bear and now recognized to provide significant benefit in liver disease. In normal dogs and cats UDCA is only present in small quantities as a secondary bile acid formed in the intestines from the primary bile acid chenodeoxycholic acid. While initially developed for the dissolution of gallstones, global appreciation of its clinical benefit in humans who have chronic hepatitis has led to a frenzy of research of its medicinal properties. Benefits in the context of necroinflammatory and cholestatic liver disease include (1) replacement/displacement of toxic endogenous bile acids, (2) cytoprotection of hepatocytes and biliary epithelium, (3) antioxidant effects, (4) immunomodulatory effects, (5) suppression of aberrantly expressed major histocompatibility foci, (6) attenuation of bile acid-induced mitochondrial toxicity and apoptosis, (7) stimulation of bile secretion, and (8) enhanced biliary elimination of toxic substances (Fig. 11).

Given orally to humans who have cholestatic liver disease (13–15 mg/kg/d), conjugated UDCA becomes the predominant serum bile acid (up to 60%), enriching liver tissue (30% of bile acids) and bile (30–40% of biliary bile acids), replacing the more hydrophobic and toxic endogenous bile acids; however, the total bile acid pool size is not altered significantly [318–322]. The cytoprotective effects of UDCA have been demonstrated in vitro and in vivo against membranocytolytic bile acids, with direct membrane-stabilizing and antiapoptotic influences linked mechanistically with modulated cell Ca^{2+} flux, protein kinase C-dependent secretory functions, and membrane transporters [322,323]. Cytoprotective effects are specific for bile acid-induced cell injury and do not confer protection against injury derived from direct or indirect toxins or exposure to ischemic–reperfusion insult [321,322]. Antiapoptotic effects of UDCA relate to its cytoprotective influence on mitochondrial membranes (dysfunction, MPT induction) and have been shown in a number of liver injury models (eg, hepatotoxicity derived from ethanol, membranocytolytic bile acids, Fas-receptor binding, TGF-β, and ROS) [6,7,89,321,323–326]. Its ability to mitigate mitodondrial MPT induced by toxic bile acids rationalizes its therapeutic use in cholestatic liver disease because the antiapoptotic effects can be realized with physiologically achievable UDCA concentrations. It has been predicted that UDCA will

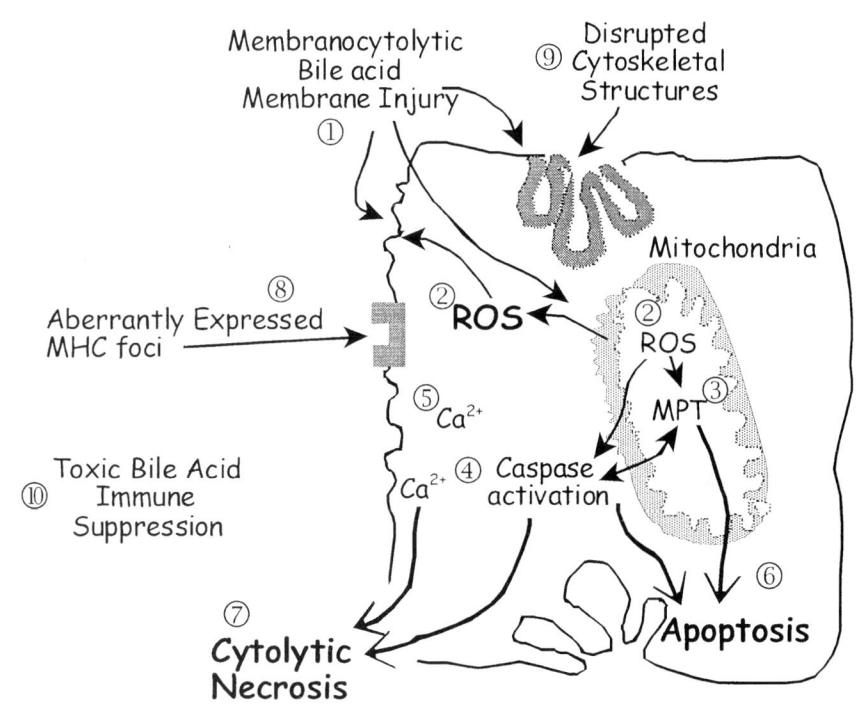

Fig. 11. Mechanisms relating to hepatocellular bile acid toxicity that can be ameliorated by therapeutic administration of ursodeoxycholic acid. As numbered (not sequential or prioritized): (1) membrane injury, (2) ROS dispersing in mitochondria and cytosol, (3) induction of MPT changes, (4) elaboration of proteases amplifying cell and organelle injury, (5) loss of control of cell calcium flux, (6, 7) induction of apoptotic or necrolytic cell death signals depending on bile acid concentration and specific bile acid, (8) aberrantly expressed major histocompatibility foci in chronic liver disease, (9) disrupted cytoskeletal elements and membrane transporters worsening cholestasis, and (10) systemic immunosuppression.

be one of the first therapeutic agents licensed for prevention of apoptosis. The antioxidant effects of UDCA have also been clearly demonstrated in vitro, where physiologically relevant concentrations mitigate Fe- and ROS-induced biomolecular injury [326]. Studies demonstrating the direct cytoprotective effects of UDCA are complicated by the high concentrations required in vitro for this phenomenon. Such concentrations are only achieved biologically near biliary epithelia but not in the hepatic parenchyma [327]. Direct cytoprotection might therefore be more relevant for disorders primarily focused on or near biliary structures (eg, feline cholangitis/cholangiohepatitis syndrome, injury incurred from major bile duct occlusion). UDCA also has an inhibitory influence on fibrogenesis simulated by PDGF, and this might impose an antifibrotic influence on Stellate cells [328,329].

Diverse immunomodulatory effects of UDCA have been described [330–341]. Cholestasis is known to induce abnormal expression of major histocompatibility foci (major histocompatibility class [MHC] I and II receptors on hepatocytes and biliary epithelia normally not bearing these foci), and this is thought to render cells vulnerable to immune targeting [330–332]. This phenomenon has been documented primarily in zone 1 in certain forms of hepatobiliary disease in humans, in whom injury is focused on the biliary tree (primary biliary cirrhosis [PBC] and primary sclerosing cholangitis [PSC]). Aberrant expression of MHC foci can evolve from hydrophobic bile acid-stimulated synthesis or unmasking of membrane structures. Some work has verified that UDCA downregulates aberrant MHC expression [321,330–333]. Direct immunosuppressive effects are mediated at the level of immunoglobulin and cytokine production and by interaction with the glucocorticoid receptor (possibly through mediation of protein kinase C or modulation of nitric oxide production, inhibiting induction of the rate controlling enzyme nitric oxide synthase) [321,334–340]. UDCA also appears to rectify immunosuppressive effects associated with toxic bile acids and to improve Kupffer cell phagocytic function [340]. These influences might have benefit for infectious hepatobiliary disorders, in cholestasis (known to increase the risk for infection), and in hepatic dysfunction associated with portal hypertension/shunting, in which an increased risk for gut bacterial translocation is surmised [339–341]. UDCA also has been shown to enhance endotoxin disposal, an effect that might be beneficial in liver injury associated with inflammatory bowel disease [321]. Preliminary work also suggests that it might limit inflammation and oxidant injury in inflammatory bowel disease through its influence on nitric oxide production [338].

Choleresis induced by UDCA augments elimination of substances normally excreted in bile, thereby facilitating removal of certain toxins (including Cu), endogenous metabolites (steroid hormones), bacterial organisms, and other potentially noxious substances. In vitro work has described that UDCA stimulates vesicular exocytosis, transporter gene expression, and ductal bicarbonate secretion by way of cholehepatic bile acid shunting and other complex mechanisms [322,342,343]; however, UDCA-induced hypercholeresis remains controversial because pharmacologic effects are achieved only with high unconjugated UDCA concentrations. Most UDCA in patients is conjugated before reaching the biliary epithelium. Nevertheless, induction of canalicular transporter proteins can independently initiate brisk choleresis, explaining the ability of UDCA to facilitate cholelith dissolution.

The pharmacodynamics of UDCA have been examined in rodents, humans, and dogs. After oral administration of unconjugated UDCA, 30% to 60% of it is absorbed passively in the small and large intestines, thereafter undergoing hepatic uptake ($>60\%$ of the absorbed dose). Like other bile acids, UDCA is conjugated with glycine or taurine (shown to be taurine in the cat and dog) [344–346]. Accumulation in bile and liver depends on whether or not the individuals studied have cholestatic liver disease. In normal dogs and cats little UDCA accumulates in serum (dose 10–15 mg/kg/d); however, in cholestasis (in human and animal models) daily oral pharmacologic administration (10–15 mg/kg/d) results in UDCA becoming a predominant bile acid in the liver and systemic circulation, where it contributes 40% to 60% of the circulating bile acid pool [318–320,327,346,347]. In rats, but not in humans, oral administration of taurine-conjugated UDCA results in higher UDCA enrichment in the liver than with unconjugated UDCA [347]. In humans, dividing the total daily dose of UDCA into two treatments increases the total enteric uptake. Bioavailability studies suggest that enteric coated tablets have higher UDCA availability than capsules [347,348,500]. UDCA capsules and tablets contain crystals of the acid form, which are poorly soluble at a pH less than 7. Enteric uptake occurs by dissolution-limited passive nonionic diffusion in the small intestine [347,348]. Because the critical micellization pH of UDCA is near 8, enteric dissolution is enhanced by solubilization in mixed micelles containing other bile acids. The absence of enteric bile acids deters uptake of unconjugated UDCA, and administration with food is thought to enhance its absorption.

Clinical evidence confirms that UDCA protects against bile acid-mediated hepatocellular injury but that it has limited effects in injury induced by toxins (eg, acetaminophen) or injury derived from ischemic–reperfusion mechanisms. A number of clinical trials in humans who had a variety of chronic necroinflammatory and cholestatic liver disorders have assessed its therapeutic effects. It has proven clinical benefit in children who have genetic abnormalities causing severe cholestasis, for managing bile flow aberrations in cystic fibrosis, and as adjunctive therapy in immunomodulatory protocols in humans who have immune-mediated liver disease and after liver transplantation [321,322]. Patients that have PBC and immune-mediated chronic hepatitis show best responses when UDCA is combined adjunctively with corticosteroids [321]. In humans who have a variety of organ transplants UDCA appears to deter cyclosporine-induced cholestasis [321]. It also reduces iatrogenic cholestasis associated with prolonged total parenteral nutrition, improves liver function tests and histologic status in humans who have hepatosteatosis, and deters hepatic triglyceride accumulation in rats fed a choline-deficient diet [184,322]. Even in animal models of liver injury induced by extrahepatic bile duct occlusion UDCA has provided substantial improvement in the extent of histologic injury; however, in clinical patients such treatment is used concurrent with biliary tree decompression and restitution of bile flow. Many studies in human clinical patients have focused on the therapeutic response to UDCA as a single therapeutic intervention. It is unlikely that any monotherapy protocol can modify the course of liver disease substantially considering the pathophysiologic complexities involved, and especially when the initiating cause of the liver disorder cannot be identified or eliminated. Thus, it is no surprise that beneficial responses are not associated with total control of the disease process. Improvement in patient status is inconsistent, variably including beneficial responses in clinicopathologic and histologic features and delayed disease progression. Collective evidence thus substantiates that UDCA should be used in an adjunctive capacity with other means of modifying disease pathobiology. Several studies (in vivo and in vitro) have already shown synergistic benefit from combination with SAMe (estradiol associated cholestasis, bile acid-induced hepatocyte injury) [25,26,325,343].

Considering the clinical benefits acknowledged in humans who have a multitude of liver disorders it is prudent to consider UDCA for necroinflammatory/cholestatic liver disorders in dogs and cats. Combined use of UDCA with other agents attenuating bile acid toxicity, inflammatory signaling, oxidant injury, and fibrogenesis is recommended for necroinflammatory and cholestatic liver injury for which a definitive cause cannot be identified or eliminated. This recommendation assumes a thorough diagnostic evaluation (including liver biopsy, tissue culture for aerobic and anaerobic bacteria, and metal analysis) and elimination of biliary tree occlusion as an underlying cause. A dose of 10 to 15 mg/kg/day of UDCA given orally in one or two divided treatments is recommended for animals that have liver disease. Administration with food is advised for best uptake.

A special circumstance might exist in cats that have severe HL. These animals have remarkable metabolic derangements and nutritional deficiencies, significantly increased bile acid concentrations, and serum bile acid profiles consistent with major bile duct occlusion (indicating impaired enterohepatic bile acid circulation) [178]. Whether UDCA is beneficial or detrimental in this disorder is unclear. Caution is warranted because any bile acid can be cytotoxic at high concentrations and this disorder can be accompanied by profound systemic and liver antioxidant depletions that might aggravate bile acid cytotoxicity. Further, this disorder is unique to most other cholestatic disorders in that it has no necroinflammatory disease component. Morbidly obese children who have hepatosteatosis demonstrate improved biochemical profiles with vitamin E supplementation and appropriate nutritional support, but not with UDCA [182,183]. Rats that have steatohepatitis do not have recovery assisted by UDCA [184].

Selenium

Selenium's function as an antioxidant is exerted by its inclusion in selenoproteins; more than 20 of these are currently recognized [349,350]. Selenoproteins contain one or more selenium atoms per protein molecule; the most common form in animals is as selenocysteine, which is structurally analogous to cysteine with the exception that selenium replaces the sulfur molecule. Most dietary selenium is derived as selenomethionine and is metabolized to selenocysteine in the hepatic transsulfuration pathway. Selenium participates in a number of antioxidant enzymes. Incorporation of selenocysteine compared with cysteine in the active site of a selenoenzyme increases its activity approximately 100- to 1000-fold. Being a major constituent of GSH-Pxs and Trx-reductases, selenium has important interactions with vitamin E assisting with rejuvenation of the reduced form from the tocopheroxy radical and in reducing lipid hydroperoxides to their equivalent hydroxy acids. Intracellular GSH-Px is thought to reserve selenium for plasma and phospholipid hydroperoxide GSH-Px [349]. Approximately 65% of total body selenium is bound to selenoprotein P [351]. Selenium bound to this protein appears in plasma as a hepatic secretory product and is also present in cell membranes, where it functions as a free radical scavenger [349–351]. Total plasma or serum selenium measurements reflect selenium incorporated in selenoproteins: selenoprotein P (6.4 ug selenium/dL plasma in humans), GSH-Px (1.7 ug selenium/dL plasma in humans), selenomethionine in albumin, and a small amount in small molecules [351]. A decline in selenoprotein synthesis due to hepatic failure reduces circulating selenoproteins; however, plasma selenium values do not represent body selenium status reliably (ie, cirrhosis in humans is associated with low plasma selenium but normal tissue selenium resources) [352].

Selenium deficiency increases risk for oxidative injury if other antioxidants are concurrently depleted (notably vitamin E); however, selenium deficiency is assumed to be rare in animals consuming commercially prepared diets that are supplemented according to federal guidelines. Using pharmacologic dosing of selenium as an antioxidant has no foundation in animals that have liver disease at the present time unless they have chronically been fed imbalanced diets or demonstrate long-term inappetence to the extent of starvation.

Zinc

Zinc, an essential trace element required for many normal homeostatic functions, has central importance in the liver. It is required for normal protein metabolism, the function of more than 200 zinc metalloenzymes, and for membrane integrity [353,354]. Zinc provides three basic functions in its dependent metalloenzymes: catalytic, coactive or cocatalytic, and structural [355]. Owing to its pivotal essentiality, zinc adequacy has impact on numerous physiologic reactions including (but not limited to) normal immune function, neurosensory functions (eg, cognition, night vision), protein metabolism, detoxification pathways (including ammonia detoxification), antioxidant availability, wound healing, and even appetite [353–355]. Zinc antioxidant functions are described by in vitro assessments and the in vivo association of oxidative stress with zinc deficiency [356–359]. Zinc is thought to exert direct antioxidant protection by occupying/displacing iron or Cu from binding sites in lipids, proteins, and DNA [356–359]. Competition of zinc for iron binding sites is particularly relevant considering that zinc deficiency develops in chronic liver disease, facilitating intracellular iron accumulation [357–360].

Zinc absorption approximates 25% of its dietary provision; however, the amount absorbed varies with many factors including competing substances in the enteric canal (eg, phytic acid, phytates) and the zinc status of the individual, enteric disease (which can impair uptake), portal hypertension, and the form of zinc ingested [361,362]. Phytates such as inositol hexaphosphates and pentaphosphates exert a negative effect on zinc availability, whereas lower phosphates have little to no effect [361,362]. Zinc intake correlates directly with protein intake because foods containing high protein content are generally rich in zinc. Uptake occurs mainly in the small bowel and excretion occurs mainly in feces. Pancreatic secretions are rich in zinc and contribute to enteric losses. In health, urinary excretion of zinc is negligible; however, it can increase remarkably in the setting of portosystemic shunting [353].

Many forms of liver disease in human and animal models of chronic liver disease are associated with zinc deficiency. Because serum zinc concentrations do not dependably reflect reduced hepatic zinc status they cannot be used to monitor liver zinc adequacy [363–365]. The author routinely measures zinc concentrations in liver biopsies to quantitatively appraise the patient's zinc status. Approximately 50% of dogs that have necroinflammatory liver disease have subnormal liver zinc concentrations. Mechanisms associated with altered zinc metabolism in liver disease involve its metabolism, distribution, urinary excretion, and enteric uptake or availability. Reduced intake might occur owing to inappetence or feeding of a novel unpalatable or undesirable diet. Increased intestinal metallothionein, portal hypertension, or mucosal edema can contribute by limiting enteric zinc uptake [353,363–365]. Zinc uptake is regulated largely by intestinal metallothionein, a cysteine-rich metal binding protein. High zinc intake induces metallothionein, which thereafter limits zinc uptake and that of other metals, notably Cu. This mechanism is capitalized upon with therapeutic use of chronic oral zinc acetate for limiting enteric Cu availability in liver disorders associated with high tissue Cu stores. Metallothionein-bound metals remain within the enterocyte, sloughing into the intestinal lumen with the senescent cell. Because metallothionein is also induced by cytokines and inflammatory mediators (eg, IL-1, TNF, IL-6), general inflammation, inflammatory liver disease, stress, and treatment with glucocorticoids might limit enteric zinc availability through enhanced metallothionein synthesis [366,367]. Metallothionein concentrations are also known to increase in the circumstance of food and water deprivation, which might aggravate onset of zinc insufficiency in the liver patient that has a poor appetite. An additional factor influencing zinc concentrations in humans, which has not yet clarified in veterinary patients, is a reduced albumin–zinc binding affinity associated with hepatic dysfunction [368,369]. Because albumin normally transports approximately 70% of circulating zinc, a reduced albumin-binding affinity might permit urinary zinc loss and impair normal tissue distribution. Increased urinary zinc loss is common in humans who have liver disease, the extent correlating with the severity of liver disease and is most extreme in the context of portosystemic shunting and diuretic therapy [368,369]. Altered zinc metabolism in liver disease also is proposed to reflect cytokine production provoked by increased exposure to enteric LPS [370].

Zinc deficiency in liver disease can worsen a patient's clinical status and permissively influence liver injury. Prominent among these effects is a tendency for increased liver accumulation of transition metals (Fe and Cu). Reduced activity of zinc metalloenzymes can impair healing and cell regeneration by limiting the rate of DNA replication and reducing amino acid use in protein synthesis [371,372]. Neutrophil function and cell-mediated immune responses might become compromised and nitrogen detoxification might become impaired (two enzymes essential for ammonia detoxification are limited by zinc deficiency) [373–383]. Subnormal zinc status has been implicated in HE by virtue of its importance in ammonia detoxification and GABAergic neurotransmission [377]; however, studies defining the role of zinc in ameliorating signs of HE have failed to show that zinc supplementation consistently improves patients, although there have been some dramatic responses.

Zinc's antioxidant effects offer protection against some, but not all, ROS-mediated injury. Its antioxidant attributes relate to several important mechanisms, the most influential involving antagonism of redox-active transition metals. By competitively displacing Fe from binding sites on negatively charged phospholipids and preventing its redox cycling, zinc protects membranes from Fe-initiated propagation reactions. Zinc repletion protects many, but not all, enzymes from Fe catalyzed oxidation and also mitigates DNA oxidative strand breaks initiated by transition metals [357]. Synergistic protection against Fe-mediated lipid peroxidation is achieved when zinc and vitamin E are used in combination [357].

Hepatocellular zinc depletion is linked with low hepatic tissue GSH concentrations, which have been proposed to reflect a zinc-sensitive step or feedback mechanism influencing the transsulfuration pathway (proximal to cysteine) rather than simply antioxidant use of GSH [383]. Altered cell thiol redox status associated with zinc deficiency is thought to influence NF-κβ signaling, favoring proinflammatory responses and cell apoptosis [359,384–387]. Thus, zinc levels might have considerable importance in a variety of necroinflammatory liver disorders given the pivotal influence of NF-κβ signaling in determining cell viability and hepatic fibrogenesis.

Metallothionein is the only protein implicated in cellular zinc distribution/storage [387]. Each metallothionein molecule binds seven zinc atoms by way of thiolated ligands. Metallothionein, a low molecular weight, cysteine-rich heavy-metal binding protein, is involved not only in zinc metabolism but also with Cu metabolism and heavy metal detoxification. It shares important features molecularly and functionally with GSH because the sulfhydryl groups of each represent major thiolated cell substrates. The thiol groups in metallothionein are preferential targets of H_2O_2 compared with GSH; on a molar basis metallothionein is nearly 39-fold more potent than GSH in preventing hydroxyl-induced DNA degradation [388,389]. While administration of cysteine donors (GSH, NAC, or methionine if it can be catabolized to cysteine) can increase liver metallothionein concentration, zinc also imposes a strong induction effect [390,391]. Metallothionein concentrations are required to maintain high concentrations of zinc in liver tissue, suggesting that the cytoprotective effects of metallothionein might be mediated by zinc [391]. Zinc that is bound to metallothionein can be released in response to stress-induced changes in cell redox state, and such release likely mediates at least some of metallothionein's cytoprotection [392,393]. Thus, high values of metallothionein in the liver are desirable because they are associated with high zinc levels and hepatoprotection. Administration of zinc has been shown to provide hepatoprotection in a number of models of liver diseases and against certain hepatotoxins and xenobiotics (acetaminophen, doxorubicin, CCl_4, bromobenzene, and heavy metals). Hepatoprotection has also been shown in the circumstance of hepatic GSH depletion; however, zinc associated hepatoprotection does not always correlate with increased tissue metallothionein concentrations [391]. Zinc modulates metabolism of some hepatotoxins, reducing the quantity of toxic adduct produced, accelerating biotransformation to a nontoxic moiety, or facilitating elimination.

Zinc deficiency can lead to a marked increase in membrane oxidation and intracellular iron concentrations [360], so tissue zinc concentrations should be determined concurrent with Cu and Fe measurements in biopsy specimens. Therapeutic zinc supplementation is appropriate when tissue zinc concentrations are low, especially when Fe or Cu values are concurrently high. Based on the author's experience, portosystemic shunting (acquired or congenital) and feeding a nitrogen-restricted diet are commonly associated with subnormal liver zinc concentrations. Because zinc uptake is linked to dietary protein intake, it is reasonable to suspect that dietary protein restriction might predispose to zinc deficiency. The concerning low tissue zinc concentrations in dogs that have severe liver disease—and especially in dogs that have acquired portosystemic shunting—might implicate a greater risk for oxidant tissue damage from transition metals coincident with their tendency to have subnormal hepatic GSH stores [77].

A number of beneficial clinical and biochemical improvements have been shown with zinc supplementation in liver disease. Treatment with zinc is proposed by some clinicians for management of Cu storage hepatopathy. It remains controversial as to whether or not this treatment provides optimal first-line therapy. The recommendation to use zinc for management of Cu storage hepatopathy in dogs is based on a single report describing findings in a few dogs (Bedlington terriers, n = 3; West Highland White Terriers, n = 3). Four dogs were studied for 2 years and two dogs were studied for 1 year [394]. Additional information is derived from management of copper storage hepatopathy in humans (Wilson's disease). Clinical data substantiate that zinc supplementation can improve metabolism (ammonia) and disease status in humans who have copper storage hepatopathy [395–399]. While many studies suggest a benefit in mild and acute HE, contradictive findings are also reported, in which plasma zinc values remained subnormal despite supplementation [374,379,396–398]. In a rat model of cirrhosis, zinc induction of ornithine transcarbamylase (an essential urea cycle enzyme) increased nitrogen detoxification [399]. Long-term treatment of humans who have chronic liver disease and subnormal plasma zinc concentrations (zinc sulfate given at a dose of 200 mg orally three times daily for 3 months) increased hepatic conversion of amino acids to urea, objectively improved clinical and biochemical parameters, and normalized serum zinc concentrations. Zinc induction of glutamine synthesis might also assist ammonia detoxification by enhancing skeletal muscle ammonia uptake and storage; however, consistent daily zinc administration is necessary to sustain a positive effect because plasma zinc values decline rapidly when supplements are discontinued. Whether zinc supplementation improves cognitive function by reducing ammonia or through a direct action on the central nervous system remains unclear. Supplemental zinc also has improved appetite and taste abnormalities in some humans who have liver disease [398,501].

The optimal dose of elemental zinc for supplementing dogs that have low liver zinc concentrations has not been verified. The author prescribes oral daily elemental zinc only for dogs that have confirmed subnormal liver zinc concentrations; 1.0 to 5.0 mg/kg of elemental zinc is given daily, divided into two doses. Elemental zinc is calculated based on the molecular weight of the zinc source and percentage of that formula weight contributed by zinc (zinc acetate = 30%, zinc gluconate = 14%, zinc sulfate = 23%); zinc acetate seems to be best tolerated. Zinc supplementation is titrated to achieve an increase in baseline plasma zinc values. Blood samples are collected 10 to 12 hours after dosing. Cautious monitoring is undertaken to avoid plasma zinc greater than or equal to 800 ppm, which indicates systemic toxicity and likelihood of hemolysis. While this treatment strategy appears to be safe, whether or not it provides a clinical benefit has not been evaluated because it is typically incorporated with other polypharmacy measures (eg, UDCA, vitamin E, and SAMe in animals that have necroinflammatory liver disease) and optimized nutritional support. The efficacy of supplemental zinc for normalizing tissue zinc concentrations has also not been evaluated rigorously in these patients. Whether chronic induction of metallothionein as a consequence of zinc supplementation has the potential to induce Cu or Fe deficiency remains undetermined. A small number of dogs are unable to tolerate oral zinc therapy in any form or dose, demonstrating inappetence, nausea, and emesis. In dogs that have Cu-associated hepatotoxicity, chronic chelation therapy with d-penicillamine or trientine is alternatively used. In dogs that have low tissue zinc concentrations associated with necroinflammatory/cholestatic liver disease or portosystemic shunting, dietary supplementation is provided using an alternative form of zinc or a vitamin mineral supplement. It is important to avoid use of zinc methionine as a zinc source in patients that have hepatic insufficiency and are prone to HE.

Probiotics used in the management of liver disease

Certain microbial-enriched food supplements claim to influence health beneficially, and some of these products are advertised for use in patients that have liver disease [400]. Probiotics containing microorganisms combined with fermented foods are proposed to optimize intestinal microbial balance. This concept has advanced beyond the simple belief that probiotics function as local immunomodulators, enhancing mucosal defense and reducing bacterial translocation. A large body of circumstantial evidence declaring healthful benefits is diverse in scope, species studied, and scientific rigor. The topic is pertinent to management of liver disease because these patients might be predisposed to bacterial translocation that might be averted by probiotics, and certain probiotics might be useful for attenuating HE.

Three lines of gastrointestinal host defense protect against opportunistic microbial invasion from the splanchnic circulation into mesenteric lymph nodes and liver. The first involves the enteric microbial populations located in different gut regions. The second involves the multilayered mucosal barrier that selectively filters absorbed water, nutrients, and electrolytes, excluding pathogens and potentially injurious substances. The third involves systemic mechanisms that recognize and eliminate potentially harmful organisms, toxins, or other agents transcending the mucosal barrier including the innate immune system (IgA production, lamina propria resident immunocytes) and enteric enzymes metabolizing/detoxifying injurious xenobiotics and enteric toxins that are unlikely to be recognized or eliminated by the immune system [400]. In health, rapid mucosal turnover, mucin secreted by enterocytes, immunoglobulin A (IgA), antimicrobial peptides, and a complex of glycosylated proteins prohibit pathogen adherence to epithelium [400–403]. Villi on the epithelial apical surface of enterocytes are covered in mucus coated with a biofilm of anaerobic bacteria that prevent adherence by other bacteria and limit overgrowth of aerobic gram-negative organisms, mainly Enterobacteria [404]. Enterically produced antimicrobial peptides that repel opportunistic microorganisms can be manipulated by diet or modulated by change in microbial flora. Gastric acidity, pancreatobiliary secretions, gastrointestinal motility, and bacterial regulation of various immune functions of the gastrointestinal tract work in concert with these mechanisms.

A number of these normally protective mechanisms can become abnormal in chronic liver disease. Hepatic cirrhosis and liver injury produced by chronic extrahepatic bile duct occlusion have been specifically studied. Impaired coordinated motor function of the small bowel might develop from a number of factors, resulting in delayed intestinal transit favoring bacterial overgrowth [404]. Implicated mechanisms include oxidative bowel damage associated with portal splanchnic hypertension, enhanced enteric nitric oxide production, coexistent inflammatory bowel disease, and increased activity of the sympathetic nervous system [404–413]. Such changes in enteric motility, coupled with altered immune defenses involving mesenteric lymph nodes, impaired opsonic capacity in serum and ascitic effusion, reduced function of macrophages and neutrophils, and impaired effector function of immune cells increases hepatic risk for infectious, oxidant, and toxic alimentary challenge. Increased uptake of endotoxin from the gut owing to increased gut permeability or altered enteric microflora contributes to liver injury in certain circumstances. For instance, circulating endotoxin has been demonstrated in dogs that have cirrhosis accompanied by portosystemic shunting, but not in dogs that have congenital portosystemic shunts but lack parenchymal liver dysfunction [414,415]. Increased gut permeability and endotoxin delivery is thought to aggravate Kupffer cell-mediated events, thereby potentiating liver injury, inflammation, and fibrosis. While only limited work regarding endotoxin and liver injury has been specifically completed in dogs or cats, Kupffer cell-mediated cytotoxicity induced by LPS in dogs has been documented and exceeds the response shown in rodent and primate models [416]. Acute fulminant hepatic failure in the dog (induced with galactosamine) increases blood endotoxin concentrations within 12 hours. This toxin notably impairs multiple organs, which undoubtedly contributes to the severity of the subsequent endotoxemia and sepsis.

Bacterial translocation from the alimentary canal is a key mechanism in development of infections in humans who have cirrhosis complicated by ascites. The phenomenon of spontaneous bacterial peritonitis, frequently asymptomatic in the early stages, is controlled by chronic administration of antibiotics (in most cases a fluorinated quinolone) suppressing aerobic intestinal flora. An alternative nonantibiotic approach, microbial interference therapy, is receiving greater attention owing to the increasing appearance of antibiotic-resistant organisms. Microbial interference therapy consists of maintaining or restoring health by introducing live microorganisms from a probiotic to stabilize the balance of intestinal flora. Because probiotics might decrease intestinal bacterial overgrowth, improve immunological host defenses, increase neutrophil phagocytic function, and inhibit enterovirulence of natural gut microbes, they have been proposed to reduce risk for spontaneous infection relating to gut translocation. Whether or not this management is appropriate for dogs and cats that have spontaneous liver disease remains unproven.

The ability of a probiotic to modulate endotoxin exposure has been demonstrated in numerous studies using chronic oral *Lactobacilli* or

Bifidobacterium infantis [417,418]. Most work has been completed using rodent models, which might not be directly applicable to other species. Combined oral administration of a probiotic with antioxidants or certain antioxidants alone can also significantly reduce bacterial translocation, the concentration of disadvantageous bacterial strains (eg, Enterobacteria and Enterococci in the lower bowel), levels of peroxidative lipid products in the bowel wall, and endotoxemia [410,418]. Enteric bacterial translocation has been reduced with a variety of antioxidants including vitamin C, vitamin E, allopurinol (50 mg/kg twice weekly), and supplemental glutamine (1 gm/kg/d) in various test systems [410–412]. Nondigestible carbohydrates and aminoglycosides (notably neomycin and pauromycin) and UDCA also have been shown in various systems to ameliorate mechanisms or clinical signs mediated by endotoxin [406,419,420].

Experimental evidence and limited information in humans who have liver disease suggests that certain probiotics can have a prophylactic and therapeutic effect in HE and in patients that have acute hepatic failure or necrosis and are predisposed to endotoxemia or sepsis, and can modify the enteric inflammation that may coexist with liver disease. Nondigestible carbohydrates that serve as microbial substrates are commonly used to ameliorate clinical signs of HE by encouraging bacterial nitrogen fixation and by providing a cathartic effect that might also ameliorate endotoxemia by modifying the microbial ecosystem, reducing the bacterial pool size, or through other antiendotoxic influences [401,419,420]. Lactulose is the prototype nondigestible carbohydrate studied in liver disease. Probiotics combining the benefit of a fermentable carbohydrate are available, and they can assist in alleviating constipation known to augment development of HE (many enteric substances contributing to this syndrome are derived from the colon). Carbohydrates with low digestibility reduce intestinal transit time, providing a cathartic influence. In animals unable to digest lactose, supplemental lactose can achieve the same effect.

Bacteria thought to benefit the host include Bifidobacteria, Eubacteria, and Lactobacillus. When combined with a fermentable carbohydrate, these bacteria are commonly referred to as liver probiotics. Because different lactic acid bacterial strains can have different probiotic effects, results obtained with a single strain cannot be expected for all others. Lactobacilli are considered to be an integral part of normal enteric microecology and have received the greatest investigation. These organisms have been capitalized on for their demonstrated effects on local enteric flora, immune response, and host metabolism. Adherence of Lactobacilli to enterocyte receptors can induce expression of genes coding for variants of intestinal mucins that inhibit enteropathogen adherence (ie, *E coli*) [421]. They also impose antimicrobial effects through production of bacteriocin and other products.

Acute fulminant hepatic failure is often associated with signs of multiple organ failure and is frequently complicated by sepsis or endotoxemia derived from bacterial translocation. Probiotics studied in models of this syndrome have examined responses to orally and rectally administered Lactobacilli. Oral or rectal administration of *Lactobacillus* increases the quantity of Lactobacilli in feces in humans and rats, and significantly reduces cecal and colonic population of Enterobacteriaceae (the family of enteric organisms most likely to function as opportunistic pathogens); however, continued treatment is necessary to sustain this effect because it is impossible to alter enteric flora without continued inoculation. Some work recommends coadministration with arginine as a metabolic nutraceutical. Because arginine can be synthesized and catabolized by microbes (including *Lactobacillus*) and it enhances bacterial numbers and diversity, it might impose detrimental effects [422].

Iatrogenic infection with bacterial probiotic strains causing endocarditis and liver abscessation has been reported in humans [423,424]. Probiotic strains turned pathologic have a greater ability to produce faciliatory enzymes, aggregate platelets, and bind collagen and fibrinogen than nonpathologic stains. Certain *Lactobacillus* species (eg, *L rhamnosus*) used in probiotic products are known to produce an enzyme that facilitates enteric translocation (phosphatidyl inositol-specific phospholipase C). While cases of confirmed *Lactobacillus* bacteremia are rare in humans, they are nearly always associated with a severe underlying disease or immunosuppression. The potential for opportunistic infection in the circumstance of immunomodulation, which is commonly imposed on dogs and cats that have chronic necroinflammatory and cholestatic liver disease, must therefore be considered carefully before recommending probiotic administration. Furthermore, not all studies (using rodent models) of chronic liver injury show that probiotic bacteria deter enteric translocation. Some studies have documented the opposite—that the probiotic bacteria itself undergoes translocation [423,424].

Glutamine: hazards of supplementation in liver disease

Glutamine is an important constituent of proteins and a central metabolite for amino acid transamination by way of α-ketoglutarate and glutamic acid (Fig. 12). It serves as a substrate for hepatic gluconeogenesis, it is used extensively in the renal tubules for handling ammonia, it has immunoregulatory and cell regulative functions, and it plays an important role in enterocyte metabolism. Glutamine by way of glutamate serves as a precursor amino acid for GSH synthesis and is essential for handling ammonia in the central nervous system. It facilitates ammonia transport in the systemic circulation and provides for temporary ammonia storage in muscle. Increased blood ammonia concentration has the potential to increase hepatic glutamine accumulation and its systemic distribution.

Glutamine has been proposed to be a conditionally essential amino acid in a number of disease conditions including cirrhosis [425–427]. Critically ill

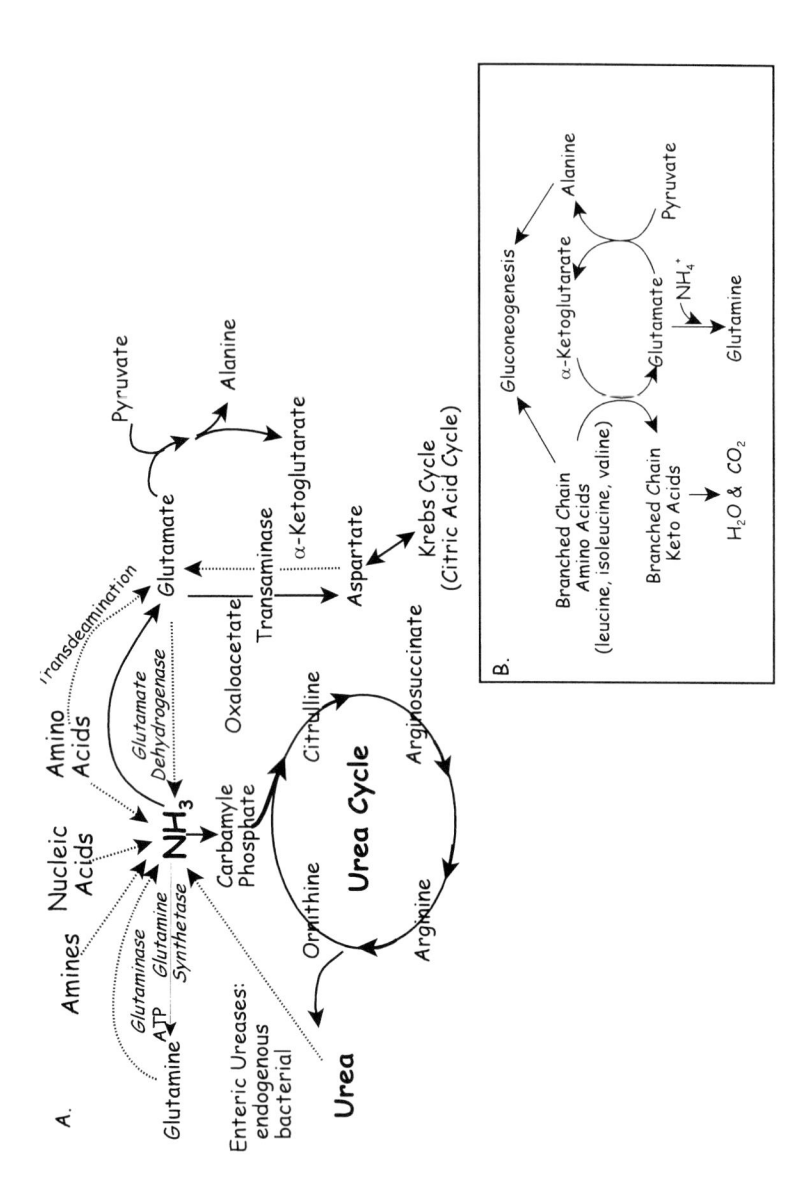

Fig. 12. Metabolic functions of glutamate and glutamine in their relationship with ammonia dispersal, storage, and metabolism. Interaction with the hepatic urea cycle (*A*) and mobilization of amino acids and glutamine after prolonged fasting or in catabolism (*B*). Mechanisms involved with potentiated ammonia toxicity in the patient that has hepatic insufficiency can be deduced. In (*A*) dotted lines denote pathways of ammonia formation; solid lines denote pathway of ammonia utilization.

patients, including those that have severe liver disease, can develop low tissue glutamine concentrations, especially in skeletal muscle; however, many other amino acids also decline, so the clinical importance of this observation remains unclear. Dietary glutamine and glutamate have been proposed as preferred fuels in catabolism and for enteral processing of nutrients. Glutamine and nutrients supplying glutamine induce unique effects in the alimentary canal that are proposed to improve metabolic response to sepsis and enteric host defense. Consequently, glutamine has undergone numerous studies investigating these effects, but few of these involve dogs or cats. There is a large body of data and few consensus conclusions.

Glutamine is absorbed efficiently in the small intestine (especially the jejunum) and has high splanchnic extraction in humans. In the small bowel it provides a multitude of beneficial effects, including enhanced mucosal protein synthesis and positive nitrogen balance, improved intestinal immune function (mucosal associated lymphocytes, immunoglobulin IgA secretion), an ability to sustain villus height (as an indicator of enterocyte health, vitality, and function in parenterally fed patients), improved enteric mucin production, and tight junction permeability (reducing permeability to macromolecules and, ostensibly, to bacterial translocation). These changes are considered to be advantageous in critically ill patients fed parenterally. These effects have been promoted zealously as reasoning behind the nutraceutical use of glutamine given in pharmacologic and microenteral amounts. Emphasis is given to collective influences reducing risk for enteric translocation (pertinent in sepsis, trauma, and shock, in which it has been studied extensively). In some disease models glutamine reduces bacterial translocation and improves gut barrier functions (mucosal permeability and immunity). A study in dogs subjected to a 70% hepatectomy (modeling the high risk for bacterial translocation shown in humans who have had liver transplants) addressed the issue of whether or not supplemental parenteral glutamine provides a significant treatment effect against enteric translocation and endotoxemia. Treatment promoted hepatocyte regeneration and gut protein synthesis and significantly reduced bacterial and endotoxin translocation; however, dogs were not provided with balanced nutritional support [428]. Similar work in rodents showed that balanced nutritional support rather than supplemental glutamine improves recovery [429]. There are a limited number of studies in rodents suggesting that enteral or parenteral glutamine supplementation can augment plasma and tissue GSH concentrations [430,431]; however, other work in dogs and cats has not supported measurable outcome effects on gut or metabolic changes with glutamine supplementation. Cats supplemented with glutamine (7% wt/wt diet) in a model of chemotherapeutic enterotoxicosis failed to achieve enteric advantage compared with control-fed cats [432]. Dogs fed a protein-restricted diet and treated concurrently with dexamethasone, which is similar to the clinical scenario imposed by management of dogs that have severe necroinflammatory liver disease, were used to study whether or not short-term glutamine administration could improve protein catabolism [433]. Treated dogs demonstrated no benefit from glutamine compared with control animals, when outcome was measured by amino acid kinetics [433].

In health, large amounts of ammonia are detoxified rapidly in peripheral tissues (mainly in skeletal muscle) by the ATP-dependent glutamine synthetase catalyzed reaction (Fig. 12). Skeletal muscle is the primary site for temporary peripheral ammonia detoxification; approximately 50% of arterial ammonia in muscle is converted into glutamine and stored temporarily [434,435]. Muscle capacity for glutamine synthesis and ammonia detoxification correlates with total muscle mass, underscoring the importance of maintaining lean body mass in hepatic insufficiency. Because there is an uptake of between 35% to 50% of arterial ammonia by the brain during a first-pass circulation, altered peripheral ammonia detoxification can have direct adverse affects on the central nervous system (HE) [436]. Neither glutamine nor glutamate cross the blood–brain barrier rapidly; rather, they are synthesized in the central nervous system, where they are involved with neurotransmission. There is a considerable body of work that suggests that brain exposure to high ammonia concentrations has serious adverse effects on the glutamate neurotransmitter system [437]. The issue of whether or not enteric or parenterally administered glutamine is relevant, safe, or effective in the patient that has liver disease has not been clarified; however, there is concern that glutamine administration to patients that have hepatic dysfunction and ammonia intolerance might not be innocuous [438–440]. Administration of as little as 0.4 to 0.6 g/kg oral or intravenous glutamine to normal humans and humans who had cirrhosis raised blood ammonia values significantly. In some patients who had liver disease, this dosage worsened cognitive function. While it is unlikely that therapeutically administered glutamine can be shared directly with the CNS, it is concerning that generated ammonia can readily cross the blood–brain barrier. Recommendations for glutamine therapy by parenteral or enteral routes of 0.24 to 0.32 g/kg/day for dogs and up to 1.08 mg/kg/day for cats have been cited in the veterinary literature [427]. This therapy has not been tested in animals that have liver disease. While there is some intriguing evidence that glutamine supplementation mixed with balanced enteral or parenteral nutrition might be useful in recovery from hepatocellular necrosis, the role in other forms of liver disease remains unestablished.

There is no information that substantiates glutamine microenteronutrition, the oral administration of miniscule amounts of glutamine to achieve responses ordinate with the complex biologic role played by glutamine/glutamate. The clinical use of glutamine in human medicine as a means of enhancing enterocyte function and health remains controversial and is hotly debated as responses and benefits in patients who have spontaneous disease remain equivocal with the exception of reduced length of hospitalization (mostly by 1 week) [426,441]. Rather, nutritional support with a species-specific balanced diet, providing enough nitrogen to minimize protein catabolism while minimizing encephalopathic effects of nitrogenous waste products, is a more reasonable approach.

Taurine: do cats that have liver disease need extra taurine?

Taurine, a β-amino acid, is found in all tissues. It differs from other amino acids containing a sulfonic acid group in place of the carboxylic acid group and an amino group attached to the second carbon (β carbon). Most amino acids have the amino group attached to the first carbon (α carbon). Unlike other amino acids, taurine is not commonly incorporated into proteins, but rather appears free in tissues, biological fluids, and, rarely, in low molecular weight peptides [442]. Taurine is acquired from dietary sources and also can be synthesized from cysteine or methionine in most species except cats, in which it is considered to be an essential amino acid. Cats can metabolize cystic acid to taurine but are unable to metabolize cysteinesulfinate, a normal intermediate of cysteine catabolism and taurine precursor in other species [443]. Rather than decarboxylating cysteinesulfinate to taurine, cats transaminate cysteine to β-sulfinylpyruvate, which decomposes spontaneously (Fig. 13). Cysteate (cysteic acid), on the other hand, undergoes reversible transamination to β-sulfopyruvate, a relatively stable product metabolized to taurine. In cats given purified diets deficient in taurine or its precursors, 800 mg of taurine or 2 g cysteic acid/kg diet met taurine requirements [443]. Enteric microbial metabolism of dietary taurine and certain dietary constituents are known to influences dietary taurine availability in cats and can unexpectedly increase requirements [444].

Taurine plays a number of well substantiated roles in the liver. It is used for bile acid conjugation in dogs and cats having an obligatory role for this function in the cat. It is thought to provide an in situ antioxidant effect against neutrophil oxidative burst products and to protect hemoglobin from oxidation. Collective studies in liver tissue in vitro and in vivo support a threshold or curvilinear response: a certain amount is good; exceeding that amount might be injurious. In vitro, taurine mitigates lipid peroxidation induced by hyperoxygenation and protects against cytotoxicity imposed by certain hepatotoxins. A body of work has shown that taurine can be used as a conjugation substrate for xenobiotics, although there is no work confirming this role in dogs or cats. Amino acid profiles in anorectic cats that have HL and cats subjected to long-term fasting disclose low plasma taurine concentrations [177].

Taurine's role in the CNS has been studied using a rodent model [445]. Findings suggest that it interacts with gamma aminobutyric acid (GABA) receptors, hyperpolarizing neuronal membranes. This finding coordinates with other findings that show that taurine can mediate neuronal excitability

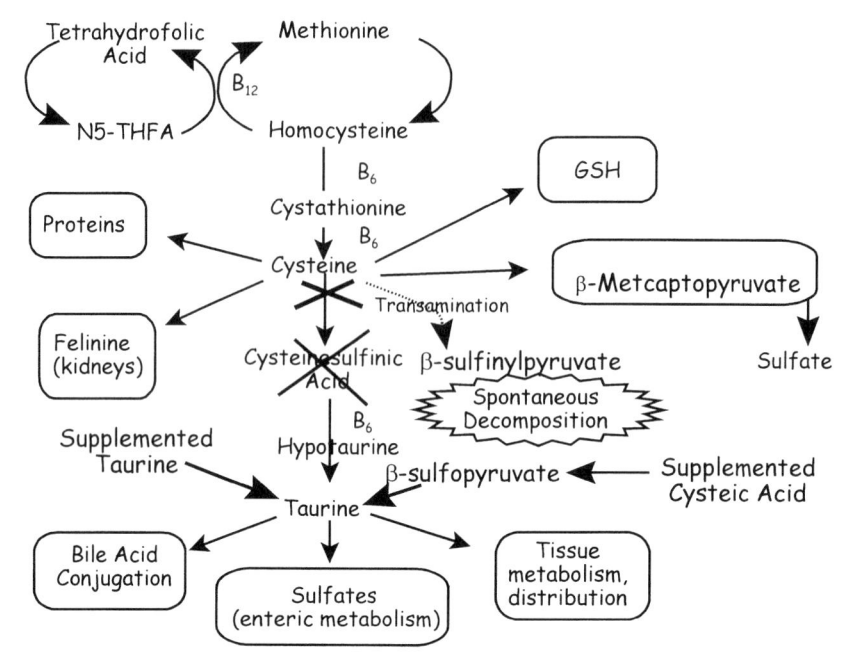

Fig. 13. Pathways involved in feline taurine synthesis. Cats consuming a balanced feline diet should not require supplemental taurine; however, owing the obligatory use of taurine for bile acid conjugation, inappetent cats that have severe liver disease and high serum bile acids might derive a benefit. Pathways operative in mammals—but not in cats—for taurine synthesis are shown, highlighting the feline inability to derive taurine from the transsulfuration pathway (consult text for further discussion).

(anticonvulsant effects). Although anorectic cats that have HL might develop low plasma taurine values concurrent with central neurologic signs, the relevance of taurine to these phenomena has not been documented. Taurine functions as an osmolar solute in cells, influencing osmotic pressure and intracellular ion balance. In conjunction with glutamic acid, it plays a role in transport of metabolically generated water from the brain. Several studies implicate a role for low taurine concentrations in brain tissue in acute HE in humans and rodents, which might have relevance to brain edema and intracranial hypertension, recognized as a fatal complication of HE. Ammonia, well recognized as a major neurotoxin implicated in HE, also is associated with brain edema through a number mechanisms, some of which might be augmented by local taurine insufficiency. It has been speculated that by contributing to brain edema in acute HE and complicating the effects of ammonia on cerebral perfusion and neuronal excitability, low taurine availability may augment oxidant injury. However, whether altered concentrations of brain taurine are an epiphenomenon of neuronal cell edema or whether they are important metabolically remains unclarified [446–449].

Nevertheless, taurine deficiency must be avoided in cats that have hepatic insufficiency, cholestatic liver disease, and those treated with UDCA, which requires taurine conjugation. Balanced feline rations should provide enough taurine to ensure repletion. Whether or not extra supplementation is essential or beneficial is unknown in feline liver patients; however, supplementation of cats that have HL during the initial week of refeeding might be appropriate as the desired total food and protein intake might not be initially achieved because of vomiting or feeding appliance intolerance. A dose of 250 to 500 mg per cat per day is considered to be adequate.

L-carnitine

L-Carnitine (3-hydroxy-4-N-trimethylaminobutyrate; L-CN) is a conditionally essential and vitamin-like nutrient involved in intermediary metabolism, in which it plays a crucial role in fat and carbohydrate metabolism. It is most discussed regarding its role as a facilitator of fatty acid oxidation, where it assists in the interorganelle translocation of fatty acids [450–453]. L-CN is synthesized in vivo or absorbed preformed through the gastrointestinal tract. The majority is synthesized, primarily in the liver, and most is distributed to skeletal muscle and the heart. Biosynthesis requires six primary precursors and a series of five enzymatic steps, the rate-limiting reaction being the conversion of γ-butyrobetaine to L-CN (Fig. 14A) [454]. This final reaction can occur in canine and feline liver and feline kidney. It remains undetermined whether or not CN precursors can provide a benefit equivalent to presynthesized CN in disease conditions. Enteric CN undergoes slow uptake into the enterocyte and slow release into portal circulation [455]. A significant amount of absorbed CN is secreted into bile, presumably by a passive process, and some of this undergoes an enterohepatic circulation. Much of it is in the form of long-chain acyl CNs that might permit removal of fatty acids from the liver. Enteric degradation of L-CN is directly proportional to the amount ingested and varies with the species studied. Carnitine and CN-bound to fatty acids (esters) are eliminated primarily by glomerular filtration [456]. Renal elimination is balanced against dietary CN intake; removal of CN from the diet resulting in a 75% decline in its urinary elimination [457]. The best dietary sources of preformed CN are minimally processed meat and dairy source proteins; however, the concentration of CN in processed and preserved foods is highly variable [453,457,458].

The bioavailability of oral CN, in pharmacologic amounts or as a dietary supplement, is complexly influenced by the quantity ingested, the extent of its enteric degradation, the metabolic status of the host, and the diet composition. As such, no supplementary doses have been firmly established across species lines. When a team of experts reviewed data accumulated from clinical trials of CN supplementation and dietary intake in humans, a conclusion was reached that L-CN dosages up to 20 mg/kg body weight

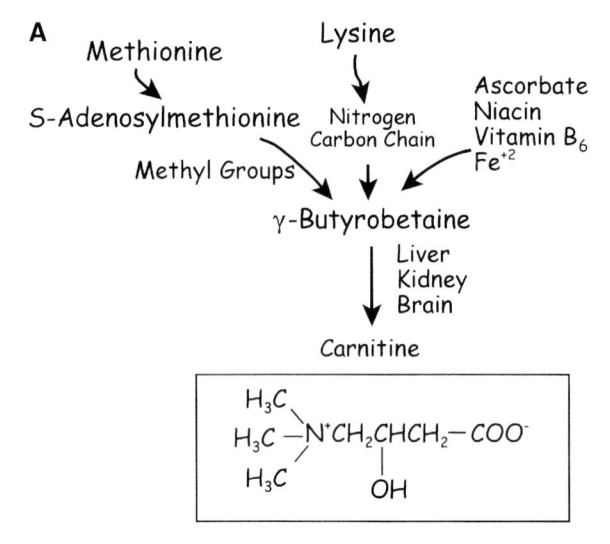

Fig. 14. Substrates and cofactors essential for L-carnitine (CN) synthesis (A) and metabolic role (B) of L-CN in fatty acid oxidation and sharing of acyl-CN moieties with the systemic circulation. Free fatty acids are activated to acyl-CoA and shuttled across the inner mitochondrial membrane. Thereafter, CN is removed and can diffuse back into the hepatocellular cytosol. Carnitine can be transported across the cell and canalicular membranes with acyl-esterification, sharing energy substrates and theoretically providing alternative routes for removal of fatty acids from the liver. This mechanism might have therapeutic value in the cat that has hepatic lipidosis. Protective effects thought to derive from CN in the brain are highlighted (protection against hyperammonemia) along with its influence facilitating nitrogen conservation, maintenance of lean body mass, and enhanced fatty acid oxidation. Acyl = fatty acid group esterified to CN; LCFA = long chain fatty acids in peroxisome.

(1–2 g/d for 50–100 kg body weight persons) were safe and served the physiologic purpose of nutrition. In humans, to cover an increased L-CN requirement and to optimize metabolism, most studies used a daily intake of 1000 to 5000 mg, representing 20 to 50 mg L-CN/kg body weight per day, which resulted in physiologic and pharmacologic effects that cannot be separated clearly. Dosages of more than 50 mg/kg body weight are mainly reserved for medical treatment, such as to remove excessive acids associated with metabolic acidemias caused by inborne errors of fatty acid oxidation. A summary of dose ranges is provided in Table 1. Studies of the influence of supplemental CN have been complicated by inconsistency in the formulations of over-the-counter CN preparations. In a study of 12 over-the-counter CN formulations, the actual mean CN content was only 52% of that indicated on the label [459]. Furthermore, 5 of 12 preparations had unsatisfactory pharmaceutical dissolution characteristics under careful evaluation. Bioavailability data are available only for pharmaceutical-grade products, and comparative data are not available between products.

Carnitine and acyl-CNs (fatty acids esterified to CN) are transported across cell and organelle membranes (two-way flux) by way of specific

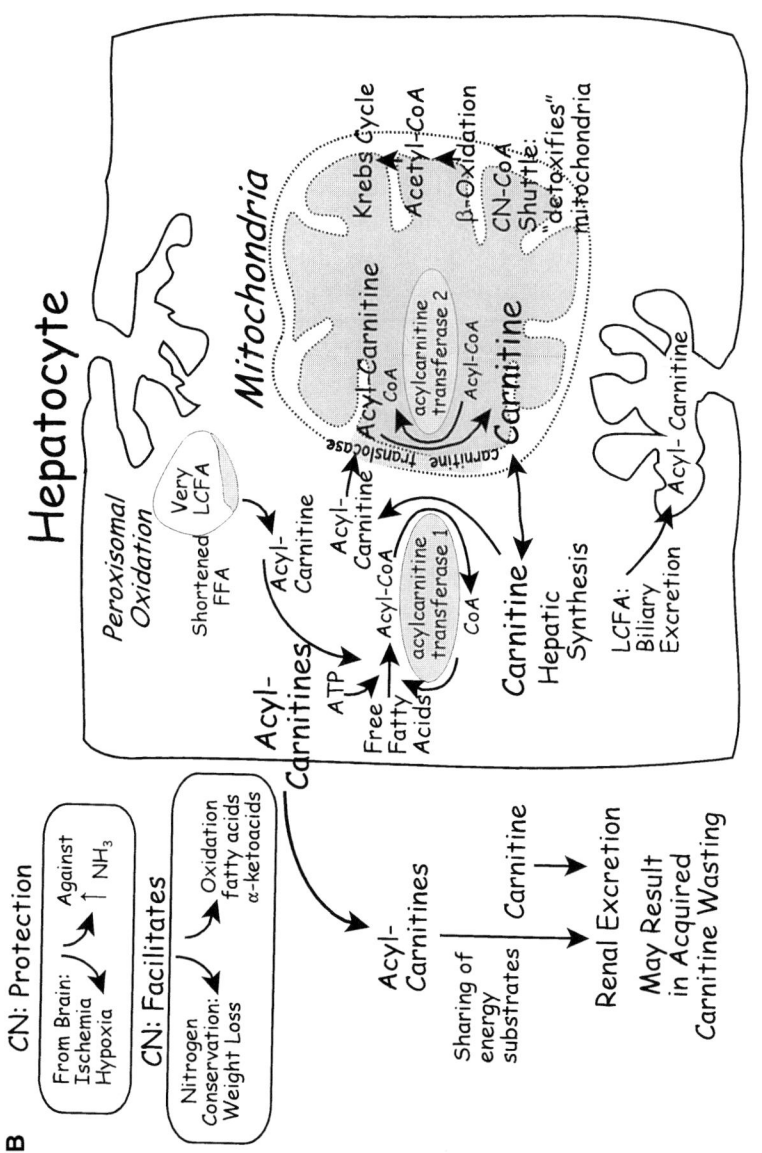

Fig. 14 (continued)

Table 1
Dose-effective scale for L-carnitine suggested for human beings

≤20 mg/kg	Physiologic effects	Foods
20–50 mg/kg	Physiologic and pharmacologic effects	Dietary supplements
50–100 mg/kg	Pharmacologic effect	Drug supplement

saturable transport systems and by passive diffusion. Because tissues differ in their complement of these transport systems, there are substantial differences in tissue CN concentrations, turnover rates, and metabolic availability of CN. Marked differences in CN concentrations among and between tissues and plasma compromises the utility of peripheral sampling to assess CN adequacy.

The best-known activity of CN is its pivotal role in fatty acid metabolism as an essential cofactor for transport of long chain fatty acids across the inner mitochondrial membrane (Fig. 14B). Fatty acid transport can be subdivided into three enzymatic steps (see Fig. 14B). Intramitochondrial CN can subsequently diffuse into the cell cytosol or locally act to bind potentially toxic acyl groups and transport them to the cytosol. In this way, CN functions to buffer/export acetyl-CoA molecules from mitochondria, where they impose an inhibitory influence on β oxidation [451,460–462]. In the presence of excess CN, this buffering or "dumping" action depletes intramitochondrial acetyl-CoA, releasing free CoA plus acetyl-CN. Because acetyl-CoA is an end-product inhibitor of pyruvate dehydrogenase while CoA is one of its substrates, this activity enhances pyruvate oxidation diverting it from reduction into lactate and acetate and the tendency for lactic acidosis and ketogenesis [463,464]. This effect may assist in the management of lactic acidosis during and after maximal muscle exercise and in the circumstance of hepatic failure. Raising the cell/organelle CN concentration not only increases free CoA and reduces acetyl-CoA concentrations in mitochondria but also increases the efflux of acyl-CNs from the organelle and from the hepatocyte, facilitating the sharing of metabolic energy (short-chain acyl-CN including acetyl-CN) between organelles (eg, mitochondria, peroxisomes, cytosol) and tissues and permitting renal excretion of CN-esterified fatty acids. Thus, CN stores and facilitates the transport of activated acyl compounds having an energy value similar to ATP. The ability of acyl-CNs to escape the hepatocyte is a proposed advantage provided by administration of pharmacologic amounts L-CN to cats that have HL, in which it might facilitate dumping of fatty acids into plasma and urine, detoxify mitochondria, and assist hepatocyte health by removal of excess triglyceride. Recent work in obese cats suggests that L-CN also can facilitate the rate of fatty acid oxidation, conserve lean body mass, and also protect against development of HL [465–467].

Other metabolic effects attributed to CN include an influence on mitochondrial enzymes, an inhibitory effect on branched chain keto-dehydrogenase (a nitrogen sparing effect), an ability to facilitate the "shuttling" of shortened very-long-chain fatty acids from peroxisomes to mitochondria, and a prophylactic effect protecting the CNS against ammonia-precipitated encephalopathy [451,461,468–474]. The latter influence remains controversial but might involve direct and indirect mechanisms including increased ammonia detoxification in the urea cycle, blocking the adverse influence of high ammonia concentrations on mitochondrial structure and function (deviation of ketoglutarate to glutamate) or by indirectly modifying the influence of high ammonia on metabolism. Furthermore, acetyl-L-carnitine hydrochloride, a physiological active metabolite of L-CN, plays an important role in the nervous system as a precursor of acetylcholine and by enhancing acetylcholine release.

There is scientific evidence in a variety of species, including the cat, that increasing CN in the cell can promote energy production from fatty acids. These findings have intrigued a variety of researchers and clinicians about the advantages offered by L-CN supplementation in weight loss and management and also in potential for L-CN to assist in recovery of cats from HL. Providing obese cats undergoing weight loss with 250 mg L-CN per day in a double-blinded study resulted in higher plasma concentrations of total and percentage of L-CN as acetylcarnitine, suggesting an enhanced rate of β-oxidation [465]. L-CN concentration in liver and plasma increase in obese humans and cats and in cats undergoing a prolonged fast as an appropriate physiologic response [465,467,475,476]. High-fat diets are associated with increased urine carnitine excretion in humans and dogs, which might also be true in cats and might similarly extend to the anorectic cat suffering from HL. Study of the influence of supplemental L-CN on the rate of fatty acid oxidation and lean body mass retention during rapid weight loss in obese cats has proven that L-CN can facilitate fatty acid oxidation in circumstances that commonly precede development of clinical HL [466].

Nutritional support is the cornerstone of treatment in HL; without adequate protein and energy intake, and provision of essential water-soluble vitamins there is little hope of recovery. Immediate provision of vitamin K_1 is recommended to avert occult bleeding tendencies (0.5 to 1.5 mg/kg given by subcutaneous or intramuscular injection, three doses at 12-hour intervals) that can complicate minor surgical procedures involving esophagostomy or gastrostomy feeding tube placement, hepatic aspiration biopsy, or insertion of jugular catheters [477]. Initial feeding is accomplished in most cats using a nasogastric route until hydration status and electrolyte balance are improved and an opportunity for response to vitamin K has been allowed. Fluid therapy is supplemented with B soluble vitamins providing thiamine and cobalamin. Thiamine is provided to achieve 100 mg per day; intramuscular injection should be avoided owing to rare vasovagal response and neuromuscular paralysis. If enteric malassimilation/maldigestion is suspected, a plasma sample for B_{12} should be collected and a 1 mg dose of B_{12} administered subcutaneously, repeated at 7 days only if plasma vitamin concentrations confirm deficiency, with treatment titrated to response using weekly monitoring and interval dosing. Because low hepatic and whole blood GSH values have been measured in severely affected HL cats, and because of the close similarity of this syndrome to kwashiorkor (documented antioxidant deficiency), vitamin E (α-tocopherol; 10 IU/kg with food) and SAMe (180 mg orally per day to an average-sized cat) are provided routinely. Intravenous NAC (as described previously) is used if hemolytic crisis or high numbers of Heinz bodies are recognized. Enteral L-CN supplementation (250 to 500 mg/d) is continued until full recovery.

Chinese herbal medicines

Chinese herbal products have been established over thousands of years of use based on clinical experience and practice; benefits derived from these medications result from synergistic interactions of multiple ingredients. Effective ingredients in most of these preparations have not been identified or studied. The exception is sho-saiko-to, which has been studied extensively. The Chinese herbal medicine approach is consistent with the current view in Western medical practice: that no single agent is capable of controlling the complex pathobiology of liver disease. It is clear that there is no simple single universal remedy for the control or management of chronic liver disease. Sho-saiko-to has received credible clinical investigation in humans and appears to have efficacy in certain hepatobiliary disorders, including carcinogenicity.

A major problem with Chinese herbal preparations is their heterogeneity. Approximately 7000 plant species are used in China, and preparations are not standardized in regard to composition or dose [478]. In traditional Chinese medicine, it is common for a treatment to be composed or tailored to an individual's needs, so a variety of combinations can be prepared [479]. The frequency with which Chinese herbs provoke adverse reactions involving the liver are unclear because there is no central registry for such reactions and only a few case reports have made their way to publication. Hepatotoxicity ascribed to Chinese herbal products is divided into two categories: (1) single-agent toxicity, and (2) combination toxicity. Of products most incriminated, jin bu huan is most prominent, which is a tablet product prescribed for its sedative and analgesic properties with active ingredients extracted from *Lypocodium serratum*. Acute and chronic hepatitis, hepatocellular necrosis, and fibrosis have been documented as toxic responses. A second single-agent preparation with hepatotoxic effects is ma-huang, a remedy used for weight control.

Sho-saiko-to

Sho-saiko-to or xiano-chai-hu-tang (Chinese name) is presently the most common drug used for outpatient treatment of humans who have chronic hepatitis and cirrhosis in Japan [478–485]. A number of clinical reports suggest that this preparation can improve laboratory abnormalities and liver function and subjectively, clinical signs associated with chronic liver disease. While the long history of sho-saiko-to use in humans in Japan is reassuring, there has been little observational work or otherwise in dogs and cats. The ingredients of a commonly used preparation are shown in Table 2 [486–490]. Active components of sho-saiko-to are derived from Scutellaria root, the most important being baicalein and balicalein. Each of these flavonoids has a chemical structure similar to silybinin and quercetin, flavonoids well studied and established as being antifibrotic [483]. Baiclein suppresses cell proliferation through inhibition of 12-lipoxygenase and protein kinase C [485]. In vitro and in vivo studies have proven that sho-saiko-to can reduce/prevent hepatic fibrosis by inhibiting hepatic Stellate cell activation through antioxidant suppression of TNF-α release, modulation of interferon-γ release/effects, inhibition of PDGF (a strong stimulant of Stellate cell transformation), and by virtue of its potent antioxidant and free radical scavenging abilities [483]. The customary daily dose for humans is 5.0 to 7.5 g given orally in three divided doses. Sho-saiko-to also is reported to reduce development of hepatocellular carcinoma in humans who have chronic hepatitis or cirrhosis secondary to hepatitis C virus [480,483]. A number of studies have documented its preventive and therapeutic effects against different hepatotoxins. Administration preceding toxin challenge appears to provide

Table 2
Sho-saiko-to composition

Herbal constituent	Amount (g)	Main active ingredient	Approximate concentration (%)
Bupleurum root	7.0	Saikosaponin-a	0.2
		Saikosaponin-b1,b2	—
		Saikosaponin-c	0.2
		Saikisaponin-d	—
Pinella tuber	5.0	Ephedrine	—
Scutellaria root	3.0	Baicalin	3.5
		Baicalein	0.3
		Wogonin	0.04
		Viscidulin III	<0.1
JuJube fruit	3.0	Cyclic AMP	—
Ginsing root	3.0	Ginsenoside RB1	0.2
		Ginsenoside RG1	1.0
Glycyrrhiza root	2.0	Glycyrchizin	—
		Liquiriti	—
Ginger rhizome	1.0	6-Gingerol	—
		6-Shogaol	—
		Zingerone	—

—, not determined.

a protective influence on hepatocellular membranes and hepatic Stellate cells.

Herbal hepatotoxicity

Herbal derivatives are used commonly in routine health care and in the context of liver disease in human and veterinary patients, irrespective of the lack of scientific work clarifying therapeutic effects and risks. Patients that have liver disease might have increased risk for toxins administered inadvertently in or with these products. Multiple reports describe circumstances in which contamination of herbal products with toxic plant derivatives or biologic products unrelated to the intended agent or substitution or adulteration of products with toxic herbs and heavy metals have caused illness in humans [486]. Furthermore, certain products have the potential to cause inadvertent drug interactions, compromising response and promoting toxicity of prescription medications.

Patterns of liver injury are emerging among known herbal agents; however, several considerations are critical for clinical identification of hepatotoxicity related to administration of natural or herbal agents, including: (1) maintaining a high index of suspicion, (2) collecting an accurate and thorough medical history, (3) awareness of the spectrum of possible hepatotoxicities, and (4) access to product contents and manufacturer. Because clients do not always readily acknowledge or offer information regarding natural and herbal therapies, it is important to specifically investigate this possibility. In humans, an estimated one third of patients attending an academic liver clinic failed to disclose concurrent herbal therapy [487]. Owing to the lack of specific diagnostic tests for hepatotoxins derived from such products, it is important to consider the temporal relationship of illness to product ingestion and withdrawal while considering other causes of liver disease. It should be emphasized to the client that while the label "natural product" is reassuring, it does not necessarily mean that it is harmless [489].

In some exceptional circumstances, unique zonal injury motivates a clinical search for a hepatotoxic agent (eg, zonal necrosis, unusual bile duct or vascular injuries [consult the following section on pyrrolizidine alkaloids]). There is a paucity of information regarding the histologic lesions associated with most herbal hepatotoxicities owing to the low rate of liver biopsy when clinical signs resolve after treatment discontinuation. Types of liver specific abnormalities recognized in humans treated with different natural remedies are summarized in Table 3 [485–496].

Pyrrolizidine alkaloid toxicity

Substances containing pyrrolizidine alkaloids are well known as being hepatotoxic. Nearly every veterinary student in North America is aware of

Table 3
Summary of reported herbal agents causing hepatobiliary toxicity, toxic ingredient where known, and type of tissue injury

Agent/product name	Toxic ingredient	Evidence/type hepatobiliary injury
African remedy (Mediterranean/African regions)	*Atractylic gummifera*	Diffuse hepatic necrosis; acute onset within hours
	Callilepsis laureola	Mitochondrial toxins
Baiaolian	Podophyllotoxin	Abnormal liver tests
Chaparral leaf	*Larrea tridentate* (nordihydroguaiaretic acid)	Fulminant hepatic necrosis, zone 3 necrosis, chronic hepatitis, cholestasis, cirrhosis
Chinese herbal medicine	Glycyrrhizin	Vanishing bile duct syndrome
Chinese herbal tea	*T'u san-chi'I* (Compositae)	Venooclusive disease
Comfrey (*Symphytum officinale*) (gordolobo yerba, tea, matè tea)	Pyrrolizidine alkaloid	Venooclusive disease
Dai-saiko-to (differs from Sho-saiko-to in proportion of components)		Acute and chronic hepatitis
European remedy	*Chelidonium majus*, other	Hepatitis, fibrosis, eosinophilic inflammation
Germander	Neoclerodan diterpenes	Zone 3 hepatitis, necrosis, fibrosis, cirrhosis
	Teucrium chamaedrys	Toxicity enhanced by p450 cytochrome induction and GSH depletion
Herbal teas (*Comfrey, Heliotroprium, Senecio, Crotalaria, Symphytum,*	Pyrrolizidine alkaloid	Venooclusive disease
	T'u-san-chi'I (Compositae)	
Jin bu huan	*Lycopodium serratum*	Acute/chronic hepatitis, fibrosis, steatosis
Kombucha 'mushroom'	Yeast-bacterial aggregate	Abnormal liver tests
Ma-huang	Ephedrine Many other ingredients	Acute hepatitis
Margosa oil	*Azadirachta indica*	Hepatic lipidosis associated with diffuse mitochondrial failure (Reye's syndrome)
Mediterranean traditional remedy	*Tecrium polium*	Zone 3 necrosis, fibrosis, acute liver failure
Mixed preparations (mistletoe, valerian, skullcap)	Unknown	Hepatic injury, laboratory abnormalities
Natural laxatives	Senna, podophyllin, aloin	Liver laboratory abnormalities
Oil of cloves	Eugenol	Direct-dose hepatotoxin

(*continued on next page*)

Table 3 (continued)

Agent/product name	Toxic ingredient	Evidence/type hepatobiliary injury
Pennyroyal oil (homemade tea)	Labitae (mint)	Zone 3 necrosis, liver test abnormalities
	Mentha pulegium; pulegone → menthofuran	Pulegone depletes GSH
Prostata	Saw palmetto	Hepatitis, fibrosis, cholestasis
(*Serenoa serrulate, Pygeum africanum*, other ingredients)		
Sassafras	*Sassafras albidum*	Hepatic carcinogen (animals)
Sho-saiko-to (TJ-9) (Chinese name: xiano-chai-hu-tang)	*Scutellaria*, others	Zonal, bridging necrosis, fibrosis, microvesicular steatosis, cholestasis
Venencapsan	Many components	Acute hepatitis, focal steatosis
(Horse chestnut leaf, sweet clover, celandine, milk thistle, dandelion root, milfoil)		
Zulu remedy	*Callilepsis laureola*	Hepatic necrosis

yellow star thistle poisoning in the horse caused by this toxin. The major liver injury produced by pyrrolizidine alkaloids is a venooclusive lesion. The venooclusive lesion involves zone 3 of the hepatic lobule, specifically a nonthrombotic obliteration of the terminal or centrilobular hepatic veins resulting in hepatic congestion and gradual development of centrilobular necrosis and fibrosis. Signs of inflammation might be uniquely lacking [491–493]. Pyrrolizidine content might vary in different plants, and the clinical course of toxicity might differ markedly owing to varying amounts of ingested toxin. Consumption of small doses over a long time span culminates in insidious liver damage [491]. While the hepatotoxicity of many pyrrolizidine-containing herbal products has been recognized and thus limited, insidious pyrrolizidine hepatotoxicosis still continues to occur in North America through continued availability of herbal products containing comfrey [495]. Comfrey reportedly contains at least nine hepatotoxic pyrrolizidine alkaloids [495]. The mechanism of injury is toxic rather than immunologic (as proposed for several other herbal agents) and is derived from cytochrome p450 biotransformation of alkaloids, which function as alkylating agents. Toxicity of many pyrrolizidines can be increased by co-administration with phenobarbital, which induces cytochrome p450 oxidases [496].

References

[1] Hrobjartsson A, Gotzsche PC. Is the placebo powerless? An analysis of clinical trials comparing placebo treatment with no treatment. N Engl J Med 2001;344:1594–604.
[2] Kaplowitz N. Mechanisms of liver cell injury. J Hepatol 2000;32:39–47.
[3] Jaeschke H, Gores GJ, Cederbaum AI, et al. Mechanisms of hepatotoxicity. Toxicol Sci 2002;65:166–76.

[4] Jaeschke H. Inflammation in response to hepatocellular apoptosis. Hepatology 2002;35: 964–6.
[5] Kaplowitz N, Tsukamoto H. Oxidative stress and liver disease. Prog Liver Dis 1996;X1V: 131–59.
[6] Lemasters JJ, Nieminen AL, Qian T, et al. The mitochondrial permeability transition in cell death: a common mechanism in necrosis, apoptosis and autophage. Biochim Biophys Acta 1998;1366:177–96.
[7] Lemasters JJ. The mitochondrial permeability transition: from biochemical curiosity to pathophysiological mechanism. Gastroenterology 1998;115:783–6.
[8] West MA, Keller GA, Cerra FB, et al. Killed *Escherichia coli* stimulate macrophage-mediated alterations in hepatocellular function during in vitro coculture: a mechanism of altered liver function in sepsis. Infect Immun 1985;49:563–70.
[9] West MA, Billiar TR, Mazuski JE, et al. Endotoxin modulation of hepatocyte secretory and cellular protein synthesis is mediated by Kupffer cells. Arch Surg 1988;123:1400–5.
[10] Billiar TR, Curran RD, Stuehr DJ, et al. An l-arginine dependent mechanism mediates Kupffer cell inhibition of hepatocyte protein synthesis in vitro. J Exp Med 1989;169:1467–72.
[11] Wang P, Ba BF, Chaudry IH. Hepatocellular dysfunction occurs earlier than the onset of hyperdynamic circulation during sepsis. Shock 1995;3:21–6.
[12] Peck MD, Alexander JW. Survival of septic guinea pigs is influenced by vitamin E but not by vitamin C in enteral diets. J Parenter Enteral Nutr 1990;15:433–6.
[13] Henderson A, Hayes P. Acetylcysteine as a cytoprotective antioxidant in patients with severe sepsis: potential new use for an old drug. Ann Pharmacother 1994;28:1086–8.
[14] Fox ES, Brower JS, Bellezzo JM, et al. N-acetylcysteine and α-tocopherol reverse the inflammatory response in activated rat kupffer cells. J Immunol 1997;158:5418–23.
[15] Betaller R, Brenner D. Hepatic stellate cells as a target for the treatment of liver fibrosis. Sem Liv Dis 2001;21:437–51.
[16] Poli G. Pathogenesis of liver fibrosis: role of oxidative stress. Mol Aspects Med 2000;21:49–98.
[17] Kawada N, Seki S, Inoue M, et al. Effect of antioxidants resveratrol, quercetin, and N-acetylcysteine, on the function of cultured rat hepatic stellate cells and Kupffer cells. Hepatology 1998;27:1265–74.
[18] Schuppan D, Porov Y. Hepatic fibrosis: From bench to bedside. J Gastroenterol Hepatol 2002;17(Suppl 3):S300–5.
[19] Benyon RC, Arthur MJ. Extracellular matrix degradation and the role of hepatic stellate cells. Sem Liv Dis 2001;21:373–84.
[20] Iredale JP. Hepatic stellate cell behavior during resolution of liver injury. Sem Liv Dis 2001;21:427–36.
[21] Sokol RJ, Devereaux M, Khandwala R, et al. Evidence for involvement of oxygen free radicals in bile acid toxicity to isolated rat hepatocytes. Hepatology 1993;17:869–81.
[22] Sokol RJ, Devereaux M, Khandwala RA. Effect of dietary lipid and vitamin E on mitochondrial lipid peroxidation and hepatic injury in the bile duct-ligated rat. J Lipid Res 1991;32:1349–57.
[23] Sokol RJ, McKim JM Jr, Goff MC, et al. Vitamin E reduces oxidant injury to mitochondria and the hepatotoxicity of taurochenodeoxycholic acid in the rat. Gastroenterology 1998;114:164–74.
[24] Yerushalmi B, Dahl R, Devereaux MW, et al. Bile acid-induced rat hepatocyte apoptosis is inhibited by antioxidants and blockers of the mitochondrial permeability transition. Hepatology 2001;33:616–26.
[25] Benz C, Angermuller S, Kloters-Plachky P, et al. Effect of S-adenosylmethionine versus tauroursodeoxyhcolic acid on bile acid-induced apoptosis and cytolysis in rat hepatocytes. Eur J Clin Invest 1998;28:577–83.
[26] Milkiewicz P, Roma MG, Cardenas R, et al. Effect of tauroursodeoxycholate and S-adenosyl-L-methionine on 17β-estradiol glucuronide-induced cholestasis. J Hepatol 2001; 34:184–91.

[27] Gumpricht E, Devereaux MW, Dahl RH, et al. Glutathione status of isolated rat hepatocytes affects bile acid-induced cellular necrosis but not apoptosis. Toxicol Appl Pharm 2000;164:102–11.
[28] Lin Y, Havinga R, Verkade HJ, et al. Bile acids suppress the secretion of very-low-density lipoprotein by human hepatocytes in primary culture. Hepatology 1996;23:218–28.
[29] Lin Y, Havinga R, Schippers IJ, et al. Characterization of the inhibitory effects of bile acids on very-low-density lipoprotein secretion by rat hepatocytes in primary culture. Biochem J 1996;316(Pt 2):531–8.
[30] Cales P. Apoptosis and liver fibrosis: antifibrotic strategies. Biomed Pharmacother 1998; 52:259–63.
[31] Van de Casteele M, Zaman Z, Zeegers M, et al. Blood antioxidant levels in patients with alcoholic liver disease correlate with the degree of liver impairment and are not specific to alcoholic liver injury itself. Aliment Pharmacol Ther 2002;16:985–92.
[32] Leo MA, Rosman AS, Lieber CS. Differential depletion of carotenoids and tocopherol in liver disease. Hepatology 1993;17:977–86.
[33] Yadav D, Hertan HI, Schweitzer P, et al. Serum and liver micronutrient antioxidants and serum oxidative stress in patients with chronic hepatitis C. Am J Gastroenterol 2002;97: 2634–9.
[34] Orlando R, Fragasso A, Lampertico M, et al. Silybin kinetics in patients with liver cirrhosis: comparative study between silybin–phosphatidylcholine complex and Silymarin. Med Sci Res 1990;18:861–3.
[35] Orlando R, Fragasso A, Lampertico M, et al. Pharmacokinetic study of silybin-phosphatidylcholine complex in liver cirrhosis after multiple doses. Med Sci Res 1990;19: 827–8.
[36] Arora AS, Gores GJ. The role of metals in ischemia/reperfusion injury of the liver. Sem Liv Dis 1996;16:31–8.
[37] Sokol RJ, Devereaux MW, O'Brien K, et al. Abnormal hepatic mitochondrial respiration and cytochrome C oxidase activity in rats with long-term copper overload. Gastroenterology 1993;105:178–87.
[38] Sokol RJ, Twedt D, McKim JM, et al. Oxidant injury to hepatic mitochondria in patients with Wilson's disease and Bedlington terriers with copper toxicosis. Gastroenterology 1994;107:1788–98.
[39] Sokol RJ. Antioxidant defenses in metal-induced liver damage. Sem Liv Dis 1996;16: 39–46.
[40] Sokol RJ, McKim JM Jr., Devereaux MW. Alpha-tocopherol ameliorates oxidant injury in isolated copper-overloaded rat hepatocytes. Pediatr Res 1996;39:259–63.
[41] Frage CG, Oteiza PI. Iron toxicity and antioxidant nutrients. Toxicology 2002;180: 23–32.
[42] Center SA, Warner KL. Copper, iron, and zinc concentrations in liver tissue from dogs with various liver disorders. J Vet Intern Med 2001;15:295.
[43] Schultheiss PC, Bedwell CL, Hamar D, et al. Canine liver iron, copper, and zinc concentrations and association with histologic lesions. J Vet Diagn Invest 2002;14: 396–402.
[44] Pietrangelo A. Iron, oxidative stress and liver fibrogenesis. J Hepatol 1998;28:8–13.
[45] Pietrangelo A. Iron, friend or foe? "Freedom" makes the difference. J Hepatol 2000;32: 862–4.
[46] Paradis V, Mathurin P, Kollinger M, et al. In situ detection of lipid peroxidation in chronic hepatitis C: correlation with pathological features. J Clin Pathol 1997;50: 401–6.
[47] Adams PC. Iron overload in viral and alcoholic liver disease. J Hepatol 1998;28(Suppl 1): 19–20.
[48] Bonkovsky HL. Iron as a comorbid factor in chronic viral hepatitis. Am J Gastroenterol 2002;97:1–4.

[49] Carthew P, Edwards RE, Dorman BM. Hepatic fibrosis and iron accumulation due to endotoxin-induced haemorrhage in the gerbil. J Comp Pathol 1991;104:303–11.
[50] Pietrangelo A, Gualdi R, Casalgrandi G, et al. Molecular and cellular aspects of iron-induced hepatic cirrhosis in rodents. J Clin Invest 1995a;95:1824–31.
[51] Kent G, Volini FI, Minick OT. Effect of iron loading upon the formation of collagen in the hepatic injury induced by carbon tetrachloride. Am J Pathol 1964;45:129–55.
[52] MacKinnon M, Clayton C, Plummer J, et al. Iron overload facilitates hepatic fibrosis in the rat alcohol/low-dose carbon tetrachloride model. Hepatology 1995;21:1083–8.
[53] Madra S, Mann F, Francis JE, et al. Modulation by iron of hepatic microsomal and nuclear cytochrome p450, and cytosolic glutathione S-transferase and peroxidase in C57BL/10ScSn mice induced with polychlorinated biphenyls (Aroclor 1254). Toxicol Appl Pharmacol 1996;136:79–86.
[54] Dawson EB, Albers JH, McGanity WJ. The apparent effect of iron supplementation on serum selenium levels in teenage pregnancy. Biol Trace Elem Res 2000;77:209–17.
[55] Sharma BK, Bacon BR, Britton RS, et al. Prevention of hepatocytes injury and lipid peroxidation by iron chelators and α-tocopherol in isolated iron-loaded hepatocytes. Hepatology 1990;12:31–9.
[56] Wagner BA, Buettner GR, Burns CP. Vitamin E slows the rate of free radical-mediated lipid peroxidation in cells. Arch Biochem Biophys 1996;334:261–7.
[57] Iqbal M, Rezazadeh H, Ansar S, et al. Alpha-tocopherol (vitamin E) ameliorates ferric nitrilotriacetate (Fe-NTA)-dependent renal proliferative response and toxicity: diminution of oxidative stress. Hum Exp Toxicol 1998;17:163–71.
[58] Milchak LM, Douglas Bricker J. The effects of glutathione and vitamin E on iron toxicity in isolated rat hepatocytes. Toxicol Lett 2002;126:169–77.
[59] Muraoka K, Shimizu K, Sun X, et al. Flavonoids exert diverse inhibitory effects on the activation of NF-kappaB. Transplant Proc 2002;34:1335–40.
[60] Pietrangelo A, Borella F, Casalgrandi G, et al. Antioxidant activity of sylibinin *in vivo* during chronic iron overload in rats. Gastroenterology 1995;109:1941–9.
[61] Arrigo AP. Gene expression and the thiol redox state. Free Rad Biol Med 1999;27:936–44.
[62] Li Q, Verma IM. NF-κβ regulation in the immune system. Nature Rev 2002;2:725–34.
[63] Peristeris P, Clark BD, Gatti S. N-acetylcysteine and glutathione as inhibitors of tumor necrosis factor production. Cell Immunol 1992;140:390–9.
[64] Houglum K, Venkataramani A, Lyche K, et al. A pilot study of the effects of d-α-tocopherol on hepatic stellate cell activation in chronic hepatitis C. Gastroenterology 1997;113:1069–73.
[65] Fox ES, Leingang KA. Inhibition of LPS-mediated activation in rat Kupffer cells by N-acetylcysteine occurs subsequent to NF-kappaB translocation and requires protein synthesis. J Leukoc Biol 1998;63:509–14.
[66] Scheinman RI, Cogswell PC, Lofquist AK, et al. Role of transcriptional activation of I kappa B alpha in mediation of immunosuppression by glucocorticoids. Science 1995;270:283–6.
[67] Cole WC, Prasad KN. Contrasting effects of vitamins as modulators of apoptosis in cancer cells and normal cells: a review. Nutr Cancer 1997;29:97–103.
[68] Droge W, Kinscherf R, Mihm S, et al. Thiols and the immune system. Meth Enzy 1995;251:255–70.
[69] Meister A. On the biochemistry of glutathione. In: Taniguchi N, Higashi R, Sakamoto Y, et al, editors. Glutathione centennial. San Diego: Academic Press; 1989. p. 3–21.
[70] Anderson ME. Glutathione: an overview of biosynthesis and modulation. Chem Biol Interact 1998;111–112:1–14.
[71] Meister A, Anderson ME. Glutathione. Ann Rev Biochem 1983;52:711–60.
[72] Aw TK, Ooktens M, Kaplowitz N. Mechanism of inhibition of glutathione efflux by methionine from isolated rat hepatocytes. Am J Physiol 1986;14:G354–61.

[73] Fernandez-Checa J, Lu SC, Ookhtens M, et al. The regulation of hepatic glutathione. In: Tavoloni N, Berk PD, editors. Hepatic anion transport and bile secretion: physiology and pathophysiology. New York: Marcel Dekker; 1992. p. 363–95.
[74] Deleve LD, Kaplowitz N. Glutathione metabolism and its role in hepatotoxicity. Pharm Ther 1991;52:287–305.
[75] Griffith OW. Biologic and pharmacologic regulation of mammalian glutathione synthesis. Free Rad Biol Med 1999;27:922–35.
[76] Lu SC. Regulation of hepatic glutathione synthesis. Sem Liv Dis 1998;18:331–43.
[77] Center SA, Warner KL, Erb HN. Liver glutathione concentrations in dogs and cats with naturally occurring liver disease. Am J Vet Res 2002;63:1187–97.
[78] Kehrer JP, Lund LG. Cellular reducing equivalents and oxidative stress. Free Rad Biol Med 1994;17:65–75.
[79] Akerboom TP, Bilzer M, Sies H. The relationship of biliary glutathione disulfide efflux and intracellular glutathione disulfide content in perfused liver. J Biol Chem 1982;257:4248–52.
[80] Suzuki H, Sugiyama Y. Excretion of GSSG and glutathione conjugates mediated by MRP1 and cMOAT/MRP2. Sem Liv Dis 1998;18:359–76.
[81] Ballatori N, Truong AT. Glutathione as a primary osmotic driving force in hepatic bile formation. Am J Physiol 1992;263:G617–24.
[82] Ballatori N, Truong AT. Relation between biliary glutathione excretion and bile acid-independent bile flow. Am J Physiol 1989;38:G22–30.
[83] Niu N, Smith BF. Addition of N-acetylcysteine to aqueous model bile systems accelerates dissolution of cholesterol gallstones. Gastroenterology 1990;98:454–63.
[84] Wosiewitz U, Gulduturna S, Fischer H, et al. Pigment gallstone dissolution in vitro. Solubilization of brown bilirubinate and black polybilirubinate stone material by buffered solvents containing EDTA, bile salts, and reducing thiols. Scan J Gastroenterol 1989;24:373–80.
[85] Griffith OW, Meister A. Origin and turnover of mitochondrial glutathione. Proc Natl Acad Sci USA 1985;82:4668–72.
[86] Griffith OW, Meister A. Glutathione: interorgan translocation, turnover, and metabolism. Proc Natl Acad Sci USA 1979;76:5606–10.
[87] Fernandez-Checa JC, Kaplowitz N, Garcia-Ruiz C, et al. Mitochondrial glutathione: importance and transport. Sem Liv Dis 1998;18:389–401.
[88] Fernandez-Checa JC, Kaplowitz N, et al. GSH transport in mitochondria: defense against TNF-induced oxidative stress and alcohol-induced defect. Am J Physiol 1997;273:G7–17.
[89] Rodrigues CMP, Fan G, Ma X, et al. A novel role for ursodeoxycholic acid in inhibiting apoptosis by modulating mitochondrial membrane perturbation. J Clin Invest 1998;101:2790–9.
[90] Rodrigues CMP, Fan G, Wong PY, et al. Ursodeoxycholic acid may inhibit deoxycholic acid-induced apoptosis by modulating mitochondrial transmembrane potential and reactive oxygen species production. Mol Med 1998;4:165–78.
[91] Lieber CS, Casini A, DeCarli LM, et al. S-adenosyl-L-methionine attenuates alcohol-induced liver injury in the baboon. Hepatology 1990;11:165–72.
[92] Lieber CS. Alcoholic liver disease: new insights in pathogenesis lead to new treatments. J Hepatol 2000;32(Suppl):113–28.
[93] Lieber CS. S-adenosyl-L-methionine: its role in the treatment of liver disorders. Am J Clin Nutr 2002;76(Suppl):1183–7s.
[94] Garcia-Ruiz C, Morales A, Colell A, et al. Feeding S-adenosylmethionine attenuates both ethanol-induced depletion of mitochondrial glutathione and mitochondrial dysfunction in periportal and perivenous rat hepatocytes. Hepatology 1995;21:207–14.
[95] Arias-Diaz J, Vara E, Garcia C, et al. S-adenosylmethionine protects hepatocytes against the effects of cytokines. J Surg Res 1996;62:79–84.

[96] Chawla RK, Watson WH, Eastin CE, et al. S-adenosylmethione deficiency and TNF-α in lipopolysaccharide-induced hepatic injury. Am J Physiol 1998;38:G125–9.
[97] Fernandez-Checa JC, Colell A, Garcia-Ruiz C. S-adenosyl-L-methionine and mitochondrial reduced glutathione depletion in alcoholic liver disease. Alcohol 2002;27:179–83.
[98] Shao LE, Tanaka T, Gribi R, et al. Thioredoxin-related regulation of NO/NOS activities. Ann N Y Acad Sci 2002;962:140–50.
[99] Powis G, Montfort WR. Properties and biological activities of thioredoxins. Annu Rev Biophys Biomol Struct 2001;30:421–55.
[100] Sen CK, Packer L. Thiol homeostasis and supplements in physical exercise. Am J Clin Nutr 2000;72(Suppl):653S–69S.
[101] Anderson ME. Glutathione and glutathione delivery compounds. Adv Pharmacol 1997;38:65–78.
[102] Anderson ME, Luo J-L. Glutathione therapy: from prodrugs to genes. Sem Liv Dis 1998;18:415–29.
[103] Puri RN, Meister A. Transport of glutathione, as γ-glutamylcysteinylglycyl ester, into liver and kidney. Proc Natl Acad Sci USA 1983;80:5258–60.
[104] Sies H. Glutathione and its role in cellular functions. Free Radic Biol Med 1999;27:916–21.
[105] Watanabe A, Okada K, Shimizu Y, et al. Nutritional therapy of chronic hepatitis by whey protein (non-heated). J Med 2000;31:283–302.
[106] Micke P, Beeh KM, Schlaak JF, et al. Oral supplementation with whey proteins increases plasma glutathione levels of HIV-infected patients. Europ J Clin Invest 2001;31:171–8.
[107] Olsson B, Johansson M, Gabrielsson J, Bolme P. Pharmacokinetics and bioavailability of reduced and oxidized N-acetylcysteine. Eur J Clin Pharmacol 1988;34:77–82.
[108] Sjodin K, Nilsson E, Hallberg A, et al. Metabolism of N-acetyl-l-cysteine. Biochem Pharm 1989;38:3981–5.
[109] Pastor A, Collado PS, Almar M, Gonzalez-Gallego J. Antioxidant enzyme status in biliary obstructed rats: effects of N-acetylcysteine. J Hepatol 1997;27:363–70.
[110] Corcoran GB, Wong BK. Role of glutathione in prevention of acetaminophen-induced hepatotoxicity by N-acetyl-L-cysteine in vivo: studies with N-acetyl-D-cysteine in mice. J Pharm Exp Ther 1986;238:54–61.
[111] Pratt S, Ioannides C. Mechanism of the protective action of N-acetylcysteine and methionine against paracetamol toxicity in the hamster. Arch Toxicol 1985;57:173–7.
[112] Harrison PM, Wendon JA, Gimson AE, et al. Improvement by acetylcysteine of hemodynamics and oxygen transport in fulminant hepatic failure. N Engl J Med 1991;324:1852–7.
[113] Nakano H, Boudjema K, Alexandre E, et al. Protective effects of N-Acetylcysteine on hypothermic ischemia–reperfusion injury of rat liver. Hepatology 1995;22:539–45.
[114] Walsh TS, Lee A. N-acetylcysteine administration in the critically ill. Intensive Care Med 1999;25:432–4.
[115] Neuschwander-Tetri BA, Bellezzo JM, Britton RS, et al. Thiol regulation of endotoxininduced release of tumour necrosis factor alpha from isolated rat Kupffer cells. Biochem J 1996;320:1005–10.
[116] Suter PM, Domenighetti G, Schaller MD, et al. N-acetylcysteine enhances recovery from acute lung injury in man: a randomized, double-blind, placebo-controlled clinical study. Chest 1994;105:190–4.
[117] Spies C, Giese C, Meier-Hellmann A, et al. The effect of prophylactically administered N-acetylcysteine on clinical indicators for tissue oxygenation during hyperoxic ventilation in cardiac risk patients. Der Anesthesist 1996;45:343–50.
[118] Devlin J, Ellis AE, McPeake J, et al. N-acetylcysteine improves indocyanine green extraction and oxygen transport during hepatic dysfunction. Crit Care Med 1997;25:236–42.

[119] Heller AR, Groth G, Heller SC, et al. N-acetylcysteine reduces respiratory burst but augments neutrophil phagocytosis in intensive care unit patients. Crit Care Med 2001;29: 272–6.
[120] Koch T, Heller S, Heissler S, et al. Effects of N-acetylcysteine on bacterial clearance. Eur J Clin Invest 1996;26:884–92.
[121] Smilkstein MJ, Knapp GL, Kulig KW, et al. Efficacy of oral N-acetylcysteine in the treatment of acetaminophen overdose. Analysis of the national multicenter study (1976 to 1985). N Engl J Med 1988;319:1557–62.
[122] Droge W, Holm E. Role of cysteine and glutathione in HIV infection and other diseases associated with muscle wasting and immunological dysfunction. FASEB J 1997;11: 1077–89.
[123] Breitkreutz R, Pittack N, et al. Improvement of immune functions in HIV infection by sulfur supplementation: two randomized trials. J Mol Med 2000;78:55–62.
[124] Kleinveld HA, Demacker PN, Stalenhoef AF. Failure of N-acetylcysteine to reduce low-density lipoprotein oxidizability in healthy subjects. Eur J Clin Pharmacol 1992;43:639–42.
[125] Oikawa S, Yamada K, Yamashita N, et al. N-acetylcysteine, a cancer chemopreventive agent, causes oxidative damage to cellular and isolated DNA. Carcinogenesis 1999;20: 1485–90.
[126] Aruoma OI, Halliwell B, Hoey BM, et al. The antioxidant action of N-acetylcysteine: its reaction with hydrogen peroxide, hydroxyl radical, superoxide, and hypochlorous acid. Free Radic Biol Med 1989;6:593–7.
[127] Kelly GS. Clinical applications of acetylcysteine. Alt Med Rev 1998;3:114–27.
[128] Bulger EM, Maier RV. Antioxidants in critical illness. Arch Surg 2001;136:1201–7.
[129] Bottiglieri. S-adenosyl-L-methionine (SAMe): from the bench to the bedside-molecular basis of a pleiotrophic molecule. Am J Clin Nutr 2002;76(Suppl):1151S–7S.
[130] Friedel HA, Goa KL, Benfield P. S-adenosyl-L-methionine. A review of its pharmacological properties and therapeutic potential in liver dysfunction and affective disorders in relation to its physiological role in cell metabolism. Drugs 1989;38:389–416.
[131] Chawla RK, Bonkovsky HL, Galambos JT. Biochemistry and pharmacology of S-adenosyl-L-methionine and rationale for its use in liver disease. Drugs 1990;40(Suppl 3): 98–110.
[132] Mato JM, Ortiz P, Pajares MA. S-adenosylmethionine synthesis: molecular mechanisms and clinical implications. Pharmacol Ther 1997;73:265–80.
[133] Mato JM, Corrales FJ, Lu SC, et al. S-adenosylmethionine: a control switch that regulates liver function. FASEB J 2002;16:15–26.
[134] Mudd SH, Poole JR. Labile methyl balances for normal humans of various dietary regimens. Metabolism 1975;24:721–35.
[135] Finkelstein JD. Methionine metabolism in mammals. J Nutr Biochem 1990;1:228–36.
[136] Martinez-Chantar ML, Garcia-Trevijano ER, Latasa MU, et al. Importance of a deficiency in S-adenosyl-L-methionine synthesis in the pathogenesis of liver injury. Am J Clin Nutr 2002;76(Suppl):1177S–82S.
[137] Kinsell LW, Harper HA, Marton HC, et al. Rate of disappearance from plasma of intravenously administered methionine in patients with liver damage. Science 1947;106: 589–90.
[138] Mato JM, Corrales F, Martin-Duce A, et al. Mechanisms and consequences of the impaired trans-sulphuration pathway in liver disease. Part I. Biochemical implications. Drugs 1990;40:58–64.
[139] Ansorena E, Garcia-Trevijano ER, Martinez-Chantar ML, et al. S-adenosylmethionine and methylthioadenosine are antiapoptotic in cultured rat hepatocytes but proapoptotic in human hepatoma cells. Hepatology 2002;35:274–80.
[140] Watson WH, Zhao Y, Chawla RK. S-adenosylmethione attenuates the lipopolysaccharide-induced expression of the gene for tumour necrosis factor alpha. Biochem J 1999;342: 21–5.

[141] Pascale RM, Simile MM, DiMiglio MR, et al. Chemoprevention of hepatocarcinogenesis: s-adenosyl methionine. Alcohol 2002;27:193–8.
[142] Ponsoda X, Jover R, Gomez-Lechon MJ, et al. Intracellular glutathione in human hepatocytes incubated with S-adenosyl-L-methionine and GSH-depleting drugs. Toxicology 1991;70:293–302.
[143] Lieber CS. Role of S-adenosyl-L-methionine in the treatment of liver diseases. J Hepatol 1999;30:1155–9.
[144] Vendemiale G, Altomare E, Trizio T, et al. Effect of oral S-adenosyl-L-methionine on hepatic glutathione in patients with liver disease. Scan J Gastroenteol 1989;24:407–15.
[145] Frezza M, Surrenti C, Manzillo G, et al. Oral S-adenosylmethionine in the symptomatic treatment of intrahepatic cholestasis: a double-blind placebo controlled study. Gastroenterology 1990;99:211–5.
[146] Pisi E, Marchesini G. Mechanisms and consequences of the impaired trans-sulphuration pathway in liver disease: part II. Clinical consequences and potential for pharmacological intervention in cirrhosis. Drugs 1990;40:65–72.
[147] Frezza M. A meta-analysis of therapeutic trials with ademethionine in the treatment of intrahepatic cholestasis. Ann Ital Med Int 1993;8(Suppl):48S–51S.
[148] Loguercio C, Nardi G, Argenzio F, et al. Effect of S-adenosyl-L-methionine administration on red blood cell cysteine and glutathione levels in alcoholic patients with and without liver disease. Alcohol 1994;29:597–604.
[149] Mato JM, Camara J, Fernandez de Paz J, et al. S-adenosylmethionine in alcoholic liver cirrhosis: a randomized, placebo-controlled, double-blind, multicenter clinical trial. J Hepatol 1999;30:1081–9.
[150] Cabrero C, Martin Duce A, Ortiz P, et al. Specific loss of the high-molecular-weight form of S-adenosyl-L-methionine synthetase in human liver cirrhosis. Hepatology 1988;88:1530–4.
[151] Kakimoto H, Kawata S, Imai Y, et al. Changes in lipid composition of erythrocyte membranes with administration of S-adenosyl-L-methionine in chronic liver disease. Gastroenterol Jpn 1992;27:508–13.
[152] Bray GP, Tredger M, Williams R. S-adenosylmethionine protects against acetaminophen hepatotoxicity in two mouse models. Hepatology 1992;15:297–301.
[153] Duce AM, Ortiz P, Cabrero C, et al. S-adenosyl-L-methionine synthetase and phospholipid methyltransferase are inhibited in human cirrhosis. Hepatology 1988;8:65–8.
[154] Wallace K, Center SA, Hickford F, et al. S-adenosylmethionine treatment of Tylenol toxicity in a dog. J Am Anim Hosp Assoc 2002;38:246–54.
[155] Webb CB, Twedt DC, Fettman MJ. S-Adenosylmethionine (SAMe) in a feline model of acetaminophen-induced oxidative damage. J Feline Med Surg 2003;5:69–75.
[156] Colell A, Garcia-Ruiz C, Morales A, et al. Transport of reduced glutathione in hepatic mitochondria and mitoplasts from ethanol-fed treated rats: effect of membrane physical properties and S-adenosyl-L-methionine. Hepatology 1997;26:699–708.
[157] Gonzalez-Correa JA, De La Cruz JP, Martin-Auricles E, et al. Effects of S-adenosyl-L-methionine on hepatic and renal oxidative stress in an experimental model of acute biliary obstruction in rats. Hepatology 1997;26:121–7.
[158] Jeon BR, Lee SM. S-adenosylmethionine protects post-ischemic mitochondrial injury in rat liver. J Hepatol 2001;34:395–401.
[159] Lee YB, Lee SM. Effect of S-adenosylmethionine on hepatic injury from sequential cold and warm ischemia. Arch Pharm Res 2000;23:495–500.
[160] Dunne JB, Piratvisuth T, Williams R, et al. Treatment of experimental ischemia/reperfusion injury with S-adenosylmethionine: evidence that donor pretreatment complements other regimens. Transplantation 1997;63:500–6.
[161] Giudici GA, Le Grazie C, Di Padova C. The use of ademethionine (SAMe) in treatment of cholestatic liver disorders: meta-analysis of clinical trials. In: Mato JM, Lieber C,

Kaplowitz N, Caballero A, editors. Methionine metabolism: molecular mechanism and clinical implications. Madrid: CSIC Press; 1992. p. 211–5.
[162] Kaplotwitz N. Biochemical and cellular mechanisms of toxic liver injury. Sem Liv Dis 2000;22:137–44.
[163] Tsukamoto H, Kim CW, Luo ZZ, et al. Role of lipid peroxidation in *in vivo* and *in vitro* models of liver fibrogenesis. Gastroenterology 1993;104:A1012.
[164] Frezza M, Pozzato G, Chiesa L, et al. Reversal of intrahepatic cholestasis of pregnancy in women after high dose S-adenosyl-L-methionine administration. Hepatology 1984;4: 274–8.
[165] Watson WH, Chawla RK. S-adenosylmethionine (SAMe) modulates biosynthesis of tumor necrosis factor a (TNF) in murine macrophage cells [abstract]. Hepatology 1997;26: 227.
[166] Schulze-Osthoff K, Bakker AC, Vanhaesebroeck B, et al. Cytotoxic activity of tumor necrosis factor is mediated by early damage of mitochondrial functions. Evidence for the involvement of mitochondrial radical generation. J Biol Chem 1992;267:5317–23.
[167] Simile MM, Banni S, Agioni E, et al. 5′-Methylthioadenosine administration prevents lipid peroxidation and fibrogenesis induced in rat liver by carbon-tetrachloride intoxication. J Hepatol 2001;34:386–94.
[168] Garcea R, Daino L, Pascale R, et al. Inhibition of promotion and persistent nodule growth by s-adenosyl-L-methionine in rat liver carcinogenesis: role of remodeling and apoptosis. Cancer Res 1989;49:1850–6.
[169] Muriel P. S-adenosyl-L-methionine prevents and reverses erythrocyte membrane alterations in cirrhosis. J Appl Toxicol 1993;13:179–82.
[170] Lu SC, Gukovsky I, Lugea A, et al. Role of S-adenosylmethionine in two experimental models of pancreatitis. FASEB J 2002;77:56–8.
[171] Laudanno OM. Cytoprotective effect of S-adenosylmethionine compared with that of misoprostol against ethanol, aspirin- and stress-induced gastric damage. Am J Med 1987; 20(Suppl 5A):43–7.
[172] Stramentinoli G. Ademethionine as a drug. Am J Med 1987;83(Suppl):35–42.
[173] Center SA, Warner K, Hoffman WE, et al. Influence of s-adenosylmethionine on metabolic and morphologic hepatocellular features induced by chronic glucocorticoid administration in dogs [abstract]. J Vet Intern Med 1999;13:253.
[174] Center SA, Warner K, Hoffman WE. Influence of SAMe on erythrocytes and liver tissue in healthy cats [abstract]. J Vet Intern Med 2000;14:357.
[175] Horne DW, Holloway RS, Wagner C. Transport of S-adenosylmethionine in isolated rat liver mitochondria. Arch Biochem Biophys 1997;343:201–6.
[176] Trainor D, Center SA, Randolph JF, et al. Urine sulfated and non-sulfated bile acids as a diagnostic test for liver disease in cats. J Vet Intern Med 2003;17:145–53.
[177] Biourge V, Groff JM, Fisher C, et al. Nitrogen balance, plasma free amino acid concentrations and urinary orotic acid excretion during long-term fasting in cats. J Nutr 1994;124:1094–103.
[178] Center SA, Thompson M, Guida L. 3 Alpha-hydroxylated bile acid profiles in clinically normal cats, cats with severe hepatic lipidosis, and cats with complete extrahepatic bile duct occlusion. Am J Vet Res 1993;54:681–8.
[179] Nakano H, Yamaguchi M, Kaneshiro Y. S-adenosyl-L-methionine attenuates ischemia–reperfusion injury of steatotic livers. Transpl Proc 1998;30:3735–6.
[180] Grattagliano I, Vendemiale G, Caraceni P, et al. Starvation impairs antioxidant defense in fatty livers of rats fed a choline-deficient diet. J Nutr 2000;130:2131–6.
[181] Abdelmalek MF, Angulo P, Jorgensen RA, et al. Betaine, a promising new agent for patients with nonalcoholic steatohepatitis: results of a pilot study. Am J Gastroenterol 2001;96:2711–7.
[182] Lavine JE. Vitamin E treatment of nonalcoholic steatohepatitis in children: a pilot study. J Pediatr 2000;136:734–8.

[183] Sokol R. The sleeping giant has awakened. J Pediatr 2000;136:711–3.
[184] Okan A, Astarcioglu H, Tankurt E, et al. Effect of ursodeoxycholic acid on hepatic steatosis in rats. Dig Dis Sci 2002;47:2389–97.
[185] Danson MJ. Dihydrolipoamide dehydrogenase: a "new" function for an old enzyme? Biochem Soc Trans 1988;16:87–9.
[186] Chen HJ, Chen YM, Chang CM. Lipoyl dehydrogenase catalyzes reduction of nitrated DNA and protein adducts using dihydrolipoic acid or ubiquinol as the cofactor. Chem Biol Int 2002;140:199–213.
[187] Reed LJ. Multienzyme complex. Acc Chem Res 1974;7:40–6.
[188] Bustamente J, Lodge JK, Marcocci L, et al. α-Lipoic acid in liver metabolism and disease. Free Rad Biol Med 1998;24:1023–39.
[189] Packer L, Witt EH, Tritschler HJ. Alpha-lipoic acid as a biological antioxidant. Free Rad Biol Med 1995;19:227–50.
[190] Han D, Handelman G, Marcocci L, et al. Lipoic acid increases de novo synthesis of cellular glutathione by improving cystine utilization. Biofactors 1997;6:321–38.
[191] Zicker SC, Hagen TM, Joisher C, et al. Safety of long-term feeding of dl α-lipoic acid and its effect on reduced glutathione: oxidized glutathione ratios in beagles. Vet Therap 2002; 3:157–66.
[192] Gal EM. Reversal of selective toxicity of (−)-alpha-lipoic acid by thiamine in thiamine-deficient rats. Nature 1965;207:535.
[193] Packer L, Weber SU, Rimbach G. Molecular aspects of tocotrienol antioxidant action and cell signalling. J Nutr 2001;131:369S–73S.
[194] Ricciarelli R, Zingg J-M, Azzi A. Vitamin E 80th anniversary: a double life, not only fighting radicals. Life 2001;52:71–6.
[195] Brigelius-Flohe R, Kelly FJ, Salonen JT, et al. The European perspective on vitamin E: current knowledge and future research. Am J Clin Nutr 2002;76:703–16.
[196] Burton GW, Traber MG, Acuff RV, et al. Human plasma and tissue α-tocopherol concentrations in response to supplementation with deuterated natural and synthetic vitamin E. Am J Clin Nutr 1998;67:669–84.
[197] Azzi A, Stocker A. Vitamin E: non-antioxidant roles. Prog Lipid Res 2000;39:231–55.
[198] Azzi A, Ricciarelli R, Zingg J-M. Non-antioxidant molecular functions of α-tochopherol (vitamin E). FEBS Let 2002;519:8–10.
[199] Chojkier M, Houghum K, Lee KS, et al. Long- and short-term D-alpha-tocopherol supplementation inhibits liver collagen alpha (I) gene expression. Am J Physiol 1998;275: G1480–5.
[200] Ricciarelli R, Maroni P, Ozer N, et al. Age-dependent increase of collagenase expression can be reduced by alpha-tocopherol via protein kinase C inhibition. Free Radic Biol Med 1999;27:729–37.
[201] Brigelius-Flohe R, Traber MG. Vitamin E: function and metabolism. FASEB J 1999;13: 1145–55.
[202] Von Herbay A, de Groot H, Hegi U, et al. Low vitamin E content in plasma of patients with alcoholic liver disease, hemochromatosis, and Wilson's disease. J Hepatol 1994;20: 41–6.
[203] Canturk NZ, Canturk Z, Utkan NZ, et al. Cytoprotective effects of alpha tocopherol against liver injury induced by extrahepatic biliary obstruction. East Afr Med J 1998;75: 77–80.
[204] Deulofeu R, Pares A, Rubio M, et al. S-adenosylmethionine prevents hepatic tocopherol depletion in carbon tetrachloride-injured rats. Clin Sci 2000;99:315–20.
[205] Jewell DE, Toll PW, Wedeking KJ, et al. Effect of increasing dietary antioxidants on concentrations of vitamin E and total alkenals in serum of dogs and cats. Vet Ther 2000;1: 264–72.
[206] Twedt DC, Webb CB, Tetrick MA. The effect of dietary vitamin E on the clinical laboratory and oxidant status of dogs with chronic hepatitis [abstract]. J Vet Int Med 2003;17:418.

[207] Traber MG, Rader D, Acuff RV, et al. Vitamin E dose–response studies in humans with use of deuterated RRR-alpha-tochopherol. Am J Clin Nutr 1998;67:669–84.
[208] Muggli R. Physiological requirements of vitamin E as a function of the amount and type of polyunsaturated fatty acid. World Rev Nutr Diet 1994;75:166–8.
[209] Alexander DW, McGuire SO, Cassity M, et al. Fish oils lower rat plasma and hepatic, but not immune cell alpha-tocopherol concentration. J Nutr 1995;125:2640–9.
[210] McGuire SO, Alexander DW, Fritsche KL. Fish oil source differentially affects rat immune cell alpha-tocopherol concentration. J Nutr 1997;127:1388–94.
[211] Bendich A, Machlin LJ. Safety of oral intake of vitamin E. Am J Clin Nutr 1988;48:612–9.
[212] Kappus H, Diplock A. Tolerance and safety of vitamin E: a toxicological position report. Free Rad Biol Med 1992;13:55–74.
[213] National Research Council. Vitamin E: vitamin tolerance of animals. Washington DC: National Academy Press; 1987.
[214] Combs GF. Vitamin E. In: Combs GF, editor. The vitamins: fundamental aspects in nutrition and health. San Diego: Academic Press; 1992. p. 179–204.
[215] Rapola JM, Virtamo J, Ripatti S, et al. Effects of alpha tocopherol and beta carotene supplements on symptoms, progression, and prognosis of angina pectoris. Heart 1998;79:454–8.
[216] Jacob RA, Sotoudeh G. Vitamin C function and status in chronic disease. Nutr Clin Care 2002;5:66–74.
[217] Gerster H. High-dose vitamin C: a risk for persons with high iron stores? Internat J Vit Nutr Res 1999;69:67–82.
[218] Lynch SR. Interaction of iron and other nutrients. Nutr Rev 1997;55:102–10.
[219] Hoffman KE, Yanelli K, Bridges KR. Ascorbic acid and iron metabolism: alternations in lysosomal function. Am J Clin Nutr 1991;54:1188S–92S.
[220] Wellington K, Jarvis B. Silymarin: a review of its clinical properties in the management of hepatic disorders. BioDrug 2001;15:465–89.
[221] Hammouda FM, Ismail SI, Hassan NM, et al. Evaluation of the Silymarin content in Silybum marianum (L) Gaertn. Cultivation under different agricultural conditions. Phytother Res 1993;7:90–1.
[222] Simanek V, Kren V, Ulrichova J, et al. Silymarin: what is in the name...? An appeal for a change of editorial policy. Hepatology 2000;32:442–3.
[223] Saller R, Meier R, Brignoli R. The use of Silymarin in the treatment of liver diseases. Drugs 2001;61:2035–63.
[224] Lucena MI, Andrade RJ, de la Cruz JP, et al. Effects of Silymarin MZ-80 on oxidative stress in patients with alcoholic cirrhosis. Results of a randomized, double blind, placebo-controlled clinical study. In t J Clin Pharmacol Ther 2002;40:2–8.
[225] Jacobs BF, Dennehy C, Ramirez G, et al. Milk thistle for the treatment of liver disease: a systematic review and meta-analysis. Am J Med 2002;113:506–15.
[226] Flora K, Hahn M, Rosen H, et al. Silybum marianum for the therapy of liver disease. Am J Gastroenterol 1998;93:139–43.
[227] Patrick D. Hepatitis C: epidemiology and review of complementary/alternative medicine treatments. Altern Med Rev 1999;4:220–38.
[228] Locher R, Suter PM, Weyhenmeyer R, et al. Inhibitory action of Silibinin on low density lipoprotein oxidation. Arzneimittelforschung 1998;48:236–9.
[229] Masini A, Ceccarelli D, Giovannini F, et al. Iron-induced oxidant stress leads to irreversible mitochondrial dysfunctions and fibrosis in the liver of chronic iron-dosed gerbils. The effect of silybin. J Bioenergy Biomembr 2000;32:175–82.
[230] Pietrangelo A, Montosi G, Garuti C, et al. Iron-induced oxidant stress in nonparenchymal liver cells: mitochondrial derangement and fibrosis in acutely iron-dosed gerbils and its prevention by silybin. Bioenerg Biomembr 2002;34:67–79.
[231] De Groot H, Dehmlow C, Rauen U. Tissue injury by free radicals and the protective effects of flavonoids. Methods Find Exp Clin Pharmacol 1996;18(Suppl B):23–5.

[232] Sonnenbichler J, Mattersberger J, Rosen H. Stimulation of RNA synthesis in the rat liver and isolated hepatocytes by silybin, an antihepatotoxic agent from Silybum marianum. Hoppee Seyler's Z Physiol Chem 1976;357:1171–80.
[233] Machicao F, Sonnenbichler J. Mechanism of the stimulation of RNA synthesis in rat liver nuclei by silybin. Hoppe Seylers Z Physiol Chem 1977;358:141–7.
[234] Sonnenbichler J, Zeti I. Mechanism of action of Silibinin. V. Effect of Silibinin on the synthesis of ribosomal RNA, mRNA, and tRNA in rat liver in vivo. Hoppe Seylers Z Physiol Chem 1984;365:555–66.
[235] Sonnenbichler J, Goldberg M, Hane L, et al. Stimulatory effect of Silibinin on the DNA synthesis in partially hepatectomized rat livers: non-response in hepatoma and other malignant cell lines. Biochem Pharm 1986;35:538–41.
[236] Sonnenbichler J, Zetl I. Biochemical effects of the flavoligand silybin on RNA, protein and DNA synthesis of macromolecules in liver cells. In: Cody V, Middleton E Jr, Harborne JB, editors. Plant flavanoids in biology and medicine: biochemical, pharmacological, and structure-activity relationships. New York: Liss; 1986. p. 319–31.
[237] Mourelle M, Muriel P, Favari L, et al. Prevention of CCl_4-induced liver cirrhosis by silymarin. Fundam Clin Pharmacol 1989;3:183–91.
[238] Favari L, Perez-Alvarez V. Comparative effects of colchicine and silymarin on CCl_4-chronic liver damage in rats. Arch Med Res 1997;28:11–7.
[239] Boigk G, Stroedter L, Herbst H, et al. Silymarin retards collagen accumulation in early and advanced biliary fibrosis secondary to complete bile duct obliteration in rats. Hepatology 1997;26:643–9.
[240] Gonzalez-Correa JA, de la Cruz JP, Gordillo J. Effects of silymarin MZ-80 on hepatic oxidative stress in rats with biliary obstruction. Pharmacology 2002;64: 18–27.
[241] Fuchs EC, Weyhenmeyer R, Weiner OH. Effects of silibinin and of a synthetic analogue on isolated rat hepatic stellate cells and myofibroblasts. Arzneimittelforschung 1997;47: 1383–7.
[242] Jia JD, Bauer M, Cho JJ, et al. Antifibrotic effect of Silymarin in rat secondary biliary fibrosis is mediated by down regulation of procollagen α1(I) and TMP-1. J Hepatology 2001;35:392–8.
[243] Crocenzi FA, Pellegrino JM, Sanchez Pozzi EJ, et al. Effect of silymarin on biliary bile salt secretion in the rat. Biochem Pharmacol 2000;59:1015–22.
[244] Gasbarrini A, Borle AB, Farghali H, et al. Effect of anoxia on intracellular ATP, Na^+, c Ca^{2+}, and cytotoxicity in rat hepatocytes. J Biol Chem 1992;267:6654–63.
[245] Dehmlow C, Erhard J, de Groot H. Inhibition of Kupffer cell functions as an explanation for the hepatoprotective properties of Silibinin. Hepatology 1996;23:749–54.
[246] Saliou C, Rihn B, Cillard J, et al. Selective inhibition of NF-kappaB activation by the flavonoid hepatoprotector Silymarin in HepG2. Evidence for different activating pathways. FEBS Lett 1998;440:8–12.
[247] Manna SK, Mukhopadhyay A, Van NT, et al. Silymarin suppresses TNF-induced activation of NF-kappa B, c-Jun N-terminal kinase, and apoptosis. J Immunol 1999;163: 6800–9.
[248] Faulstich H, Jahn W, Wieland T. Silybin inhibition of amatoxin uptake in the perfused rat liver. Arzneimittelforschung 1980;30:452–4.
[249] Zhao J, Sharma Y, Argarwal R. Significant inhibition by the flavonoid antioxidant Silymarin against 12-O-tetradecanoylphorbol 13-acetate-caused modulation of antioxidant and inflammatory enzymes, and cyclooxygenase 2 and Interleukin-1α expression in SENCAR mouse epidermis: implications in the prevention of stage 1 tumor promotion. Mol Carc 1999;26:321–33.
[250] Zhao J, Agarwal R. Tissue distribution of silibinin, the major active constituent of silymarin, in mice and its association with enhancement of phase II enzymes: implications in cancer chemoprevention. Carcinogenesis 1999;20:2101–8.

[251] Bartholomaeus AR, Bolton R, Ahokas JT. Inhibition of rat liver cytosolic glutathione S-transferase by silybin. Xenobiotica 1994;24:17–24.
[252] Kroncke KD, Ficker G, Meiers PJ, et al. α-Amanitin uptake into hepatocytes. J Biol Chem 1986;261:12562–7.
[253] El-Bahay C, Gerber E, Horbach M, et al. Influence of tumor necrosis factor-α and Silibinin on the cytotoxic action of α-Amanitin in rat hepatocyte culture. Toxicol App Pharm 1999;158:253–60.
[254] Vogel G, Tuchweber B, Trost W, et al. Protection by Silibinin against *Amanita phalloides* intoxication in beagles. Toxicol Appl Pharmacol 1984;73:355–62.
[255] Desplaces A, Choppin J, Vogel G, et al. The effects of Silymarin on experimental phalloidine poisoning. Arzneimittelforschung 1975;25:89–96.
[256] Wu CG, Chamuleau RA, Bosch KS. Protective effect of Silymarin on rat liver injury induced by ischemia. Virchows Arch B Cell Pathol Incl Mol Pathol 1993;64:259–63.
[257] Kropacova K, Misurova E, Hakova H. Protective and therapeutic effect of Silymarin on the development of latent liver damage. Radiats Biol Radioecol 1998;38:411–5.
[258] Chrungoo VJ, Singh K, Singh I. Silymarin mediated differential modulation of toxicity induced by carbon tetrachloride, paracetamol, and D-galactosamine in freshly isolated rat hepatocytes. Indian J Exp Biol 1997;35:611–7.
[259] Muriel P, Garciapina T, Perez-Alvrez V, et al. Silymarin protects against paracetamol-induced lipid peroxidation and liver damage. J Appl Toxicol 1992;12:439–42.
[260] Szilard S, Szentgyorgyi D, Demeter I. Protective effect of Legalon in workers exposed to organic solvents. Acta Med Hung 1988;45:249–56.
[261] Valenzuela A, Guerra R. Protective effect of the flavonoid silybin dihemisuccinate on the toxicity of phenylhydrazine on rat liver. FEBS Lett 1985;181:291–4.
[262] Campos R, Garrido A, Guerra R, et al. Silybin dihemisuccinate protects against glutathione depletion and lipid peroxidation induced by acetaminophen on rat liver. Planta Med 1989;55:417–9.
[263] Zuber R, Modriansky M, Dvorak Z, et al. Effect of silybin and its congeners on human liver microsomal cytochrome p450 activities. Phytother Res 2002;16:632–8.
[264] Beckmann-Knopp S, Rietbrock S, Weyhenmeyer R, et al. Inhibitory effects of silibinin on cytochrome p-450 enzymes in human liver microsomes. Pharm Tox 2000;86:250–6.
[265] Down WH, Chasseaud LF, Grundy RK. Effect of silybin on the hepatic microsomal drug-metabolizing enzyme system in the rat. Arzneimittelforsch 1974;24:1986–8.
[266] Koch H, Insberger ZG. Loslichkeitsparameter von Silybin, Silydianin und Silychristin. Arch Pharm 1980;313:526–33 [in German].
[267] Morazzani P, Montalbetti A, Malandrino S. Comparative pharmacokinetics of silipide and Silymarin in rats. Europ J Drug Metabl Pharmacokinet 1993;18:289–97.
[268] Gatti G, Perucca E. Plasma concentrations of free and conjugated silybin after oral intake of a silybin-phosphatidylcholine complex (silipide) in healthy volunteers. Int J Clin Pharmacol Ther 1994;32:614–7.
[269] Barzaghi N, Crema F, Gatti G, et al. Pharmacokinetic studies on IdB 1016, a silybin-phosphatidylcholine complex, in healthy human subjects. Eur J Drug Metab Pharmacokinet 1990;15:333–8.
[270] Schandalik R, Gatti G, Perucca E, et al. Pharmacokinetics of silybin in bile following administration of silipide and Silymarin in cholecystectomy patients. Arzneimittelforschung 1992;42:964–8.
[271] Lorenz D, Lucker PW, Mennicke WH, et al. Pharmacokinetic studies with silymarin in human serum and bile. Methods Find Exp Clin Pharmacol 1984;6:655–61.
[272] Weyhenmeyer R, Mascher H, Birkmayer J, et al. Study on dose-linearity of the pharmacokinetics of Silibinin diastereomers using a new stereospecific assay. Int J Clin Pharmacol Ther Toxicol 1992;30:134–8.
[273] Flory PJ, Krug G, Lorenz D, Mennicke WH. Studies on elimination of silymarin in cholecystomized patients. I. Biliary and renal elimination after a single oral dose. Planta Med 1980;38:227–37.

[274] Bulles H, Bulles J, Krumbiegel G, Mennicke WH, Nitz D. Studies of the metabolism and excretion of silybin in the rat. Arzneimittelforschung 1975;25:902–5.
[275] Rickling B, Hans B, Kramarczyk R, et al. Two high-performance liquid chromatographic assays for the determination of free and total silibinin diastereomers in plasma using column switching with electrochemical detection and reversed-phase chromatography with ultraviolet detection. J Chromatogr B Biomed Appl 1995;670:267–77.
[276] Nassuato G, Iemmolo RM, Strazzabosco M, et al. Effect of Silibinin on biliary lipid composition. Experimental and clinical study. J Hepatol 1991;12:290–5.
[277] Nassuato G, Iemmolo RM, Lirussi F, et al. Effect of Silybin on biliary lipid composition in rats. Pharmacol Res Commun 1983;15:337–46.
[278] Lorenz D, Mennicke WH, Behrendt W. Elimination of silymarin by cholecystectomized patients. 2. Biliary elimination after multiple oral doses. Planta Med 1982;45:216–23.
[279] Parthasarathy S, Subbaiah PV, Ganguly J. The mechanism of intestinal absorption of phosphatidylcholine in rats. Biochem J 1974;140:503–8.
[280] Zierenberg O, Grundy SM. Intestinal absorption of polyenephosphatidylcholine in man. J Lip Res 1982;23:1136–42.
[281] Galli C, Sirtori CR, Mosconi C, et al. Prolonged retention of doubly labeled phosphatidylcholine in human plasma and erythrocytes after oral administration. Lipids 1992;27:1005–12.
[282] Navder KP, Baraona E, Lieber CS. Polyenylphosphatidylcholine decreases alcoholic hyperlipemia without affecting the alcohol-induced rise of HDL-cholesterol. Life Sci 1997; 61:1907–14.
[283] Navder KP, Baraona E, Leo MA, et al. Oxidation of LDL in baboons is increased by alcohol and attenuated by polyenylphosphatidylcholine. J Lipid Res 1999;40:983–7.
[284] Navder KP, Baraona E, Lieber CS. Dilinoleoylphosphatidylcholine protects human low density lipoproteins against oxidation. Atherosclerosis 2000;152:89–95.
[285] Marathe GK, Harrison KA, Murphy RC, et al. Role of oxidation in atherosclerosis: bioactive phospholipids oxidation products. Free Rad Biol Med 2000;28:1762–70.
[286] Lieber CS, Leo MA, Aleynik SI, et al. Polyenyl-phosphatidylcholine decreases alcohol-induced oxidative stress in the baboon. Alcohol Clin Exp Res 1997;21:375–9.
[287] Aleynik SI, Leo MA, Ma X, et al. Polyenylphosphatidylcholine prevents carbon tetrachloride-induced lipid peroxidation while it attenuates liver fibrosis. J Hepatol 1997;27:554–61.
[288] Navder KP, Baraona E, Lieber CS. Polyenylphosphatidylcholine attenuates alcohol-induced fatty liver and hyperlipemia in rats. J Nutr 1997;127:1800–6.
[289] Baraona E, Zeballos GA, Shoichet L, et al. Ethanol consumption increases nitric oxide production in rats, and its peroxynitrite-mediated toxicity is attenuated by polyenylphosphatidylcholine. Alcohol Clin Exp Res 2002;26:883–9.
[290] Leiber CS, Robins SJ, Li J, et al. Phosphatidylcholine protects against fibrosis and cirrhosis in the baboon. Gastroenterology 1994;106:152–9.
[291] Aleynik SI, Leo MA, Takeshige U, et al. Dilinoleoylphosphatidylcholine is the active antioxidant of polyenylphosphatidylcholine. J Investig Med 1999;47:507–12.
[292] Ma X, Zhao J, Lieber CS. Polyenylphosphatidylcholine attenuates non-alcoholic hepatic fibrosis and accelerates its regression. J Hepatol 1996;24:604–13.
[293] Gigliozzi A, Romeo R, Fraioli F, et al. Effect of s-adenosyl-L-methionine and dilinoleoyl-phosphatidylcholine on liver lipid composition and ethanol hepatotoxicity in isolated perfused rat liver. Dig Dis Sci 1998;43:2211–22.
[294] Cao Q, Mak KM, Lieber CS. DLPC decreases TGF-beta1-induced collagen mRNA by inhibiting p38 MAPK in hepatic stellate cells. Am J Physiol Gastrointest Liver Physiol 2002;283:G1051–61.
[295] Cao QI, Mak K, Lieber CS. Dilinoleoylphosphatidylcholine (DLPC) decreases transforming growth factor-B1-mediated collagen production by rat hepatic stellate cells. J Lab Clin Med 2002;139:202–10.

[296] Mi L-J, Mak MK, Lieber CS. Attenuation of alcohol-induced apoptosis of hepatocytes in rat livers by polyenylphosphatidylcholine (PPC). Alcohol Clin Exp Res 2000;24:207–12.
[297] Poniachik J, Baraona E, Zhao J, et al. Dilinoleoylphosphatidylcholine decreases hepatic stellate cell activation. J Lab Clin Med 1999;133:342–8.
[298] Holecek M, Mraz J, Koldova P, et al. Effect of polyunsaturated phosphatidylcholine on liver regeneration onset after hepatectomy in the rat. Arzneimittelforschung 1992;42:337–9.
[299] Oneta CM, Mak KM, Lieber CS. Dilinoleoylphosphatidylcholine selectively modulates lipopolysaccharide-induced Kupffer cell activation. J Lab Clin Med 1999;134:433–46.
[300] Aleynik SI, Leo MA, Ma X, Aleynik MK, et al. Polyenylphosphatidylcholine prevents carbon tetrachloride-induced lipid peroxidation while it attenuates liver fibrosis. J Hepatol 1997;27:554–61.
[301] Aleynik SI, Leo MA, Aleynik MK, et al. Polyenylphosphatidylcholine protects against alcohol but not iron-induced oxidative stress in the liver. Alcohol Clin Exp Res 2000;24:196–206.
[302] Aleynik MK, Lieber CS. Dilinoleoylphosphatidylcholine decreases ethanol-induced cytochrome p4502E1. Biochem Biophys Res Commun 2001;288:1047–51.
[303] Fassati P, Horejsi J, Fassati M, et al. Essential choline phospholipids and their effect on HbsAG and selected biochemical tests in cirrhosis of the liver. Gas Lek Cesk 1981;120:56–60.
[304] Jenkins PJ, Portmann BP, Eddleston ALWF, et al. Use of polyunsaturated phosphatidylcholine in HbsAg negative chronic active hepatitis: results of prospective double-blind controlled trial. Liver 1982;2:77–81.
[305] Bird GLA, Panos MZ, Polson R, et al. Activity of polyunsaturated phosphatidylcholine in HbsAG negative active chronic active hepatitis and acute alcoholic hepatitis. Z Gastroenterol 1991;29(Suppl 2):21–4.
[306] Schuller-Perez A, Conzalez-San Martin F. Kontrollierte studie mit mehrfach ungesttigtem phosphatidylcholine im vergleich zu plazebo bei alkoholscher lebersteatose Med Welt 1985;36:517–21 [in German].
[307] Singh ND, Prasad RC. A pilot study of polyunsaturated phosphatidyl choline in fulminant and subacute hepatic failure. J Assoc Physicians India 1998;46:530–2.
[308] Niederau C, Strohmeyer G, Heintges T, et al. Polyunsaturated phosphatidyl-choline and interferon alpha for treatment of chronic hepatitis B and C: a multi-center, randomized, double-blind, placebo-controlled trial. Hepatogastroenterology 1998;45:797–804.
[309] Kishi T, Takahashi T, Usui A, et al. Cytosolic NADPH-UQ reductase, the enzyme responsible for cellular ubiquinone redox cycle as and endogenous antioxidant in the rat liver. Biofactors 1999;9:189–97.
[310] Ernster L, Dallner G. Biochemical, physiological and medical aspects of ubiquinone function. Biochem Biophys Acta 1995;1271:195–204.
[311] Nohl H, Gille L, Staniek K. Endogenous and exogenous regulation of redox-properties of coenzyme Q. Mol Aspects Med 1997;18:s33–40.
[312] Xia L, Bjornstedt T, Nordman LC, et al. Reduction of ubiquinone by lipoamide dehydrogenase. An antioxidant regenerating pathway. Eur J Biochem 2001;268:1486–90.
[313] Willis RA, Anthony M, Loop R, et al. The effect of ethanol and/or food restriction on coenzyme Q in liver in rats. Mol Aspects Med 1997;18:s205–11.
[314] Yamamoto Y, Yamashita S, Fujisawa A, et al. Oxidative stress in patients with hepatitis, cirrhosis, and hepatoma evaluated by plasma antioxidants. Biochem Biophys Res Commun 1998;247:166–70.
[315] Weis M, Mortensent SA, Rassing MR, et al. Bioavailability of four oral coenzyme Q10 formulations in healthy volunteers. Mol Aspects Med 1994;15(Suppl):s273–80.
[316] Weber C, Bysted A, Holmer G. Intestinal absorption of coenzyme Q10 administered in a meal or as capsules to healthy subjects. Nutr Res 1997;17:941–5.

[317] Weber C, Bysted A, Holmer G. Coenzyme Q10 in the diet—daily intake and relative bioavailability. Mol Aspects Med 1997;18:s251–54.
[318] Beuers U, Spenglar U, Zwiebel FM, et al. Effect of ursodeoxycholic acid on the kinetics of the major hydrophobic bile acids in health and in chronic cholestatic liver disease. Hepatology 1992;15:603–8.
[319] Rudolph G, Endele R, Seen M, et al. Effect of ursodeoxycholic acid on the kinetics of cholic acid and chenodeoxycholic acid in patients with primary sclerosing cholangitis. Hepatology 1993;17:1028–32.
[320] Mazzella G, Parini P, Bazzoli F, et al. Ursodeoxycholic acid administration on bile acid metabolism in patients with early stages of primary biliary cirrhosis. Dig Dis Sci 1993;38: 896–902.
[321] Poupon R, Chazouilleres O, Poupon RE. Chronic cholestatic diseases. J Hepatol 2000;32: 129–40.
[322] Trauner M, Graziadei IW. Ursodeoxycholic acid in liver disease. Aliment Pharmacol Ther 2002;13:979–95.
[323] Gores GJ, Miyoshi H, Botla R, et al. Induction of the mitochondrial permeability transition as a mechanism of liver injury during cholestasis: a potential role for mitochondrial proteases. Biochim Biophys Acta 1998;1366:167–75.
[324] Benz C, Angermuller S, Otto G, et al. Effect of tauroursodeoxycholic acid on bile acid-induced apoptosis in primary human hepatocytes. Eur J Clin Invest 2000;30:203–9.
[325] Nicastri PL, Diaferia A, Tartagni M. A randomised placebo-controlled trial of ursodeoxycholic acid and S-adenosylmethionine in the treatment of intrahepatic cholestasis of pregnancy. Br J Obstet Gynaecol 1998;105:1205–7.
[326] Lapenna D, Ciofani G, Festi D, et al. Antioxidant properties of ursodeoxycholic acid. Biochem Pharm 2002;64:1661–7.
[327] Setchell KDR, Rodrigues CMP, Clerici C, et al. Bile acid concentrations in human and rat liver tissue and in hepatocyte nuclei. Gastroenterology 1997;112:226–35.
[328] Poo JL, Feldmann G, Erlinger S, et al. Ursodeoxycholic acid limits liver histologic alterations and portal hypertension induced by bile duct ligation in the rat. Gastroenterology 1992;102:1752–9.
[329] Peterson TC, Slysz G, Isbrucker R. The inhibitory effect of ursodeoxycholic acid and pentoxifylline on platelet derived growth factor stimulated proliferation is distinct from an effect by cyclic AMP. Immunopharmacology 1998;39:181–91.
[330] Calmus Y, Gane P, Rouger P, et al. Hepatic expression of class I and class II major histocompatibility complex molecules in primary biliary cirrhosis: effect of ursodeoxycholic acid. Hepatology 1990;11:12–5.
[331] Terasaki S, Nakanuma Y, Ogino H, et al. Hepatocellular and biliary expression of HLA antigens in primary biliary cirrhosis before and after ursodeoxycholic acid therapy. Am J Gastroenterol 1991;86:1194–9.
[332] Hillaire S, Boucher E, Calmus Y, et al. Effects of bile acids and cholestasis on major histocompatibility complex class I in human and rat hepatocytes. Gastroenterology 1994; 107:781–8.
[333] Calmus Y, Arvieux C, Gane P, et al. Cholestasis induces major histocompatibility complex class 1 expression in hepatocytes. Gastroenterology 1992;102:1371–7.
[334] Calmus Y, Weill B, Ozier Y, et al. Immunosuppressive properties of chenodeoxycholic and ursodeoxycholic acids in the mouse. Gastroenterology 1992;103:617–21.
[335] Yoshikawa M, Tsukii T, Matsumura K, et al. Immunomodulatory effects of ursodeoxycholic acid on immune response. Hepatology 1992;16:358–64.
[336] Tanaka H, Makino I. Ursodeoxycholic acid-dependent activation of the glucocorticoid receptor. Biochem Biophys Res Commun 1992;188:942–8.
[337] Mitsuyoshi H, Nakashima T, Inaba K, et al. Ursodeoxycholic acid enhances glucocorticoid-induced tyrosine aminotransferase gene expression in cultured rat hepatocytes. Biochem Biophys Res Commun 1997;240:732–6.

[338] Invernizzi P, Salzman AL, Szabo V, et al. Ursodeoxycholate inhibits induction of NOS in human intestinal epithelial cells and in vivo. Am J Physiol 1997;273:G131–8.
[339] Kuerktshiev D, Subat S, Adler D. Immunomodulating effect of ursodeoxycholic acid therapy in patients with primary biliary cirrhosis. J Hepatol 1993;18:373–7.
[340] Nishigaki Y, Ohnishi H, Moriwaki H, et al. Ursodeoxycholic acid corrects defective natural killer activity by inhibiting prostaglandin E2 production in primary biliary cirrhosis. Dig Dis Sci 1996;41:1487–93.
[341] Funaoka M, Komatsu M, Toyoshima I, et al. Tauroursodeoxycholic acid enhances phagocytosis of the cultured rat Kupffer cell. J Gastroenteol Hepatol 1999;14:652–8.
[342] Paumgartner G, Beuers U. Ursodeoxycholic acid in cholestatic liver disease: mechanisms of action and therapeutic use revisited. Hepatology 2002;36:525–31.
[343] Milkiewicz P, Mills CO, Roma MG, et al. Tauro UDC and S-adenosyl-L-methionine exert an additive ameliorating effect on taurolithocholate-induced cholestasis: a study in isolated rat hepatocyte couplets. Hepatology 1999;29:471–6.
[344] Day DG, Meyer DJ, Johnson SE, et al. Evaluation of total serum bile acids concentration and bile acid profiles in healthy cats after oral administration of ursodeoxycholic acid. Am J Vet Res 1994;55:1474–8.
[345] Nicholson BT, Center SA, Randolph JF, et al. Effects of oral ursodeoxycholic acid in healthy cats on clinicopathological parameters, serum bile acids and light microscopic and ultrastructural features of the liver. Res Vet Sci 1996;61:258–62.
[346] Meyer DJ, Thompson MB, Senior DF. Use of ursodeoxycholic acids in a dog with chronic hepatitis: effects on serum hepatic tests and endogenous bile acid composition. J Vet Intern Med 1997;11:195–7.
[347] Hofmann AF. Pharmacology of ursodeoxycholic acid, an enterohepatic drug. Scand J Gastroenterol 1994;29(Suppl 204):1–15.
[348] Rubin RA, Kowalski TE, Khandelwal M, Malet PF. Ursodiol for hepatobiliary disorders. Ann Intern Med 1994;89:1447–54.
[349] Burk RF, Hill KE. Regulation of selenoproteins. Annu Rev Nutr 1993;13:65–81.
[350] Burk RF. Selenium, an antioxidant nutrient. Nutr Clin Care 2002;5:75–9.
[351] Burk RF, Hill KE. Selenoprotein P. A selenium rich extracellular glycoproteins. J Nutr 1994;124:1891–7.
[352] Burk RF, Early DE, Hill KE, et al. Plasma selenium in patients with cirrhosis. Hepatology 1998;27:794–8.
[353] McClain CJ, Marsano L, Burk RF, et al. Trace metals in liver disease. Sem Liv Dis 1991;11:321–39.
[354] Prasad AS, Rabbani P, Abbasil A, et al. Experimental zinc deficiency in humans. Ann Intern Med 1978;89:483–90.
[355] Valle BL, Falchuk KH. The biochemical basis of zinc physiology. Phys Rev 1993;73:79–118.
[356] Bray TM, Bettger WJ. The physiological role of zinc as an antioxidant. Free Rad Biol Med 1990;8:281–91.
[357] Zago MP, Oteiza PI. The antioxidant properties of zinc: interactions with iron and antioxidants. Free Radic Biol Med 2001;31:266–74.
[358] Oteiza PI, Olin KL, Fraga CG, et al. Zinc deficiency causes oxidative damage to proteins, lipids and DNA in rat testes. J Nutr 1995;125:823–9.
[359] Oteiza PI, Clegg MS, Keen CI. Short-term zinc deficiency affects factor-κB nuclear binding activity in rat testes. J Nutr 2001;131:21–6.
[360] Rogers JM, Lonnerdal B, Hurley LS, et al. Iron and zinc concentrations and 59Fe retention in developing fetuses of zinc-deficient rats. J Nutr 1987;117:1875–82.
[361] Lonnerdal B. Dietary factors influencing zinc absorption. J Nutr 2000;130:1378S–83S.
[362] Hunt JR, Hohnson PE, Swan PB. Dietary conditions influencing relative zinc availability from foods to the rat and correlations with in vitro measurements. J Nutr 1987;117:1913–23.
[363] Sullivan JF, Jetton MM, Burch RE. A zinc tolerance test. J Lab Clin Med 1979;93:485–92.

[364] Karayalcin S, Areasoy A, Uzunalimoglu O. Zinc plasma levels after oral zinc tolerance test in nonalcoholic cirrhosis. Dig Dis Sci 1988;33:1096–102.
[365] Antonow DR, McClain CJ. Nutrition and alcoholism. In: Tarter RE, Thiel DH, editors. Alcohol and the brain. New York: Plenum Publishing; 1985. p. 81–120.
[366] Dunn MA, Blalock TL, Cousins RJ. Minireview: metallothionein (42525A). Proc Soc Exp Biol Med 1987;185:107–19.
[367] Cousins RJ, Leinart AS. Tissue-specific regulation of zinc metabolism and metallothionein genes by interleukin I. FASEB J 1988;2:2884–90.
[368] Vallee BL, Wacker WEC, Bartholomay AF, et al. Zinc metabolism in hepatic dysfunction. I. Serum zinc concentrations in Laennec's cirrhosis and their validation by sequential analysis. N Engl J Med 1956;255:403–8.
[369] Giroux E, Schechter PJ, Shoun J, et al. Reduced binding of added zinc in serum of patients with decompensated hepatic cirrhosis. Eur J Clin Invest 1977;7:71–3.
[370] Yoshida Y, Higashi T, Nouso K, et al. Effects of zinc deficiency/zinc supplementation on ammonia metabolism in patients with decompensated liver cirrhosis. Acta Med Okayama 2001;55:349–55.
[371] Williams RB, Chesters JK. The effects of early zinc deficiency on DNA and protein synthesis in the rat. B J Nutr 1970;24:1053–9.
[372] Hsu JM, Anthony WL, Buchanan PJ. Zinc deficiency and incorporation of ^{14}C-labeled methionine into tissue proteins in rats. J Nutr 1969;99:425–32.
[373] Chandra RK, Au B. Single nutrient deficiency and cell-mediated immune responses. I. Zinc. Am J Clin Nutr 1980;33:736–8.
[374] Rabbani P, Prasad AS. Plasma ammonia and liver ornithine transcarbamylase activity in zinc deficient rats. Am J Physiol 1978;235:E203–6.
[375] Burch RE, Williams RV, Hahn HKJ, et al. Serum and tissue enzyme activity and trace-element content in response to zinc deficiency in the pig. Clin Chem 1975;21:568–77.
[376] Van der Rijt CC, Schalm SW, Schat H, et al. Overt hepatic encephalopathy precipitated by zinc deficiency. Gastroenterology 1991;100:1114–8.
[377] Baraldi M, Caselgrandi E, Borella P, et al. Decrease of brain zinc in experimental hepatic encephalopathy. Brain Res 1982;258:170–2.
[378] Romero-Gomez M, Boza F, Garcia-Valdecasas MS, et al. Subclinical hepatic encephalopathy predicts the development of overt hepatic encephalopathy. Am J Gastroenterol 2001;96:2718–23.
[379] Bresci G, Parisi G, Banti S. Management of hepatic encephalopathy with oral zinc supplementation: a long-term treatment. Eur J Med 1993;2:414–6.
[380] Loomba V, Pawar G, Dhar KL, et al. Serum zinc levels in hepatic encephalopathy. Indian J Gastroenterol 1995;14:51–3.
[381] Reding P, Duchateau J, Bataille C. Oral zinc supplementation improves hepatic encephalopathy. Results of a randomized controlled trial. Lancet 1984;2:493–5.
[382] Riggio O, Ariosto F, Merli M, et al. Oral zinc supplementation does not improve chronic hepatic encephalopathy. Result from a double blind crossover trial. Dig Dis Sci 1991;36(9):1204–8.
[383] Nakatani T, Tawaramoto M, Opare Kennedy D, et al. Apoptosis induced by chelation of intracellular zinc is associated with depletion of cellular reduced glutathione level in rat hepatocytes. Chem Biol Interact 2000;125:151–63.
[384] Mackenzie GG, Zago MP, Keen CL, et al. Low intracellular zinc impairs the translocation of activated NF-κB to the nuclei in human neuroblastoma IMR-32 cells. J Biol Chem 2002;277:34610–7.
[385] Nodera M, Yanagisawa H, Wada O. Increased apoptosis in a variety of tissues of zinc-deficient rats. Life Sci 2001;69:1639–49.
[386] Sen CK, Packer L. Antioxidant and redox regulation of gene transcription. FASEB J 1996;10:709–20.

[387] Ye B, Maret W, Vallee B. Zinc metallothionein imported into liver mitochondria modulates respiration. Proc Natl Acad Sci USA 2001;98:2317–22.
[388] Abel J, de Ruiter N. Inhibition of hydroxyl-radical-generated DNA degradation by metallothionein. Toxicol Lett 1989;47:191–6.
[389] Quesada AT, Byrnes RW, Krezoski SO, et al. Direct reaction of H_2O_2 with sulfhydryl groups in HL-60 cells: zinc-metallothionein and other sites. Arch Biochem Biophys 1996; 334:241–50.
[390] Giralt M, Gasull T, Hernandez J, et al. Effect of stress, adrenalectomy and changes in glutathione metabolism on rat kidney metallothionein content: comparison with liver metallothionein. Biometals 1993;6:171–8.
[391] Zhou Z, Sun X, Lambert J, et al. Metallothionein-independent zinc protection from alcoholic liver injury. Am J Pathol 2002;160:2267–74.
[392] Maret W. Oxidative metal release from metallothionein via zinc-thiol/disulfide interchange. Proc Natl Acad Sci USA 1994;91:237–41.
[393] Jiang LJ, Maret W, Vallee BL. The glutathione redox couple modulates zinc transfer from metallothionein to zinc-depleted sorbital dehydrogenase. Proc Natl Acad Sci USA 1998; 95:3483–8.
[394] Brewer GJ, Dick RD, Schall W, et al. Use of zinc acetate to treat copper toxicosis in dogs. J Am Vet Med Assoc 1992;201:564–8.
[395] Marchesini G, Fabbri A, Bianchi G, et al. Zinc supplementation and amino acid-nitrogen metabolism in patients with advanced cirrhosis. Hepatology 1996;23:1084–92.
[396] Riggio O, Ariosto F, Merli M, et al. Short-term oral zinc supplementation does not improve chronic hepatic encephalopathy. Results of a double-blind crossover trial. Dig Dis Sci 1991;36:1204–8.
[397] Couinaud C. Traitement de l'encephalopathie portosystemique aigue par le zinc. Chirurgie 1985;111:575–9 [in French].
[398] Weismann K, Christensen E, Dreyer V. Zinc supplementation in alcoholic cirrhosis. Acta Med Scand 1979;205:361–6.
[399] Riggio O, Merli M, Capocaccia L, et al. Zinc supplementation reduces blood ammonia and increases liver ornithine transcarbamylase activity in experimental cirrhosis. Hepatology 1992;16:785–9.
[400] Schrezenmeir J, de Vrese M. Probiotics, prebiotics, and synbiotics—approaching a definition. Am J Clin Nutr 2001;73:2(Suppl):361S–4S.
[401] Liehr H, Heine WD. Treatment of endotoxemia in galactosamine hepatitis by lactulose administered intravenously. Hepatogastroenterology 1981;28:296–8.
[402] Spaeth G, Gottwald T, Specian RD, et al. Secretory immunoglobulin A, intestinal mucin, and mucosal permeability in nutritionally induced bacterial translocation in rats. Ann Surg 1994;220:798–808.
[403] Buddington RK, Kelly-Quagliana K, Buddington KK, et al. Non-digestible oligosaccharides and defense functions: lessons learned from animal models. Br J Nutr 2002; 87(Suppl 2):S231–9.
[404] Albillos A, de la Hera A. Multifactorial gut barrier failure in cirrhosis and bacterial translocation: working out the role of probiotics and antioxidants. J Hepatol 2002;37: 523–6.
[405] Greve JW, Gouma DJ, Buurman WA. Bile acids inhibit endotoxin-induced release of tumor necrosis factor by monocytes: an in vitro study. Hepatology 1989;10:454–8.
[406] Hattori Y, Murakami Y, Hattori S, et al. Ursodeoxycholic acid inhibits the induction of nitric oxide synthase. Eur J Pharmacol 1996;300:147–50.
[407] Perez-Paramo M, Munoz J, et al. Effect of propranolol on the factors promoting bacterial translocation in cirrhotic rats with ascites. Hepatology 2000;31:43–8.
[408] Chang CS, Chen GH, Lien HC, et al. Small intestinal dysmotility and bacterial overgrowth in cirrhotic patients and spontaneous bacterial peritonitis. Hepatology 1998; 28:1187–90.

[409] Pardo A, Bartoli R, Lorenzo-Zuniga V, et al. Effect of cisapride on intestinal bacterial overgrowth and bacterial translocation in cirrhosis. Hepatology 2000;31:858–63.
[410] Chiva M, Soriano G, Rochat I, et al. Effect of *Lactobacillus johnsonii* La1 and antioxidants on intestinal flora and bacterial translocation in rats with experimental cirrhosis. J Hepatol 2002;37:456–62.
[411] Schimple G, Pesendorfer P, Steinwender G, et al. Allopurinol and glutamine attenuate bacterial translocation in chronic portal hypertensive and common bile duct ligated growing rats. Gut 1996;39:48–53.
[412] Schimpl G, Pesendorfer P, Steinwender G, et al. The effect of vitamin C and vitamin E supplementation on bacterial translocation in chronic portal hypertensive and common-bile-duct ligated rats. Eur Surg Res 1997;29:187–94.
[413] Chang CS, Chen GH, Lien HC, et al. Small intestinal dysmotility and bacterial overgrowth in cirrhotic patients and spontaneous bacterial peritonitis. Hepatology 1998;28:1187–90.
[414] Howe LM, Boothe DM, Boothe HW. Endotoxemia associated with experimentally induced multiple portosystemic shunts in dogs. Am J Vet Res 1997;58:83–8.
[415] Peterson SL, Koblik PD, Whiting PG, et al. Endotoxin concentrations measured by a chromogenic assay in portal and peripheral venous blood in ten dogs with portosystemic shunts. J Vet Intern Med 1991;5:71–4.
[416] Kuratsune H, Koda T, Kurahori T. The relationship between endotoxin and the phagocytic activity of the reticuloendothelial system. Hepatogastroenterol 1983;30:79–82.
[417] Caplan MS, Miller-Catchpole R, Kaup S, et al. Bifidobacterial supplementation reduces the incidence of necrotizing enterocolitis in a neonatal rat model. Gastroenterology 1999;117:577–83.
[418] Kasravi FB, Adawi D, Molin G, et al. Effect of oral supplementation of lactobacilli on bacterial translocation in acute liver injury induced by D-galactosamine. J Hepatol 1997;26:417–24.
[419] Liehr H, Englisch G, Rasenack U. Lactulose, a drug with antiendotoxin effect. Hepatogastroenterology 1980;27:356–60.
[420] Scevola D, Magliulo E, Trpin L, et al. Control of endotoxemia in liver disease by lactulose and paromomycin. Boll Ist Sieroter Milan 1979;58:242–7.
[421] Mack DR, Michail S, Wei S, et al. Probiotics inhibit enteropathogenic E. coli adherence in vitro by inducing intestinal mucin gene expression. Am J Physiol 1999;276:G941–50.
[422] Adawi D, Kasravi B, Molin G, et al. Effect of *Lactobacillus* supplementation with and without arginine on liver damage and bacterial translocation in an acute liver injury model in the rat. Hepatology 1997;25:642–7.
[423] Oakey HJ, Harty DW, Knox KW. Enzyme production by lactobacilli and the potential link with infective endocarditis. J Appl Bacteriol 1995;78:142–8.
[424] Rodriguez AV, Baigori MD, Alvarez S, et al. Phosphatidyl inositol-specific phospholipase C activity in *Lactobacillus rhamnosus* with capacity to translocate. FEMS Microbiol Lett 2001;204:33–8.
[425] Buchman AL. Glutamine: commercially essential or conditionally essential: A critical appraisal of the human data. Am J Clin Nutr 2001;74:25–32.
[426] Reeds PJ, Burrin DG. Glutamine and the bowel. J Nutr 2001;131:2505S–8S.
[427] Mazzaferro E, Hackett T, Wingfield W, et al. Role of glutamine in health and disease. Comp Contin Ed Small Anim 2000;22:1094–102.
[428] Ito A, Higashiguchi T. Effects of glutamine administration on liver regeneration following hepatectomy. Nutrition 1999;15:23–8.
[429] Skullman S, Wiren M, Chu M, et al. Effects of graded glutamine intake on liver protein metabolism following partial hepatectomy. Eur J Gastroenterol Hepatol 1995;7:881–6.
[430] Hong RW, Round JD, Helton WS, et al. Glutamine preserves liver glutathione after lethal hepatic injury. Ann Surg 1992;215:114–9.
[431] Denno R, Rounds JD, Fans R, et al. Glutamine-enriched total parenteral nutrition enhanced plasma glutathione in the resting state. J Surg Res 1996;61:35–8.

[432] Marks SL, Cook AK, Reader R, et al. Effects of glutamine supplementation of an amino acid-based purified diet on intestinal mucosal integrity in cats with methotrexate-induced enteritis. Am J Vet Res 1999;60(6):755–63.
[433] Humbert B, Le Bacquer O, Nguyen P, et al. Protein restriction and dexamethasone as a model of protein hypercatabolism in dogs: effect of glutamine on leucine turnover. Metabolism 2001;50:293–8.
[434] Bessman SP, Bradley JE. Uptake of ammonia by muscle. Its implications in ammoniagenic coma. N Engl J Med 1955;253:1143–7.
[435] Hod G, Chaouat M, Haskel Y, et al. Ammonia uptake by skeletal muscle in the hyperammonemic rat. Eur J Clin Invest 1982;12:445–50.
[436] Lockwood AH, McDonald JM, Reiman RE, et al. The dynamics of ammonia metabolism in man. Effects of liver disease and hyperammonemia. J Clin Invest 1979;63:449–60.
[437] Felipo V, Butterworth RF. Neurobiology of ammonia. Prog Neurobiol 2002;67:259–79.
[438] Rudman D, DiFulco TD, Galambos JT, et al. Maximal rates of excretion and synthesis of urea in normal and cirrhotic subjects. J Clin Invest 1973;52:2241–9.
[439] Oppong K, Al-Mardini H, Thick M, et al. Oral glutamine challenge in cirrhotics awaiting liver transplantation: a psychometric and analyzed EEG study. Hepatology 1997;26:870–6.
[440] Plauth M, Roske A-E, Romaniuk P, et al. Post-feeding hyperammonaemia in patients with transjugular intrahepatic portosystemic shunt and liver cirrhosis: role of small intestinal ammonia release and route of nutrient administration. Gut 2000;46:849–55.
[441] Heyland DK, Novak F, Drover JW, et al. Should immunonutrition become routine in critically ill patients: a systematic review of the evidence. JAMA 2001;286:944–53.
[442] Hayes KC, Trautwein EA. Taurine deficiency syndrome in cats. Vet Clin North Am Small Anim Pract 1989;19:403–13.
[443] Edgar SE, Hickman MA, Marsden MA, et al. Dietary cysteic acid serves as a precursor of taurine for cats. J Nutr 1994;124:103–9.
[444] Morris JG, Rogers QR, Kim SW, et al. Dietary taurine requirement of cats is determined by microbial degradation of taurine in the gut. Adv Exp Med Biol 1994;359:59–70.
[445] Huxtable RJ. Physiological actions of taurine. Physiol Rev 1992;72:101–63.
[446] Hilgier W, Olson JE. Brain ion and amino acid contents during edema development in hepatic encephalopathy. J Neurochem 1994;62:197–204.
[447] Cordoba J, Gottstein J, Blei AT. Glutamine, myo-inositol, and organic brain osmolytes after portacaval anastomosis in the rat: implications for ammonia induced brain edema. Hepatology 1996;24:919–23.
[448] Cordoba J, Gottstein J, Blei AT. Chronic hyponatremia exacerbates ammonia-induced brain edema in rats after portacaval anastomosis. J Hepatol 1998;29:589–94.
[449] Raghavendra Rao VL, Audet RM, Butterworth RF. Selective alternations of extracellular brain amino acids in relation to function in experimental portal-systemic encephalopathy: results of an in vivo microdialysis study. J Neurochem 1995;65:1221–8.
[450] Bremer J. The role of carnitine in cell metabolism. In: De Simone C, Famularo G, editors. Carnitine today. Austin (TX): Landes Bioscience; 1997. p. 1–37.
[451] Goa KL, Brogden RN. l-carnitine: a preliminary review of its pharmacokinetics, and its therapeutic use in ischemic cardiac disease and primary and secondary carnitine deficiencies in relationship to its role in fatty acid metabolism. Drugs 1987;34:1–24.
[452] Borum PR. Carnitine function. In: Borum PR, editor. Clinical aspects of human carnitine deficiency. New York: Pergamon Press; 1985. p. 157–64.
[453] Walter P. L-carnitine, a "vitamin-like" substance for functional food. Ann Nutr Metab 2000;44:75–96.
[454] Rebouche CJ, Bosch EP, Chenard CA, et al. Utilization of dietary precursors for carnitine synthesis in human adults. J Nutr 1989a;119:1907–13.
[455] Gudjonsson H, Li BU, Shug AL, et al. In vivo studies of intestinal carnitine absorption in rats. Gastroenterology 1985a;88:1880–9.

[456] Guder WG, Wagner S. The role of the kidney in carnitine metabolism. J Clin Chem Clin Biochem 1990;28:347–50.
[457] Frohlich J, Seccombe DS, Hahn P, et al. Effect of fasting on free and esterified carnitine levels in human serum and urine: correlation with serum levels free fatty acids and β-hydroxybutyrate. Metabolism 1978;27:555–61.
[458] Cantoni C, L'Acqua V, Merlino P. Carnitine contents of meat and organs of slaughter house animals. Arch Vet Ital 1972;23:412–7.
[459] Millington DS, Dubay G. Dietary supplement L-carnitine: analysis of different brands to determine bioavailability and content. Clin Res Regul Aff 1993;10:71–80.
[460] Bohmer T. Tissue levels of activated fatty-acids (acylcarnitines) and the regulation of fatty acid metabolism. Biochim Biophys Acta 1967;144:259–70.
[461] Bremer J. Carnitine: metabolism and functions. Physiol Rev 1983;63:1420–80.
[462] Siliprandi N, Di Lisa F, Pieralisi G, et al. Metabolic changes induced by maximal exercise in human subjects following l-carnitine administration. Biochim Biophys Acta 1990a;1034:17–21.
[463] Kerbey AL, Randle PJ, Cooper RX, et al. Regulation of pyruvate dehydrogenase in rat heart. Biochem J 1976;154:327–48.
[464] Uziel G, Garvaglia B, DiDonato S. Carnitine stimulation of pyruvate dehydrogenase complex in isolated human skeletal muscle mitochondria. Muscle Nerve 1988;11:720–4.
[465] Center SA, Harte J, Watrous D, et al. The clinical and metabolic effects of rapid weight loss in obese pet cats and the influence of supplemental oral l–carnitine. J Vet Intern Med 2000;14:598–608.
[466] Center SA, Warner KL, Randolph JR, et al. Influence of L–carnitine on metabolic rate, fatty acid oxidation, body condition, and weight loss in obese cats. World Veterinary Congress, Vancouver, BC, 2001.
[467] Blanchard G, Paragon BM, Milliat F, et al. Dietary L-carnitine supplementation in obese cats alters carnitine metabolism and decreases ketosis during fasting and induced hepatic lipidosis. J Nutr 2002;132:204–10.
[468] Feller AG, Rudman D. Role of carnitine in human nutrition. J Nutr 1988;118:541–7.
[469] O'Connor JE, Costell M. New roles of carnitine metabolism in ammonia cytotoxicity. In: Grisolia S, Felipo V, Minana M-D, editors. Cirrhosis, hepatic encephalopathy, and ammonium toxicity. New York: Plenum Press; 1990. p. 182–95.
[470] Ohtsuka Y, Clark D, Griffith OW. Metabolic effects of carnitine and carnitine analogs. In: Grisolia S, Felipo V, Minana M-D, editors. Cirrhosis, hepatic encephalopathy, and ammonium toxicity. New York: Plenum Press; 1990.
[471] Siliprandi N, Di Lisa F, Menabo R. Clinical use of carnitine: past, present and future. In: Grisolia S, Felipo V, Minana M-D, editors. Cirrhosis, hepatic encephalopathy, and ammonium toxicity. New York: Plenum Press; 1990. p. 175–80.
[472] Siliprandi N, Sartorelli L, Ciman M, et al. Carnitine: metabolism and clinical chemistry. Clin Chim Acta 1989;183:3–12.
[473] Therrien G, Rose C, Butterworth J, et al. Protective effect of L-carnitine in ammonia-precipitated encephalopathy in the portocaval shunted rat. Hepatology 1997;25:551–6.
[474] Bellei M, Battelli D, Guarriero DM, et al. Changes in mitochondrial activity caused by ammonium salts and the protective effect of carnitine. Biochem Biophys Res Commun 1989;158:181–8.
[475] Hoppel CL, Genuth SM. Carnitine metabolism in normal-weight and obese human subjects during fasting. Am J Physiol 1980;238:E409–5.
[476] Jacobs G, Cornelius L, Keene B, et al. Comparison of plasma, liver, and skeletal muscle carnitine concentrations in cats with idiopathic hepatic lipidosis and in healthy cats. Am J Vet Res 1990;51:1349–51.
[477] Center SA, Warner D, Corbett J, et al. Protein invoked by vitamin K absence in clotting times in clinically ill cats. J Vet Intern Med 2000;14:292–7.
[478] Chan TYK, Chan JCN, Tomlinson B, et al. Chinese herbal medicines revisited: a Hong Kong perspective. Lancet 1993;342:1532–4.

[479] Oka H, Fujiwara K, Oda T, et al. Xiao-chai-hu-tang and gui-zhi-fu-ling-wan for treatment of chronic hepatitis; recent advances in traditional medicine in East Asia. In: Oda T, Needham J, Otsuka Y, Guo Bin I, editors. Recent advances in traditional medicine in East Asia. Amsterdam: Excerpta Medica; 1984. p. 232–7.
[480] Gibo Y, Nakamura Y, Takahashi N, et al. Clinical study of sho-saiko-to therapy to the Japanese patients with chronic hepatitis type C (CH-C). Prog Med 1994;14: 217–9.
[481] Oka H, Yamamoto A, Kuroki T, et al. Prospective study of chemoprevention of hepatocellular carcinoma with sho-saiko-to (TJ-9). Cancer 1995;76:743–9.
[482] Tajiri H, Kozaiwa K, Ozaki Y, et al. The study of the effect of sho-saiko-to on HbsAg clearance in children 8with chronic HBV infection and with abnformal liver function test. Acta Paediatr Jpn 1990;94:1811–5.
[483] Shimizu I. Sho-saiko-to: Japanese herbal medicine for protection against hepatic fibrosis and carcinoma. J Gastroenterol Hepatol 2000;15:D84–90.
[484] Hirayama C, Okumura M, Tanikawa K, et al. A multicenter randomized controlled clinical trial of Sho-saiko-to in chronic active hepatitis. Gastroenterol Jpn 1989;24: 715–9.
[485] Geerts A, Rogiers V. Sho-saiko-to: the right blend of traditional Oriental medicine and liver cell biology. Hepatology 1999;29:282–4.
[486] Tomlinson B, Chan TYK, Chan JCN, et al. Toxicity of complementary therapies: an Eastern perspective. J Clin Pharmacol 2000;40:451–6.
[487] Berk BS, Chaya C, Benner KC, et al. Comparison of herbal therapy for liver disease: 1996 versus 1999. Hepatology 1999;30:A478.
[488] Chitturi S, Farrell GC. Herbal hepatotoxicity: an expanding but poorly defined problem. J Gastroenterol Hepatol 2000;15:1093–9.
[489] Kaplowitz N. Hepatotoxicity of herbal remedies: insights into the intricacies of plant–animal warfare and cell death. Gastroenterology 1997;113:1408–12.
[490] Stedman C. Herbal hepatotoxicity. Sem Liv Dis 2002;22:195–206.
[491] Valla D, Benhamou JP. Drug-induced vascular and sinusoidal lesions of the liver. Clin Gastroenteol 1988;2:481–500.
[492] Larrey D. Hepatotoxicity of herbal remedies. J Hepatol 1997;26:47–54.
[493] Ridker PM, Ohkuma S, McDermott WV, et al. Hepatic venocclusive disease associated with the consumption of pyrrolizidine-containing dietary supplements. Gastroenterology 1985;88:1050–4.
[494] Stickle F, Egerer G, Seitz HK. Hepatotoxicity of botanicals. Public Health Nutr 2000;3: 113–24.
[495] Smith LW, Culvenor CCJ. Plant sources of hepatotoxic pyrrolizidine alkaloids. J Nat Prod 1981;44:129–52.
[496] Mattocks AR. Chemistry and toxicology of pyrrolizidine alkaloids. London: Academic Press; 1986.
[497] Schupke H, Hempel R, Peter G, et al. New metabolic pathways of α-lipoic acid. Drug Met Disp 2001;29:855–62.
[498] Weber P, Bendich A, Machlin LJ. Vitamin E and human health: rationale for determining recommended intake levels. Nutrition 1997;13:450–60.
[499] Morazzoni P, Bombardelli E. Silybum marianum (*Carduus marianus*). Fitoterapia 1995; 66:3–42.
[500] Williams CN, Al-Knawy B, Blanchard W. Bioavailability of four ursodeoxycholic acid preparations. Aliment Pharmacol Ther 2000;14:1133–9.
[501] Shay NF, Mangian H. Neurobiology of zinc-influenced eating behavior. J Nutr 2000;130: 1493S–9S.
[502] Hill AS. Effects of lipoic acid in cats: pharmacokinetics, toxicity, and antioxidant activity [PhD dissertation]. Davis (CA): University of California at Davis; 2002.

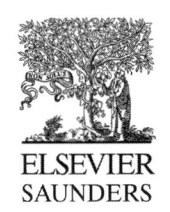

Functional foods and the urinary tract

Scott A. Brown, VMD, PhD

*Department of Physiology and Pharmacology, College of Veterinary Medicine,
University of Georgia, Athens, GA 30602, USA*

There is no universally accepted definition of a commonly used term for a functional food: nutraceutical. For the purposes of this article, a nutraceutical is any ingredient found in foods that has a demonstrated (or proposed) physiologic benefit. Although a nutraceutical is generally taken to be an ingredient that can be isolated or purified from food, plants, or marine products and made available in medicinal form [1–4], this article also considers claims of benefit to the urinary tract for foods or food supplements in which the active ingredient has not yet been characterized or isolated.

Nephrology and evidence-based medicine

Veterinarians, in general, and veterinary urologists, in particular, agree that a therapeutic agent should be accepted only on the basis of objective evidence of benefit and safety. For treatment of people, there are well-defined criteria for evaluating the quality of evidence of beneficial effects and for grading therapeutic recommendations based on this evidence (Table 1) [4–6]. Recently, this approach to therapy has been referred to as evidence-based medicine (EBM). EBM, according to David Sackett, is "the conscientious, explicit and judicious use of current best evidence in making decisions about the care of the individual patient. It means integrating clinical expertise with the best available external clinical evidence from systematic research" [4–6].

The EBM criteria originally designed for treatment of people (see Table 1) do not apply easily to veterinary urology. This is largely because they (1) do not account for the paucity of clinical studies in diseases of the urinary tract in cats and dogs and (2) do not account for the increased utility of laboratory studies in urology employing the same species as that being treated clinically. A modified classification system that takes these limitations into account can be applied to veterinary nephrology (see

---

E-mail address: sbrown@vet.uga.edu

Table 1
Levels of evidence of benefit for therapies for veterinary and human nephrology

Level of evidence	Study type	Human urology [4-6]	Veterinary urology (proposed)
1	Double-blind, randomized, controlled trial (RCT): a clinical trial involving at least one test treatment and one control treatment in which animals are randomly assigned to treatment groups and investigators and patients/pet owners are unaware of group assignments until the completion of the study	Systematic review or meta-analysis of double-blind trial RCT or an individual RCT with a clear homogeneous response	Systematic review or meta-analysis of double-blind RCT or an individual RCT with a clear homogeneous response
1.5	Type A laboratory study (TALS): laboratory research using an applicable in vivo model of the target disease in the homologous species; the study must be randomized, controlled, and blinded	Although seemingly homocentric, laboratory studies that use models of spontaneous conditions (eg, studies of obesity) are generally classified as RCT in people (level 1 study)	Systematic review or meta-analysis of TALS or an individual TALS with a clear homogeneous response
2	Cohort study: clinical study utilizing one group of animals affected with the disease, condition, or treatment being studied and a control group without the disease, condition, or treatment being studied	Systematic review or meta-analysis of cohort studies or an individual cohort study with clear homogeneous response or low-quality RCT or TALS trials	Systematic review or meta-analysis of cohort studies or an individual cohort study with a clear homogeneous response or low-quality RCT or TALS trials
3	Case-control study: animals with a certain condition or specific therapy are compared with a control group of animals without the condition or therapy being studied; usually an historical study	Systematic review or meta-analysis of case-control studies or an individual case-control study with a clear homogeneous response or low-quality RCT, TALS, or cohort trials	Systematic review or meta-analysis of case-control studies or an individual case-control study with a clear homogeneous response or low-quality RCT, TALS, or cohort trials

(*continued on next page*)

Table 1 (continued)

Level of evidence	Study type	Human urology [4–6]	Veterinary urology (proposed)
4	Case series: collection of individual animals with a disease	Case series of low-quality cohort, RCT, TALS, or case-control trials	Case series or low-quality RCT, TALS, cohort, or case-control trials
5	Expert opinion (based on physiologic principles), type B laboratory study (in vivo study in heterologous species), type C laboratory study (in vitro study)	Expert opinion, physiologic principles, type B laboratory study, type C laboratory study	Expert opinion, physiologic principles, type B laboratory study, type C laboratory study

Table 1). According to the principles of EBM in human and veterinary medicine, the best evidence for therapeutic choice is a systematic review (eg, meta-analysis) of multiple randomized clinical trials. Unfortunately, in nearly all areas of veterinary medicine, appropriate randomized controlled trials are either absent, solitary, or not conducted in a manner allowing a systematic review to be performed. Thus, for most diseases of the urinary tract in dogs and cats, a single, conclusive, randomized clinical trial, where available, is the highest (and preferred) justification for therapeutic choices.

Laboratory studies, generally model studies in rodents and in vitro studies in cell cultures and test tubes, are considered low-level evidence (level 5) for evaluating claims of beneficial effects of treatment for people (see Table 1). Similar studies provide low-level evidence for making therapeutic choices in veterinary medicine. A laboratory study of an appropriate model of urologic disease conducted in dogs or cats is inherently more valuable for managing clinical disease in the same species, however. Although of less utility than a double-blind, randomized, controlled clinical trial, a properly conducted laboratory study (blind, randomized, applicable model with a clear result) is herein referred to as a type A laboratory study; it has high predictive value and is rated as level 1.5, lying between randomized controlled trials and cohort studies in general reliability (see Table 1). Studies conducted in vivo but in a heterologous species, such as rats, are referred to as a type B laboratory study and are classified as level 5 in EBM. An in vitro study is generally even less reliable evidence of benefit and is herein referred to as a type C laboratory study (level 5 of EBM).

The EBM classification system provides clear preference for objective controlled trials as the best justification for a therapeutic recommendation for an animal with a disease of the urinary tract. Nonetheless, we routinely recommend therapy on the basis of less reliable evidence. We base these recommendations on the best and highest level of EBM (see Table 1) evidence available at the time, however. There is no place for arbitrary recommendations based on anecdotes and traditions without evidence of a physiologic rationale, which should be rejected outright. A further corollary is that absence of evidence does not imply carte blanche approval to ignore EBM principles and use a therapy to "do something" because it "might work" or "can't hurt." Nutraceuticals are not safe simply because they are "natural" or because they have been occasionally administered to an animal in the absence of grossly observable tragic results. In veterinary urology, these principles of the rational approach of EBM are, and should be, widely accepted in judging efficacy and safety of therapeutic agents.

Functional foods and evidence-based medicine

A survey of the scientific and popular literature and the Worldwide Web by the author identified a variety of claims for functional foods in diseases of the urinary tract (Tables 2 and 3). This illustrative list is by no means exhaustive. Many of these claims seem to be incredulous, contrary to our existing knowledge, or unsupported by evidence (see Table 2). Because the approach of veterinarians is based on the principles of EBM, we are appropriately skeptical of unsupported claims, and cynicism about the utility of nutraceuticals is often appropriate. There are organizations appropriately committed to careful study of these agents (eg, North American Veterinary Nutraceutical Council). Currently, evidence of benefits, safety, and quality of production is usually absent in published claims. Even in journals devoted to nutraceuticals, trials may be uncontrolled as in [7], yielding low-level EBM support for use and making results difficult to interpret. Because there is little regulation of nutritional supplements by the US Food and Drug Administration (FDA), unscrupulous advertising, impurities, and potentially dangerous reactions can occur. Veterinarians should expect to evaluate claims for nutraceuticals and other functional foods by applying the principles of EBM to evaluate evidence of benefit and safety. Nevertheless, it also follows that veterinarians should be (and generally are) open to claims of benefit for nutraceuticals when these claims are supported by EBM principles.

Functional foods and veterinary nephrology

It is important to remember that nutraceuticals are contained in or isolated from food, plants, or marine products. Many of our most effective pharmaceutical agents share a similar origin. As a recent example, a cholesterol-lowering agent derived from Chinese red rice yeast was originally an active ingredient of a commercially available nutraceutical (cholestin, 1999 formulation; Pharmanex, Simi Valley, California) [1]. The active product, lovastatin, was isolated and patented and is now commonly used in pharmacologic therapy of hypercholesterolemia, being administered on the basis of the highest EBM levels of evidence [8–10].

Table 2
Illustration of proposed benefits of nutraceuticals in urinary tract disorders for which evidence was not found

Therapeutic agent	Therapeutic claim[a]	Evidence found in support of a claim for dogs and cats[b]
Kidney "glandulars" (preparations of various endocrine and other tissues)	Induces oral tolerance of dietary allergens	None
Champex (mushroom extract)	Slows progression of chronic kidney disease (CKD)	None
Flaxseed oil (α-linolenic acid rich)	Slows rate of progression of CKD	None
Whey proteins	Inhibits angiotensin-converting enzyme	None
Dandelion	Potassium-sparing diuretic, increases glomerular filtration rate	None
Parsley	Diuretic, anti-bacterial	None
Teas (various)	Increases kidney function, antihypertensive, reduces urinary incontinence	None
Saw palmetto (*Serenoa repens*)	Prostatic anti-inflammatory agent (inhibits conversion of testosterone to dihydrotestosterone)	Negative study in dogs [33]
Plant mixtures (eg, lysimachia, knotweed, plantain seed, rhubarb, cape jasmine, cooked rehmannia, alisma, moutan, aconite, poria, cornus, pyrrosia, mallow fruit, citron fruit, caccaria seed, radish seed, rehmannia root, wolfberry fruit, dogwood fruit, achyranthes root, atractylodes rhizome, eucommia bark, cinnamon bark, pilose asiabell root, dandelion leaf, saw palmetto, climbing fern spore, kidney bean plant extracts, among many others)	Restoration of kidney function, diuresis and relieving stranguria, dissolution of uroliths, anti-inflammatory effects	None

(*continued on next page*)

Table 2 (*continued*)

Therapeutic agent	Therapeutic claim[a]	Evidence found in support of a claim for dogs and cats[b]
Plantain derivatives, akebia, vine, plantago seeds, knot weed, dianthus, pyrrosia, seeds of Job's ears, various fungal preparations, among others	Promotes urination	None

[a] List generated from a survey of the popular press, health food stores, and the Worldwide Web. The author makes no assertion that this list is exhaustive and certainly does not advocate that proposed claims are valid.

[b] To the best of the author's knowledge, on the basis of Medline, and PubMed literature searches and Yahoo and Google Internet searches. Many of these claims are novel, poorly tested, lack proof of safety, and/or are at odds with existing scientific knowledge. This does not prove they are invalid, only that the use of such agents is not warranted without further studies.

The potential utility of functional foods is no stranger to veterinary nephrology, because the first commercial "prescription" diet was developed for use in renal failure in the 1930s by Mark Morris, Sr [11]. Although the main principle behind the original formulations of "kidney diets" was restriction of nutrients, diets formulated for dogs and cats with renal failure now routinely contain nutrients with a demonstrated (or proposed) physiologic function. Common examples in nephrology include polyunsaturated fatty acids (PUFAs) and dietary fibers. Certainly these added "functional" nutrients, and perhaps even the diets themselves, can be classified as functional foods or nutraceuticals. Dietary formulations are routinely recommended for the treatment or prevention of various uroliths, providing another example of the already strong link between veterinary urology and the concept of functional foods. A web site devoted to a new diagnostic test related to renal disease recently advocated the use of nutraceuticals [12]. There are numerous other examples of potential roles for functional food in veterinary nephrology (see Table 3).

Functional foods and chronic kidney disease: the attraction

In traditional Chinese medicine, the kidney is one of five vital systems, being regarded as "the root of life." Given its numerous central functions in maintaining body homeostasis, many veterinary urologists would agree with this concept. Because of the multisystemic effects of chronic kidney disease (CKD) and the history of specialized diets in veterinary nephrology, CKD is a disease process that engenders a clinical approach incorporating the concept of functional foods. A central notion in the management of CKD is that nutritional intake is a critical determinant of an animal's general as well

Table 3
Illustration of proposed benefits of nutraceuticals in urinary tract disorders for which evidence was found

Therapeutic agent	Therapeutic claim[a]	Evidence found in support of a claim for dogs and cats
Protein or amino acid ingestion, meat-based diets	Enhances renal function; slows progression of chronic kidney disease (CKD); reduces prevalence of CKD	Ingestion of protein induces transient increase in glomerular filtration rate and renal plasma flow in many species, including dogs, [34,35]; less known in cats; rationale for this effect is unclear; author unaware of any evidence that meat ingestion has the proposed beneficial effects on CKD
Vegetable protein	Urinary alkalinization	Effect likely for most vegetable-based diets (rationale to seek this effect present only in a few select disease states); by itself, raising urine pH is of no benefit to most animals and may harm those predisposed to certain uroliths
Inulin (oligofructose), various other dietary fiber supplements, probiotics	Enhances gut nitrogen absorption; increases clearance of uremic toxins	Certain mixtures of fiber shown to enhance gut clearance of urea in dogs [36]; trials of probiotic and fiber formulations in animals in progress; evidence that uremic toxin clearance enhanced is inconclusive
Fish oil (eicosapentaenoic and docosahexaenoic acid rich, ω-3 polyunsaturated fatty acids [PUFAs] or n-3 PUFA)	Slows rate of progression of CKD; reduces proteinuria; lowers glomerular pressure	Alters renal eicosanoid production in dogs [30]; reduces glomerular hypertension in dogs [30]; slows rate of progression of CKD in dogs [29]
Vegetable oil (linoleic acid, ω-6 polyunsaturated fatty acids or n-6 PUFA)	Enhances glomerular filtration rate	Short-term benefit in dogs [31]; chronically, worsens proteinuria, reduces survival, and enhances rate of progression of CKD in dogs [29,30]

(*continued on next page*)

Table 3 (*continued*)

Therapeutic agent	Therapeutic claim[a]	Evidence found in support of a claim for dogs and cats
Antioxidants (eg, vitamin E, lycopene, vitamin C, 2-MPG)	Slows rate of progression of CKD	Preliminary results of studies in dogs support this claim (S. Brown, personal observation, 2003)
Carnitine	Reduced dosage of recombinant human erythropoietin required to maintain hematocrit	Supported in people [37]; no studies in veterinary medicine

[a] List generated from a survey of the popular press, health food stores, and the Worldwide Web. The author makes no assertion that this list is exhaustive and does not advocate that proposed claims are valid.

as "renal" health. A published survey confirms that nearly all veterinarians (>99%) recognize the importance of nutritional approaches to CKD in dogs and cats [13].

Other characteristics of CKD make it a frustrating disease to treat, thereby increasing the likelihood of seeking alternative therapies. For example, once acquired, CKD is generally present for, and limits the length of, the animal's life; specific curative treatments are usually not known. CKD is usually progressive, expensive to manage, and characterized by considerable morbidity and, eventually, mortality. Renal replacement (eg, dialysis and transplantation) is expensive and of limited availability. In the face of this frustrating scenario, claims of benefit from nutraceuticals may seem more attractive to frustrated owners (and veterinarians). Particularly attractive claims are those for palliative effects, such as enhancing kidney health or regeneration of renal tissue (see Table 2). Indeed, in one survey of pet owners, 29% had considered or tried nutraceuticals for their animal with CKD [14].

There are troubling historical characteristics of our approach to CKD that make nutraceuticals with unfounded claims difficult to refute. Since the 1930s, nutrition has been thought to play a role in protecting kidneys from damage and limiting clinical signs of affected animals. Unfortunately, the nutritional modification originally advocated for CKD in people, dogs, and cats was dietary protein restriction. This recommendation was based largely on studies in a heterologous species (rats) and thus is now taken to be a low-level evidence (see level 5 of Table 1). Dietary protein restriction in early CKD to delay disease progression is now suspect in all other species, causing a prominent medical nephrologist to recently comment: "The benefit of a low-protein diet in slowing progression of renal failure [in people] is negligible" [15,16]. It should be emphasized that veterinarians did adhere to principles of EBM by initially following the best evidence available (original evidence was a level 5 study in rodents) until new information was developed that refuted the claims for benefits in CKD of dietary protein restriction using blind, controlled, randomized laboratory studies in the homologous species (level 1.5 or type A laboratory studies) [17–19].

Nutraceuticals and chronic kidney disease: the conflict

For many reasons, nutraceuticals are met with skepticism in veterinary medicine. The language of nutraceutical claims (eg, promotes "kidney health," increases "kidney-qi," or removes "retained bladder air") varies dramatically from the more familiar terminology that describes physiologic effects of therapy mechanistically (eg, acidifying or antihypertensive agent). In part, this is artificial, because the FDA has standard policy guidelines for nutraceutical versus pharmaceutical claims, which increase this dichotomy by requiring that nutraceutical claims avoid assertions that the agent can cure or prevent a disease but generally allowing claims that nutraceuticals affect organ or body health in some nebulous manner.

Nutraceutical claims are often made in association with therapeutic modalities that are unfamiliar to veterinarians, such as acupuncture, chiropractic manipulation, and homeopathy. There is often mutual inherent distrust between those practicing traditional veterinary medicine and those offering these alternative therapies. Studies of nutraceuticals are often published in literature unfamiliar to veterinarians (eg, *Journal of the American Nutraceutical Association*). Limited regulation by the FDA permits unfounded claims, poor manufacturing processes, and safety concerns to permeate the nutraceutical market, obscuring viable products with viable claims. The incredible expense of developing a compound for approval by the FDA as a pharmaceutical agent inhibits proper development of nutraceutical claims where small markets or inadequate resources are available. Despite these differences, veterinarians are often open to nontraditional therapies and approaches to disease; they are likely to accept claims for functional foods on the basis of EBM principles. The question is straightforward: is there high-level evidence in support of therapeutic claims and safety in the treatment of urinary tract disorders in the species of interest?

Nutraceuticals and chronic kidney disease: toward a resolution

Veterinary urology has relied heavily on nutritional approaches to disease, and the claims for some nutraceuticals are supported by evidence (see Table 3). For it to be appropriate for a nutraceutical to be used in our patients, we must conduct studies of efficacy and safety and establish standards for production free from contamination with guaranteed bioavailability. Because anecdotal evidence and claims based on tradition are not acceptable evidence for making therapeutic choices in veterinary urology, there is often no support in the EBM paradigm for most nutraceutical claims (see Table 2). There is a common concept that natural products, particularly those of plant origins, are inherently safer than pharmaceutical agents. Veterinarians, being accustomed to treating herbivorous animals for plant toxicities and aware of the origins of many pharmaceutical agents, inherently recognize that such claims are nonsense. Easter Lilies are "natural" but hardly a safe food for a cat. Although it is likely that most claims of benefit for nutraceuticals will prove false, and it is at least as likely that some of these recommended therapies are toxic, there is considerable potential for a few of these health claims to provide valid therapeutic alternatives. Such claims (see Table 2) do present nephrologists with a number of testable hypotheses that can, and in some cases should, be pursued and evaluated more fully.

Polyunsaturated fatty acids and chronic kidney disease: a tale of two oils

One of the key discoveries of modern nephrology is that animals [20] (including dogs [21] and cats [22]) with renal insufficiency exhibit increased intraglomerular pressure. This "glomerular hypertension" is maladaptive and a primary cause of progressive renal injury [20,23,24]. Nath and colleagues [25] proposed that increased levels of renal eicosanoid production were responsible for these changes in glomerular hemodynamics based on their studies of various rodent models of renal insufficiency.

In 1988, on the basis of these findings and a published study in a rodent model of renal failure [26], we proposed that dietary fish oil supplementation might alter renal eicosanoid production, reducing glomerular pressure and slowing the progression of CKD in dogs. At that time, the use of dietary fish oil supplementation was not recommended, largely because of the low-level support for benefit of laboratory studies in rodents (type B laboratory studies, level 5; see Table 1) being applicable to dogs, heterogeneity of results in published work, and concerns about possible toxicity.

A study of urinary eicosanoid excretion in dogs with renal insufficiency demonstrated that there is a severalfold increase in eicosanoid excretion per nephron [27]. Thus, in an animal with CKD, remaining nephrons are characterized by hyperproduction of eicosanoids, specifically prostaglandin E2 and thromboxane A2.

Because dogs with reduced kidney function exhibit a relative increase in renal eicosanoid production, we reasoned that excessive production of vasoactive eicosanoids could play a role in the genesis of the glomerular hypertension observed in dogs with CKD. Our hypothesis is that dietary ω-6 PUFA supplementation would heighten prostaglandin E2 or thromboxane A2 production, thus exacerbating glomerular hypertension (when compared with a low-PUFA diet). In the short-term, this effect of ω-6 PUFA might increase the glomerular filtration rate, but in so doing, it would be expected to hasten the progression to end-stage renal failure. We further reasoned that ω-3 PUFA supplementation (ω-3 PUFA, approximately 1 g, for 250 kcal of metabolizable energy in the diet) would lower glomerular pressure by interfering with the production of these two-series vasoactive proinflammatory eicosanoids (the less active three-series eicosanoids are produced by renal cells from ω-3 PUFA substrates [25,28]). Our results [29,30] confirmed our hypothesis: ω-6 PUFA supplementation increased urinary eicosanoid excretion and glomerular hypertension and worsened proteinuria, renal injury, and the development of end-stage uremia. A clinical study confirmed the expected transient increases in glomerular filtration rate from ω-6 PUFA supplementation in CKD [31]. More critically, our results demonstrated that ω-3 PUFA supplementation lowered renal eicosanoid excretion, reduced intraglomerular pressure, and exerted long-term benefits for canine CKD. On the basis of the proposed EBM for veterinary nephrology (see Table 1), this constitutes level 1.5 evidence and served as a clear rationale for incorporating ω-3 PUFA into diets for dogs with CKD and for avoiding ω-6 PUFA in early canine CKD. It is important to follow-up these results with a double-blind, controlled, randomized clinical trial to ascertain more fully the applicability of these findings to our canine clinical patients (level 1 evidence is always preferred). Applicable long-term clinical trials are in progress; although not directly testing our hypothesis, results of a randomized controlled clinical trial consistent with these type A laboratory studies have recently been published [32].

Functional foods and nephrology: summary

There is clearly a link between functional foods and veterinary urology. The link between CKD and nutraceuticals is explored herein, but there are functional food approaches to many other diseases of the urinary tract, including urolithiasis in particular. Several key points characterize the relation between nutraceuticals and urinary tract disorders:

- With the continuing use of the Internet and relatively low cost of marketing and without regulatory intervention, pet owners and veterinarians will be increasingly bombarded with claims for benefits of nutraceuticals in the treatment of urinary tract disorders.
- Veterinarians are familiar with this approach and open-minded in this regard. Nutritional approaches to disorders of the urinary tract, particularly CKD and urolithiasis, have long been a standard part of veterinary therapy.
- Functional foods can have beneficial and adverse effects in managing diseases of the urinary tract. For example, there is high-level evidence that the nutraceutical fish oil, or ω-3 PUFA, has a beneficial effect in dogs with CKD. There is equally reliable evidence that ω-6 PUFA represents a nutraceutical with adverse long-term effects in dogs with CKD.

- Veterinarians have demonstrated they are open to novel therapies that use nutraceuticals in the treatment of urinary tract disorders but only if supported by reliable evidence of benefit and safety.
- Veterinary urologists should consider the myriad of nutraceutical claims and determine which claims are potentially viable enough to be treated as hypotheses worthy of further scientific evaluation.
- In making therapeutic choices for disorders of the urinary tract, veterinarians are obligated to adhere to the principles that are codified in EBM.

References

[1] Brower B. Nutraceuticals: posed for a healthy slice of the market. Nat Biotechnol 1998;16: 728–33.
[2] Bull E, Rapport L, Lockwood R. What is a nutraceutical? Pharm J 2000;265:57–8.
[3] Jack DB. Keep taking the tomatoes—the exciting world of nutraceuticals. Mol Med Today 1995;1:118–21.
[4] Sackett DL, Rosenberg W, Gray J, et al. Evidence based medicine: what is and what it isn't. BMJ 1996;312:71–2.
[5] Evidence Based Medicine Working Group. A new approach to teaching the practice of medicine. JAMA 1992;268:2420–5.
[6] Guyatt GH. Evidence-based medicine. Ann Intern Med 1991;114:576–81.
[7] Kanto I, Dfonikyan LA, Simon R, et al. Results of a study evaluating use of a dietary supplement formula in the management of age-related skin changes in women with moderate to severe wrinkling of the periorbital area. J Am Nutraceutical Assoc 2002; 5:10–9.
[8] Amsterdam EA. Lower is better: the Heart Protection Study. Prev Cardiol 2002;5:166–7.
[9] Asztalos BF, Horvath KV, McNamara JR, et al. Comparing the effects of five different statins on the HDL subpopulation profiles of coronary heart disease patients. Atherosclerosis 2002;164:361–9.
[10] Singh BK, Mehta JL. Management of dyslipidemia in the primary prevention of coronary heart disease. Curr Opin Cardiol 2002;17:503–11.
[11] Haselbush WC. Thirsty dogs and a blind man. In: Mark Morris veterinarian. Chicago: RR Donnelley & Sons; 1984. p. 81–102.
[12] Heska Corporation. ERD-screen test. Available at: http://www.heska.com/eerdscreen/questions.asp. Accessed March 12, 2003.
[13] Ralston Purina. State of the American Pet Survey. Available at: http://www.purina.com/institute/survey. Accessed March 12, 2003.
[14] Animal Protection Institute Companion Animal Nutrition Survey. Association of Veterinarians for Animal Rights. Available at: http://www.api4animals.org/doc.asp. Accessed March 15, 2003.
[15] Klahr S, Levey AS, Beck GJ, et al. The effects of dietary protein restriction and blood-pressure control on the progression of chronic renal diseases. N Engl J Med 1994;330:877–84.
[16] Ruggenenti P, Schieppati A, Remuzzi G. Progression, remission, regression of chronic renal diseases. Lancet 2001;357:1601–8.
[17] Bovee KC. High dietary protein intake does not cause progressive renal failure in dogs after 75% nephrectomy or aging. Semin Vet Med Surg (Small Anim) 1992;7:227–36.
[18] Finco DR, Brown SA, Crowell WA, et al. Effects of aging and dietary protein intake on uninephrectomized geriatric dogs. Am J Vet Res 1994;55:1282–90.

[19] Finco D, Brown S, Crowell W, Groves C, Barsanti J. Effects of dietary phosphorus and protein on dogs with chronic renal failure. Am J Vet Res 1992;53:2264–71.
[20] Brenner BM, Meyer TW, Hostetter TH, et al. Dietary protein intake and the progressive nature of kidney disease: the role of hemodynamically mediated glomerular injury in the pathogenesis of progressive glomerular sclerosis in aging, renal ablation, and intrinsic renal disease. N Engl J Med 1982;307:652–9.
[21] Brown S, Finco D, Choat D, Navar L. Single nephron adaptations to partial renal ablation in dogs. Am J Physiol Renal Fluid Electrolyte Physiol 1990;258(27):F495–F503.
[22] Brown SA, Brown CA. Single nephron adaptations to partial renal ablation in cats. Am J Physiol 1995;269:R1002–8.
[23] Brown SA, Barsanti J, Finco DR. Pathophysiology and management of progressive renal disease in dogs. Br Vet J 1996;152:1–24.
[24] Brown SA. Evaluation of chronic renal disease: a staged approach. Compend Contin Educ Pract Vet 1999;21:752–63.
[25] Nath KA, Chmielewski DH, Hostetter TH. Regulatory role of prostanoids in glomerular microcirculation of remnant nephrons. Am J Physiol 1987;252:F829–37.
[26] Scharschmidt LA, Gibbons NB, McGarry L, et al. Effects of dietary fish oil on renal insufficiency in rats with subtotal nephrectomy. Kidney Int 1987;32:700–9.
[27] Brown SA, Finco DR, Brown CA. Is there a role for dietary polyunsaturated fatty acid supplementation in canine renal disease? J Nutr 1998;128:2765–7.
[28] Hostetter TH, Nath KA. Role of prostaglandins in experimental renal disease. Contrib Nephrol 1989;75:13–8.
[29] Brown SA, Brown C, Crowell W, Barsanti J, Finco DR. Effects of dietary fatty acid composition on the course of chronic renal disease in dogs. J Lab Clin Med 1998;131: 447–55.
[30] Brown SA, Brown C, Crowell W, Barsanti J, Finco DR. Effect of dietary fatty acid supplementation in early renal insufficiency in dogs. J Lab Clin Med 2000;135:275–86.
[31] Bauer J, Crocker R, Markwell P, et al. Dietary n-6 fatty acid supplementation improves glomerular ultrafiltration in spontaneous canine chronic renal failure [abstract]. J Vet Intern Med 1997;11:126.
[32] Jacob F, Polzin DJ, Osborne CA, et al. Clinical evaluation of dietary modification for treatment of spontaneous chronic renal failure in dogs. J Am Vet Med Assoc 2002;220: 1163–70.
[33] Barsanti JA, Finco DR, Mahaffey MM, et al. Effects of an extract of Serenoa repens on dogs with hyperplasia of the prostate gland. Am J Vet Res 2000;61:880–5.
[34] Brown SA, Navar LG. Single nephron responses to parenteral administration of amino acids in dogs. Am J Physiol Renal Fluid Electrolyte Physiol 1990;259(28):F739–46.
[35] Brown S, Finco D. Characterization of the renal response to protein ingestion in dogs with experimentally induced chronic renal failure. Am J Vet Res 1992;53:569–73.
[36] Brown SA. Dietary fiber affects intestinal urea clearance in dogs with renal insufficiency. Presented at the Iams International Nutrition Symposium. Chicago, May 14, 2000.
[37] Kletzmayr J, Mayer G, Legenstein E, et al. Anemia and carnitine supplementation in hemodialyzed patients. Kidney Int 1999;55(Suppl):S93–106.

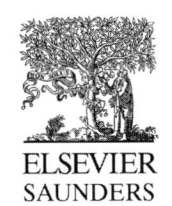

Vet Clin Small Anim
34 (2004) 187–216

Traditional and nontraditional effective and noneffective therapies for cardiac disease in dogs and cats

Paul D. Pion, DVM

Veterinary Information Network, 777 West Covell Boulevard, Davis, CA 95616, USA

Law of conservation of ignorance

> A false conclusion once arrived at and widely held is not easily dislodged and the less it is understood, the more tenaciously it is held —Georg Cantor (1845–1918) —Mathematician/philosopher, developer of concept of infinity

Veterinary cardiology has advanced greatly in the past two decades. The widespread availability of imaging technology has opened the door for greater understanding and assessment of cardiovascular disease. If one considers how little veterinary cardiovascular therapeutics have advanced during the same period, however, it becomes clear that the advances in veterinary cardiology we perceive are largely the result of improved diagnostic rather than therapeutic acumen and skill.

In the therapeutic realm, the state of the art remains largely limited to what might be called "Band-Aid therapies," which palliate the effects of cardiovascular disease for a short duration but do little to address the primary disease process. Further progress in the management of the more common cardiovascular diseases affecting dogs and cats will likely require greater focus on surgical options and greater understanding of underlying genetic, degenerative, autoimmune, metabolic, nutritional, and inflammatory causes of the primary lesions involved.

Surprisingly, many of the more exciting advances in cardiovascular therapy in the past two decades have not come from the development of new pharmaceutics. Instead, physical manipulations (balloon dilation of stenotic valves and pacemaker implantation) and nutritional management of cardiac disease have leapt forward as solutions for certain cardiac diseases affecting dogs and cats.

E-mail address: Paul@vin.com

0195-5616/04/$ - see front matter © 2004 P.D. Pion. Published by Elsevier Inc.
doi:10.1016/j.cvsm.2003.10.012

As recently as the mid-1980s, few would have believed that nutrition and biochemistry might hold the key to understanding common cardiac diseases in dogs and cats. At that time, our understanding of nutrition and cardiology was focused primarily on the sodium content of diets fed to patients suffering from congestive heart failure (CHF).

Today, we know that the amino acid taurine plays a primary role in the pathogenesis and management of what we used to classify as feline dilated cardiomyopathy (DCM) [1–5]. In addition, we strongly suspect that taurine (and possibly carnitine) have a place in the pathogenesis and treatment of some cases of canine DCM. There are also increasing (and as of yet undocumented) claims of clinical efficacy of coenzyme Q_{10}, vitamin E, fish oils, and other nutrients in the management of cardiovascular disease in dogs and cats.

The purpose of this article is to focus attention on what we know about management of cardiovascular disease in dogs with nontraditional therapeutics. In this pursuit, it is important to realize that much of the information circulating in support of common therapeutic recommendations and printed in veterinary textbooks and journals (including this one) is derived from well-meaning but weakly supported sources, including the clinical impression of influential members of our profession.

When one looks for the origin of these recommendations, many commonly accepted opinions and recommendations are found to be based on anecdotal experience and small, often poorly controlled, clinical and experimental studies in the veterinary literature; extrapolation from the human literature (a similarly imperfect and inexact scientific collection); claims by companies selling prescription diets, pharmaceutics, and nutraceuticals; and perpetuation of hearsay in unrefereed trade magazines.

Only the hindsight provided by looking back at our current state from the future will allow us to know which data, anecdotes, and hunches circulating today are correct. Therefore, our present responsibility to ourselves, our clients, our patients, and our colleagues centers on an open and honest application of therapeutics and ideas so as not to increase hope falsely for the patients of today or diminish faith in what real advances the future might hold.

Good health is the slowest rate at which one can die

From a "holistic" perspective, maintaining good health can be reduced to a simple set of rules:

Rule 1: choose your parents wisely. Start life with good genes.
Rule 2: You are what you eat. Eat a nutritionally complete and balanced diet.
Rule 3: Be careful out there. Avoid traumatic injuries.
Rule 4: Your body is a temple. Avoid exposure to metabolic or cellular toxins or toxin generators.

Rule 5: Take your medicine. When ill, take advantage of the best available evidence to cure or palliate the disease or clinical signs.

Some are within the control of our patients, their sire and dam, their owners, their veterinarian, or society as a whole. Some, such as being in the path of a natural disaster, are random and outside the control of any individual. Follow these simple rules, and the chance of the individual organism maintaining good health is improved.

Advancing from witch doctor to real doctor: how far have we come?

Individual organisms are composed of organ systems, which are composed of organs, which are composed of cells of various types. Each cell is composed of organelles. At multiple levels, these systems are designed to counter entropy, that is, to control and contain electrochemical reactions, a process we call "life."

As medical science advances, our targets for preventive, curative, and palliative care increasingly aim at more specific targets.

Initially, we focused on how the external world affects the individual. We explained disease as punishment for "insulting the Gods." As therapy, we performed sacrifices and ceremonial dances to appease the Gods or ward off evil spirits.

As we became more aware of the form (anatomy) and function (physiology and biochemistry) of life, the focus of medicine moved from blaming and attempting to appease external "Gods and Spirits" to attempts to alter the internal milieu. We did not know why, but many early therapies, such as bloodletting, applying leeches, and chewing willow bark (the first use of salicylates) or foxglove (the first use of digitalis glycosides), were truly beneficial. Like many modern day therapies, these therapies were discovered by serendipity.

Today, we understand why these therapies work at a molecular level. As we peel back the mysteries of life, we better understand (without the need to invoke "mystical spirits") why early "healers" recognized these therapies as beneficial and passed them from generation to generation.

Less easy to understand is how therapies we can now explain the toxicity of, and know to be quite harmful, survived the same "test of time." Today, it is hard for us to understand why administering heavy metals like arsenic or mercury was ever considered beneficial. Perhaps these practices survived the test of time because, at the doses used, their detrimental effects are more chronic and the practitioners of the day were unable to associate a causal effect.

Today, we read or hear about therapies from a century ago—or even as recent as one, two, or three decades ago—and are amazed at what was considered "standard practice." We think we have come so far. We think we base treatment of our patients on the best science, sticking to the facts. If that were true, this article would be much shorter. It could be summed up in one short list for veterinary cardiology.

After 20 years of focusing on veterinary cardiology, it is my conclusion that we, like our ancestors, remain highly susceptible to what I consider beliefs driven from superstition and our desire to claim victory over ailments for which we do not yet possess effective preventive treatments or therapies.

What follows are three lists of treatments that I believe encompasses the sum total of treatments that, when applied appropriately, do (list 1), likely may (list 2), or have a high theoretic probability of being proven to (list 3) prevent disease or prolong or improve the quality of life for veterinary cardiac patients. Certainly, my bias is unavoidable, and some treatments will be proven not to belong in the list I have assigned them to.

Please note that I intentionally excluded heartworm disease prevention and treatment so as to avoid confusion. Also, I have kept my descriptions nonspecific so as to avoid attempting to write an entire text on cardiovascular therapy on this single page. The reader is encouraged to consult appropriate references for details regarding appropriate indications and application of these therapies.

List 1 (strong literature documentation backed by wide-ranging clinical experience):

- Diuretics, specifically furosemide, prolong the life of patients with CHF[1]
- Calcium entry blocker (specifically amlodipine) for cats (and perhaps dogs) with systemic hypertension
- Treatment of underlying hyperthyroidism in patients with thyrotoxic heart disease
- Taurine (and perhaps carnitine) supplementation to reverse myocardial failure in cats and dogs with taurine deficiency-induced myocardial failure[2]
- Carnitine supplementation in rare cases of dogs with familial carnitine deficiency-induced myocardial failure
- Surgery or other interventions that "close" a patent ductus arteriosus
- Physical removal of pericardial effusion, pleural effusion, or ascites
- Pacemaker implantation in patients with appropriate and symptomatic bradyarrhythmias

---

[1] Interestingly, despite the widely held belief that furosemide is the most valuable therapeutic agent for the treatment of CHF in veterinary patients, there are no published studies documenting this in a placebo-controlled manner. Nonetheless, the immediate cause and effect—you give it and they urinate and breath better—unquestionably argues for inclusion in this list.

[2] One could argue whether this should be considered an effective therapy or simple "patch" that compensates for shortcomings in our ability to formulate diets for companion animals.

List 2 (anecdotal literature documentation backed by some clinical experience):

- Appropriate antiarrhythmic drugs for "clinically significant" or "life-threatening" supraventricular or ventricular arrhythmias
- Anticholinergics or β2 agonists for dogs with symptomatic bradyarrhythmias that respond to therapy or are not candidates for pacemaker implantation[3]
- Angiotensin-converting enzyme (ACE) inhibitors may reduce the dose of diuretic needed and prolong the life of patients with CHF taking diuretics
- Afterload reduction with nitroprusside (acute), hydralazine, or amlodipine in dogs with advanced mitral regurgitation
- Low-molecular-weight heparins for prevention of recurrence of feline aortic thromboemboli
- Balloon dilation of the pulmonic valve in patients with pulmonic stenosis[3]

List 3 (high theoretic probability but no direct clinical evidence in dogs or cats):

- ACE inhibitors or spironolactone may reduce fibrosis in the myocardium or improve diastolic function in patients with diseases where intramyocardial fibrosis is a significant component (eg, hypertrophic cardiomyopathy)

Before the intent of these lists is shot down because it is judged as "wrong," I go on record as freely admitting that I could argue for another set of slightly differently lists. The precise content of the lists remains open to debate and perhaps would be an interesting exercise to pursue. Nevertheless, the point remains that whatever the ultimate content and organization of the lists, the brevity of this admittedly imperfect version demonstrates that veterinary cardiology cannot currently claim to have many proven therapies based on good placebo-controlled clinical trials. Much of what we feel certain about comes from widely based clinical experience. Next comes what we believe from "some clinical experience" and then what we want to believe based on a specific need and a theoretic basis for believing a therapy should work or a strong desire to extrapolate evidence from other species.

The largest challenge associated with the latter approach, extrapolation, is to be sure that we are extrapolating between similar indications. A specific example that deserves mention is coenzyme Q_{10} (CoQ_{10}). CoQ_{10} is absent from the lists, because there is no clinical evidence or documented clinical

---

[3] The evidence for a true clinical benefit is more in question than literature-documented efficacy.

experience that supports its use in veterinary patients with cardiac disease. Yet, it is commonly mentioned as being of general benefit in cardiac patients. I believe this misplaced faith in CoQ_{10} evolved for three reasons: first, because it is the perfect substrate for theorizing a benefit; second, because there are some data in other species that provide fertile ground for inappropriate extrapolation; and, third, because there is a commercial veterinary product available.

1. CoQ_{10} is a perfect substrate for theorizing a benefit because it is central to the function of every aerobically metabolizing cell. Knowing that, how could it not be of benefit? Although on a superficial level, I would not question that it "might" be of benefit, the current reality is that CoQ_{10} has been given to many patients, and, to my knowledge, there is no demonstrable benefit that can be proven to be associated with the administration of CoQ_{10}. To be fair, I also know of no harm coming from the administration of CoQ_{10}. That is not the question we are addressing, however. If we go "there," I could continue this article with lists of tens, perhaps hundreds, of compounds found within cardiac cells with known physiologic activity that "might" be of benefit if given as a supplement. Let's not go down that "slippery slope."
2. There is inappropriate extrapolation, because although there are data demonstrating benefit from giving CoQ_{10} to human patients and experimental animals, this does not justify applying these data to our patients. The problem with this logic is that most of the data applies to human beings and animals with spontaneous or induced ischemic cardiac disease. This type of extensive ischemic damage is not believed to be a significant component of any common canine or feline cardiac diseases.
3. Finally, and perhaps most germane to motivating a bias toward CoQ_{10}, there is a commercial formulation for sale. Unfortunately, commercial availability sometimes blurs the lines between recommendations being based on the best marketing rather than on the best medicine.

   In closing this somewhat drawn out introductory section, what likely jumps out, given the focus of this monograph, is the absence of any suggestion that nontraditional therapies other than taurine, and perhaps carnitine, have a place in clinical veterinary practice. If you have taken that message to heart, you can read the next two short sections and then stop reading, because the rest of what I have to say is repetition of what has been reported many times before in many formats.

What is out there?

In three recent overviews of this topic, two veterinary and one human medical, the authors mention similar lists of nutrients or nutraceuticals as important to cardiac health (Table 1).

Table 1
Nutrients or nutraceuticals with importance to cardiac health suggested in the literature

	Keene [65]	Freeman [66]	Saff et al [67]	Proposed target	Documented evidence of benefit in canine or feline patients
Carnitine	X	X	X	FFA transport across mitochondrial membranes and facilitates carbohydrate metabolism	Improves myocardial function in rare cases of carnitine deficiency–induced myocardial failure (DCM) in dogs [68] May play a role in the therapy of dogs with taurine deficiency myocardial failure [22]
Taurine	X	X	X	Unknown	Improves myocardial function in canine and feline cases of taurine deficiency–induced myocardial failure [1,22]
Arginine		X	X	Endothelium, enhanced NO production	None
Coenzyme Q_{10}	X	X	X	Mitochondrial metabolic pathways	None
Antioxidants					
Vitamin E	X	X			None
Vitamin C	X	X			None
Beta carotene	X	X			None
Glutathione peroxidase		X			None
Selenium	X				None
Superoxide dismutase		X			None
Catalase		X			None
N-acetyl-L-upsteine			X	SH donor, free radical scavenger	None
Flavonoids			X	Free radical scavenger	None
β-sitosterol			X	Hypolipidemic	None
Creatine			X	Skeletal muscle, ADP- >ATP	None
n-3 fatty acids		X		Inflammatory mediators	May improve cachexia in dogs with stable CHF [69]

Abbreviations: ADP, adenosine diphusphate; ATP, adenosine triphosphate; DCM, dilated cardiomyopathy; FFA, free fatty acid.

Now, pay attention, here comes the main message of this entire article. This list includes compounds that are physiologically or biochemically active at various levels. Nothing in this article is intended to question the validity of the nutritional, biochemical, or metabolic function of these compounds or their metabolites. Nevertheless, being a metabolically active component, an antioxidant, part of a complete and balanced dietary formulation, or even an essential or conditionally essential nutrient does not justify elevating a compound to the level of an effective therapy. To make that leap and prevent us from leaping to the dark side of peddling "snake oil," where marketing overrides medicine, we must have documented and repeatable evidence that the proposed therapy makes a clinically significant improvement that results in a measurable improvement in quality or quantity of life in individual patients.

As noted previously, shamefully few traditional therapies meet these criteria. This realization should not justify elevating similarly unproved nontraditional therapies, however. It should motivate the elimination of false claims and hope for ineffective traditional or nutritional therapies until such time as we gain new insights providing the evidence we need to elevate their status as an effective therapy. To do otherwise is irresponsible, and those who promote other standards should be eliminated from positions of influence within our professional community.

Our current state of affairs

If the focus of this issue and this article is intended to present what we know about therapies that effectively alter cellular mechanisms of disease, there is only one story (perhaps two stories) worth documenting. They are the evidence supporting the specific indications and benefits of taurine (and perhaps carnitine) in veterinary cardiac patients. I will state one more time that there is no clinically significant evidence supporting the cardiac benefit of other nutrients or nutraceuticals beyond what is considered appropriate for a complete and balanced diet.

I may be overconcerned with semantics, but it is worth emphasizing that even when considering taurine (and perhaps carnitine), we may remain guilty of falsely assigning a higher status as "therapeutic" when, in fact, what we have documented is "phenomenology" that (1) taurine (in some way that we do not yet understand) is essential for normal myocardial function and (2) we can design commercial and homemade diets capable of messing up our patients' taurine nutrition to the degree that we create pathologic findings that seem to respond to the administration of "magic white crystals."

No doubt, observing, documenting, and experimentally reproducing this phenomenon has had a significant clinical and commercial impact on feline and canine medicine. Hopefully, we have also opened doorways to better understanding the nutrition of our patients and myocardial function at a cellular level in all species. Perhaps these will lead to effective therapeutic strategies some day. For the moment, however, we need to be careful not to let the serendipitous appearance of success dupe us into believing we have curing "powers." All we have done is to correct prior errors in our path of advancement.

Taurine and carnitine in canine and feline cardiology

The sections on taurine and carnitine are largely based on a prior article in this journal entitled "The effectiveness of taurine and L-carnitine in dogs with heart disease" [6], written in conjunction with Drs. Sherry L. Sanderson and Mark D. Kittleson. In this article, I include primarily information relating to the clinical reality of these compounds as I see them today. Please refer to the previously cited article and the references for more extensive discussions of the known and theorized physiology, biochemistry, and pharmacology of these compounds.

What is taurine?

Taurine (2-aminoethanesulfonic acid) is a sulfur containing amino acid. Taurine is primarily found in animals but is only seldom found in plants [7].

Initially identified in the bile of bovines, for which it was named, taurine plays a significant role in bile acid conjugation in many species. Most taurine is found intracellularly dissolved in the cytosolic fluid and bound to cell membranes. Tissues with the highest taurine concentrations include the heart, retina, central nervous system, and skeletal muscle [8]. Taurine is also present in high concentrations in white blood cells and platelets [9,10]. The commonalty is that taurine is important in "excitable tissues." These high tissue taurine concentrations are maintained by active transport of taurine from extracellular fluid to the intracellular space, which is modulated by the β-adrenergic receptor-adenyl cyclase system [11].

Other than conjugation of bile acids and the detoxification of xenobiotics via conjugation and excretion in bile, the function of taurine in mammals is not well understood [7]. It has been known since the mid-1970s that taurine is essential for normal retinal function in cats [12]. Clinical and experimental evidence collected in the late 1980s documents that taurine is essential for normal myocardial function [1,13–16]. Despite these and other in vivo and in vitro studies illustrating the varied and ubiquitous effects of taurine in mammals, the basis for these effects remains unknown.

After thinking about this problem for almost two decades, I conclude that the best explanation of taurine's function was communicated to me by Dr. Ryan Huxtable, whom many consider to be the father of taurine in modern biology. When asked what taurine does, Dr Huxtable responded with the question: "What does water do in the cell?" The point is that water is the most ubiquitous ingredient in living beings. Although it has specific functions, such as being the primary fluid (and solvent) both intra- and extracellularly as well as an essential nutrient and most voluminous excretory solvent, defining the specific function of water intracellularly is not currently possible.

One could spend a lifetime documenting phenomenology describing how altering water or taurine content in cells alters the function of specific receptors, macromolecules, and cellular functions within the aqueous, lipid, and proteinaceous components of cells.

What Dr Huxtable was communicating, and I believe is true, is that water and taurine alter the internal milieu for biochemical reactions. They contribute to defining the physical chemistry of cellular reactions even when they do not directly participate in them. In the case of water, this is relatively easy to document without resorting to extreme conditions, whereas in the case of taurine, the beneficial and protective effects of taurine are often not easily documented until the excitable cell, tissue, or organ under study is exposed to some form of "stress," whether the specific stress is ischemia, hypocalcemia, or exposure to doxorubicin.

Taurine and the cat

Low tissue concentration of cysteine-sulfinic acid decarboxylase (CSAD), a key enzyme in the biosynthesis of taurine [17], has been reported as the reason why cats have a limited ability to synthesize taurine from cysteine and methionine. This low synthetic ability is not unique to the cat (eg, human beings also have limited synthetic ability), however, and it is unlikely that this alone is sufficient to explain the cat's propensity for developing low plasma taurine concentrations and associated abnormalities.

Many mammals preferentially use taurine for bile acid conjugation, forming taurocholic acid; however, if taurine is in low supply, glycine can be used so that the major bile acid produced is glycocholate (the glycine conjugate). Cats are unable to conjugate significant amounts of their bile acids with glycine [18]. They use taurine exclusively for bile acid conjugation even when dietary taurine is restricted. Continued biliary taurine loss combined with a low synthetic ability predisposes the cat to becoming taurine depleted [17].

As an obligate carnivore, the feral cat has little risk of developing taurine deficiency. The modern practice of feeding pet cats commercially produced foods (many based on plant products) and our incomplete understanding of nutrition have put pet cats at risk for becoming taurine deficient. Clusters of taurine deficiency in the pet cat population resulting from dependence on commercial diets and ignorance have served to define clinical states (ie, retinal degeneration, DCM, infertility) associated with taurine deficiency.

From a global perspective, these events have served basic and medical science by unintentionally using the pet cat population as a large clinical laboratory that has helped to advance our understanding of taurine nutrition and pathobiology. Unfortunately, the costs to the pet-owning public, feline patients, and veterinary profession have been high. The silver lining in this cloud is the knowledge gained and the resultant widespread modification of standards for feline diet formulations. The most important of these modifications in our thinking is that it is now widely understood that it is not appropriate to formulate a diet based on current guidelines for nutritional requirements alone. To prove that a diet is complete and balanced for all life stages, it must be fed to a large group of animals living through the life stages that the diet is claimed to support.

Taurine and the dog

Taurine is not an essential amino acid in the dog. Normal dogs fed diets with little or no taurine maintain plasma and whole blood taurine concentrations similar to those found in the normal cat [19]. The activity of CSAD (the rate-limiting enzyme in the synthesis of taurine) is high in the dog compared with the cat [20]. Activity of this enzyme alone does not fully explain the difference in the requirement between these two species, however, because the activity of this enzyme in human beings is even lower than in the cat and taurine is not an essential amino acid in human beings. Dogs also conjugate bile acids solely with taurine [21], whereas people can conjugate with taurine or glycine. Thus, species differences in the balance between taurine synthesis and biliary taurine loss during bile acid conjugation qualitatively explain the dietary need for taurine in the cat and the lack of a dietary requirement in most healthy dogs and human beings.

Until recently, it was thought that taurine deficiency was not a clinical issue to consider when managing canine patients. Data collected in the past decade suggest that taurine deficiency should be considered when formulating a differential diagnosis for DCM in dogs [19,22,23]. To what degree pathologic findings of taurine deficiency in dogs are attributable to aberrations in the taurine metabolism of certain individual or breeds of dogs or ongoing errors in the assumptions used in formulating commercial diets remains to be determined.

Taurine and the heart: what does taurine do in the heart?

Extensive literature exists describing in vivo and in vitro physiologic phenomena related to modulation of myocardial or cardiac function associated with alterations in intracellular and extracellular taurine concentration [7,13–15,24–27].

These observations, coupled with the high concentration of taurine normally found in the heart, led many investigators to speculate that taurine depletion might lead to a clinically significant reduction in myocardial mechanical function. The identification of taurine deficiency-induced myocardial failure in pet cats, and its reversal after taurine administration [1–4], was the first direct evidence that taurine deficiency can cause a clinically significant decrement in myocardial mechanical function in vivo. The mechanisms underlying these effects remain unknown.

Taurine deficiency-induced myocardial failure

An association between DCM in pet cats, low plasma taurine concentration, and diet was reported in 1987 [1]. This phenomenon has been reproduced in experimental animals [4] and was independently confirmed in a multicenter clinical study [28]. A similar association between taurine deficiency and myocardial failure in foxes [29] and dogs [19,22] has been documented.

Taurine deficiency-induced myocardial failure should be suspected when myocardial failure is found concurrent with low plasma, whole blood, or tissue taurine concentrations or when other systemic evidence of taurine deficiency (ie, central retinal degeneration) is present. Confirmation of the causative nature of taurine deficiency in an individual patient requires documenting normalization of myocardial function after taurine supplementation.

Taurine deficiency-induced myocardial failure in cats

DCM or congestive cardiomyopathy was not widely recognized in cats until the early 1970s [30,31]. The clinical findings, response to treatment, and gross and microscopic pathologic findings of this disease have been described [32–35]. In 1987, it was determined that many cats presenting with DCM were taurine deficient and that supplementation with taurine reversed the myocardial failure. Therefore, much of the literature referring to idiopathic DCM in cats is strongly suspected to be referring to taurine deficiency-induced myocardial failure, which is a nutritional secondary cardiomyopathy rather than idiopathic DCM. To date, there are no criteria other than a lack of response to taurine in a patient that survives for a sufficient time that can conclusively differentiate between taurine deficiency-induced myocardial failure and primary idiopathic DCM in cats.

Not all taurine-deficient cats develop myocardial failure. In repeated studies performed at the University of California at Davis, approximately 25% of all (n > 100) cats depleted of taurine for more than 2 years developed overt myocardial failure. The other factor(s) required for taurine deficiency to cause overt myocardial failure are unknown. A genetic predisposition has been proposed [36]. It is reasonable to assume that nutritional taurine deficiency combined with other causes of myocardial "stress" (eg, congenital or acquired left ventricular volume overload; toxic, ischemic, nutritional, endocrine, or metabolic problems) may lead to synergistic complicating effects.

Taurine deficiency in cats is believed to be a direct result of inadequate amounts of taurine in the diet in most cases and is thus preventable. A precise requirement for taurine cannot be determined for all foods, because the requirement is dependent on many factors [17,37–39]. For this reason, no commercial diet should be assumed to be taurine sufficient until the manufacturer has provided feeding trial data documenting that the food maintains normal taurine concentrations in blood and tissue while feeding for at least 6 months. In general, supplementation of commercial cat foods with additional taurine has greatly reduced the prevalence of DCM in cats.

Clinical presentation

The presenting complaints, signalment, and physical examination findings are similar to those of other forms of feline cardiomyopathy [2]. Funduscopic evidence of taurine deficiency-induced central retinal degeneration in a cat with evidence of cardiac disease should increase suspicion of taurine deficiency-induced myocardial failure. Taurine deficiency-induced retinal lesions are permanent, however; thus, documenting retinal degeneration is evidence of taurine deficiency at some time in the cat's life but not proof of current taurine deficiency. In addition, not all taurine-deficient cats with myocardial failure develop central retinal degeneration, and absence of retinal lesions in a cat with myocardial failure does not rule out the diagnosis of taurine deficiency-induced myocardial failure.

Ancillary tests like electrocardiography and thoracic radiography cannot definitively discriminate between taurine deficiency-induced myocardial failure and other forms of feline cardiac disease. Echocardiography can detect myocardial failure but cannot confirm the underlying cause.

Diet history should be ascertained during the initial workup of any cat with myocardial failure. Many owners have managed to formulate diets with inadequate amounts of taurine and need to be educated to prevent recurrence. In addition, it is likely that a small number of cases will continue to be the result of commercial cat foods containing inadequate amounts of taurine.

The veterinary profession remains the most effective sentinel for detecting patterns with regard to diet and disease occurrence.

Cats diagnosed with any form of myocardial failure should have plasma and whole blood taurine concentrations determined on blood samples obtained before taurine administration, because a single dose of taurine makes interpretation difficult. Sample handling is critical for accurate results.

The following guidelines should be used in handling samples for taurine analysis:

1. Submit heparinized plasma and heparinized whole blood.[4]
2. Draw the sample into a syringe "wetted" with heparin.
3. Remove the needle from the syringe, and gently transfer the blood sample to an open-topped blood tube.
4. Place the sample on wet ice or immediately centrifuge the sample and separate plasma immediately.
5. Make sure samples to be used to harvest plasma contain no clots or hemolysis.
6. Store and ship samples chilled or frozen (dry ice or ice packs).

Normal values:

1. Plasma (normal) greater than 60 nmol/mL
   a. At risk: less than 30 nmol/mL
      i. Comment: plasma taurine concentration is extremely labile; 24 hours of fasting can cause plasma concentrations to fall below 30 nmol/mL.
2. Whole blood (normal) greater than 200 nmol/mL
   a. At risk: less than 100 nmol/mL
      i. Comment: whole blood taurine concentration is not as labile. Fasting does not significantly affect values.

Therapy

1. During the initial phase of therapy, proper supportive and symptomatic care for CHF is essential if CHF is present.
2. Digoxin is not an essential component of therapy, nor is it contraindicated.
3. Cats with documented taurine deficiency should be supplemented with taurine, 250 mg, orally every 12 hours until echocardiographically determined left ventricular dimensions normalize. This usually occurs within 4 months. Clinical improvement (eg, attitude, appetite) is usually evident within 2 weeks.
4. Diuretics and ACE inhibitors can be discontinued when signs of CHF resolve. The ACE inhibitor should be removed first, with the diuretic then tapered over a period of 2 weeks. While withdrawing heart failure medications, the owner should be taught to monitor respiratory rate and instructed to return to the clinic for evaluation if the respiratory rate

---

[4] If a choice must be made, the whole blood analysis is most important and likely most tolerant to "mishandling" during sample acquisition and shipment.

increases above 30 breaths per minute. Clinical and radiographic evaluation should be repeated 1 week after withdrawing medications to detect any decline in the cat's condition.
5. The diet should be altered to maintain normal plasma and whole blood taurine concentrations.
6. Taurine supplementation can be discontinued once echocardiographic values return to within normal limits.
7. Taurine concentration in plasma and whole blood should be monitored periodically to be certain that the diet fed is maintaining concentrations within acceptable limits. If taurine concentrations are depleted again, many cats will redevelop myocardial failure.

Prognosis

Because the results of taurine analysis are not immediately known, all cats with myocardial failure should be prescribed taurine supplementation and given an initially guarded to grave prognosis. In one study [3], 30% of cats with myocardial failure died within the first week after diagnosis. Hypothermia and thromboembolic disease were associated with a poor prognosis. Taurine supplementation did not provide benefit with regard to survival until 2 weeks after treatment was begun. Cats that survive 1 week and respond to treatment for CHF can be upgraded to having a fair prognosis. Cats that survive 2 weeks and are shown to be taurine deficient can be upgraded to a good prognosis.

Most taurine-responsive cats have complete reversal of echocardiographic and clinical evidence of myocardial failure after supplementation with taurine [3]. Occasionally, cats have residual mild myocardial failure (25%-30% left ventricular shortening fraction); however, these cats are generally asymptomatic and rarely require any form of therapy other than maintaining normal plasma taurine concentrations.

Does taurine play a role in canine cardiac health management?

Biology

Taurine is not an essential amino acid in the dog. Normal dogs fed diets with little or no taurine maintain plasma and whole blood taurine concentrations similar to those found in normal cats [19]. The activity of CSAD (the rate-limiting enzyme in the synthesis of taurine from cysteine and methionine) is high in the dog compared with the cat [20]. The activity of this enzyme alone does not fully explain the difference in the requirement between these two species, however, because the activity of this enzyme in human beings is even lower than in the cat and taurine is not an essential amino acid in people. Dogs, like cats, conjugate bile acids solely with taurine [21], whereas human beings can conjugate with taurine or glycine. Thus, species differences in the balance between taurine synthesis and biliary taurine loss during bile acid conjugation qualitatively explain the dietary need for taurine in the cat and the lack of a dietary requirement in most healthy dogs and human beings. Until recently, it was thought that taurine deficiency was not a clinical issue to consider when managing canine patients.

Early negative results

Soon after the identification of taurine deficiency myocardial failure in cats, the Cardiology Service at the University of California at Davis began adding taurine to the therapeutic regimen of dogs presenting with DCM. Approximately 10 dogs presenting with idiopathic DCM were treated with standard therapy plus taurine, 1 g, twice daily and followed for at least 4 months or until death (P. Pion, unpublished data). Four months was chosen as an end point, because this was the maximum time it had taken to observe improvement in the cats under study [3]. None of these dogs were found to have a low plasma taurine concentration or demonstrated marked echocardiographic improvement as had been observed in cats. In addition, feeding neither taurine-free diets nor diets with taurine but found to be taurine depleting [2] in cats was significantly taurine depleting when fed to a group of 8 laboratory Beagle dogs (P. Pion, unpublished data). As a result of these early negative results, the University of California at Davis group abandoned canine taurine studies with the exception of continuing to collect and "bank" plasma samples from dogs with DCM for potential future consideration of "unknown factors."

Collaboration between University of California at Davis and the Animal Medical Center reveals low plasma taurine concentration in some breeds of dogs with dilated myocardiopathy

Several years later, these plasma samples from dogs seen at the University of California at Davis with primarily DCM were analyzed for taurine concentration along with plasma samples collected from dogs with primarily chronic degenerative mitral valve disease seen at the Animal Medical Center in New York City. After accounting for somewhat different collection techniques, including anticoagulant used during blood collection, an interesting pattern emerged [19]. It was found that plasma taurine concentration in dogs with chronic valvular disease was slightly elevated above normal. This finding is noteworthy but likely of little clinical significance.

Of greater interest was the finding that plasma taurine concentration was low in 17% of the 75 dogs with DCM studied. Plasma taurine concentration was not decreased in the breeds that are more commonly afflicted with DCM. Instead, all the American Cocker Spaniels (three of three dogs), three of the five Golden Retrievers, and four of the seven atypical or mixed breeds with DCM in this study had a low plasma taurine concentration.

Combined with the prior anecdotal taurine treatment failures in dogs with DCM, this study provided the current belief that taurine deficiency does not seem to play an important role in the etiopathogenesis or therapy of DCM in the more commonly affected breeds.

Design, execution, results, conclusions, and lessons learned from the Multicenter Spaniel Trial study

Kramer et al's study [19] provided the impetus for examining American Cocker Spaniels with DCM for taurine deficiency and response to taurine supplementation. The first two American Cocker Spaniels treated with taurine supplementation did not respond. The next two American Cocker Spaniels presented to Kittleson et al [22] with DCM were treated with taurine and L-carnitine. Both dogs responded to this combined therapy despite the fact that plasma taurine but not plasma carnitine concentration was decreased in these dogs.

As a result of these observations, it was decided to design a study that would examine American Cocker Spaniels before and after supplementation with taurine (500 mg three times daily) and L-carnitine (1000 mg three times daily). The study was performed as a randomized, double-blind, placebo-controlled, partial crossover design. In other words, neither the investigators overseeing and performing the study nor the clients administering the medications had knowledge of which medication was being administered (double-blind) during the first segment of the study.

Eleven American Cocker Spaniels with DCM were entered into the trial (the Multicenter Spaniel Trial [MUST]). All were found to have a low plasma taurine concentration at baseline. For purposes of this study, low plasma taurine concentration was defined as less than 50 nmol/mL based on a survey of 10 normal American Cocker Spaniel dogs.

During the first segment, six dogs were randomly assigned to the taurine-carnitine treatment group and five were assigned to the placebo group. Dogs in the taurine-carnitine treatment group demonstrated echocardiographic improvement after 2 to 4 months of therapy, whereas those in the placebo pill group did not. After this initial segment, the treatment group to which each patient was assigned was made available to the investigators, and those on placebo were then crossed over to the taurine-carnitine treatment group. Those initially assigned to the taurine-carnitine treatment group were not crossed over to placebo for ethical reasons. After being crossed over to the taurine-carnitine treatment, dogs initially assigned to the placebo group similarly improved over the next 2 to 4 months. The improved myocardial performance allowed the investigators to discontinue cardiovascular drug therapy in each dog.

In summary, echocardiographic measures of myocardial performance and clinical signs improved in America Cocker Spaniel dogs with DCM after taurine-carnitine supplementation. The magnitude of echocardiographic improvement was not as dramatic as seen after treating cats with taurine deficiency myocardial failure [3]. Nevertheless, cardiovascular drug support could be removed 3 to 4 months after starting supplementation with taurine and L-carnitine.

This study illustrates important considerations with regard to research evaluating therapy in clinical patients with DCM. First, we need a hypothesis. The hypothesis usually arises from a "hunch" based on prior work in (1) nonliving systems (chemicals, membranes, cells, or tissue slices in a test tube or perfused tissues or organs), (2) experimental animals of the same or different species, or (3) clinical observations in the same or different species.

What must never be forgotten is that the answers we can derive from this type of clinical study are fully dependent on the questions we ask. In this case, the initial intent was to ask: "Is taurine supplementation beneficial to taurine-deficient American Cocker Spaniels with DCM?" After considering the poor response to taurine supplementation alone in two dogs before beginning the study, however, it was decided to add carnitine to the treatment regimen used in the MUST study. As a result, we now know that American Cocker Spaniels with DCM are taurine deficient (as defined by the investigators) but not plasma carnitine deficient and respond to taurine and carnitine supplementation.

Based on this study, we cannot conclude if taurine or carnitine alone would be sufficient to have produced a similar effect in this breed of dog. We also cannot conclude if a similar response should be expected in other "atypical" breeds developing DCM, nor can we conclusively state that similar (taurine and carnitine) therapy in Doberman Pinschers and other more "typical" breeds for developing DCM would not be similarly positive.

Since the publication of this study, there has been at least one documented report [40] of echocardiographic and clinical improvement in one taurine-deficient American Cocker Spaniel treated with only taurine supplementation, so carnitine may not be required in all American Cocker Spaniels. I have also heard a significant number of anecdotal reports from colleagues with canine patients with what appears to be taurine deficiency-induced myocardial failure that responded to taurine supplementation alone.

To determine whether taurine or L-carnitine can independently produce improvement similar to that seen in the MUST trial, a similar trial needs to be repeated using taurine or carnitine supplementation only. In the interim, it is prudent to recommend that carnitine and taurine be supplemented to American Cocker Spaniels with DCM unless the owner cannot afford carnitine. In this situation, taurine alone can be tried first. If no response is identified, the addition of carnitine supplementation should be strongly recommended.

Another important lesson from this study is in carefully considering the design of the study. When the initial studies documenting the benefits of taurine supplementation in cats with DCM and taurine deficiency were begun, the intent was to perform these in a double-blind and placebo-controlled manner. While evaluating the first few feline patients and the early data in laboratory-housed cats, however, it was decided that the preliminary evidence was too overwhelming to justify not treating clinical patients with taurine. This was an ethically based but risky decision. Had the initial positive responses and patterns not continued, the data might not have been strong enough to withstand scrutiny. In fact, had the MUST study been performed in this manner (not randomized, not placebo controlled, not a crossover design), the MUST data might have been judged inconclusive during the peer review process. The magnitude of the changes would not have been sufficient to rule out the possibility that the echocardiographic changes observed were a result of chance or the natural history of the disease.

It should also be noted that the MUST study involved only 11 dogs. The clinical experience of the authors and anecdotal reports from the veterinary community support the results and conclusions of the MUST study. Before accepting the results, however, the profession would be well served by replication by an independent group of investigators. A difficulty in the MUST study that must be considered in future studies testing these readily available nutrients relates to clients' natural desire to have their pet in the treatment group. A few dogs in the MUST study that were initially assigned to the placebo group were excluded because the recheck plasma taurine concentration was higher than that ever seen in any other unsupplemented dogs. This suggested that the owners had supplemented their pets on their own. This type of monitoring regarding compliance is essential. It should also be mentioned that the need to exclude these "contaminated" patients in a study with so few participants represents a potential weakness in the study.

Other data supporting the continued search to understand the relation between taurine deficiency and myocardial failure in dogs

For more detail, the reader is referred to an article in a prior issue of this journal [6]. As a quick review and update, the following is provided:

1. Freeman et al [41] reported nine cases of DCM diagnosed in nine male Dalmatians. Four of the dogs had a history of urate crystalluria or urate urolithiasis. Eight of the nine dogs had been fed a low-protein diet (Canine u/d Prescription Diet; Hill's Pet Nutrition, Topeka, Kansas) for all or part of their lives. Taurine concentration was measured in four of these dogs, with at least one dog having a plasma taurine level of less than 50 nmol/mL. The total myocardial carnitine concentration was normal in the one dog in which it was determined. These dogs were initially treated with standard therapeutic drugs (various combinations of furosemide, an ACE inhibitor, and digoxin) plus taurine (two dogs), coenzyme Q_{10}, (two dogs), and L-carnitine (three dogs). Seven of the

nine dogs were switched to different diets at the time of diagnosis. Significant improvement in myocardial function was reported in one dog after diet change.
2. Sanderson and her colleagues evaluated plasma taurine concentration in a population of 15 dogs with cystine and urate urolithiasis (unpublished data). Thirteen of the 15 dogs were determined to have plasma taurine deficiency (plasma taurine <41 nmol/mL), with a mean plasma taurine concentration of 13.8 nmol/mL. Four of 15 dogs had echocardiographic evidence of DCM at the time of initial observations. All 4 dogs had low plasma taurine concentrations, and 2 of 3 dogs that had an endomyocardial biopsy performed had a low myocardial carnitine concentration. Three other dogs in this group of 15 subsequently developed DCM during the observation period. Two of the 3 dogs had low plasma taurine concentrations. An endomyocardial biopsy was performed in only 1 of these dogs, and it had a low myocardial carnitine concentration. In addition, plasma carnitine was low in 1 of the 2 dogs in which an endomyocardial biopsy was not performed. After treatment with conventional therapy as needed to control CHF plus carnitine and taurine, myocardial function improved in all dogs and echocardiographic parameters normalized in 2 of these dogs. Interestingly, DCM recrudesced in 1 of these dogs after the owner stopped carnitine and taurine supplementation. Related data were published in 2001 [42].
3. Further work by Sanderson et al [43] with Beagle dogs fed high-fat low-protein diets suggest that the taurine deficiencies induced by these diets can lead to reduced myocardial function. Progress toward developing an experimental model of taurine (and possibly carnitine) deficiency that results in myocardial failure in the dog is an exciting prospect for advancing our understanding of canine and human cardiac function in health and disease.

A major gap in the MUST study is the absence of whole blood or tissue documentation of taurine deficiency. Canine plasma is not believed to be as labile with respect to taurine concentration as feline plasma [9], but true verification of taurine deficiency requires measurement of tissue taurine concentrations. One interesting finding not included in the MUST study report is that at least three American Cocker Spaniels with a low plasma taurine concentration and DCM that responded to taurine supplementation were observed to have bilaterally symmetric hyperreflective retinal lesions similar to those seen in cats with taurine deficiency (M.D. Kittleson and P. Pion, unpublished data).

Why are some dogs susceptible to taurine deficiency?

Because taurine is present in high concentrations in myocardium and, from several lines of evidence, seems to be essential to normal myocardial function, it is not surprising that a taurine-deficient dog might develop myocardial disease. The more important remaining question, however, is why some dogs seem to be conditionally susceptible to developing taurine deficiency.

Largely untested explanations for why dogs might develop taurine deficiency include reduced taurine synthesis, increased urinary loss, and increased intestinal loss. Gavaghan and Kittleson [40] examined renal clearance of taurine in one American Cocker Spaniel with DCM and found a low plasma taurine concentration. Fractional excretion of taurine in this dog was deemed to be modestly increased. Dogs, like cats, preferentially use taurine for bile acid conjugation, and they cannot readily convert to use of glycine even when taurine pools in the body are depleted. As a result, dogs have at least one known risk factor for developing taurine deficiency in common with cats, and it has recently been shown by Sanderson et al [43] that feeding a high-fat low-protein diet can result in significant reduction of taurine in plasma, whole blood, and tissues in the dog. Whether these dietary manipulations lead to taurine deficiency via setting the stage for bacterial overgrowth and interruption of normal enterohepatic circulation of taurine-conjugated bile acids with increased fecal taurine losses as documented in the cat [44] remains under study.

What we know to date is:

1. American Cocker Spaniels and a few other breeds with DCM may be taurine deficient and often respond to taurine supplementation [22].
2. Cystinuria may be a risk factor for developing taurine (and possibly carnitine deficiency) [42].
3. Feeding diets with low sulfur amino acids or containing rice (usually as a part of a lamb and rice formulation) may be a risk factor for developing taurine deficiency and myocardial failure [45–48].

What is L-carnitine

L-carnitine (β-hydroxy-γ-trimethylaminobutyric acid) is a small (molecular weight = 160) water-soluble molecule. In the dog, L-carnitine is synthesized primarily in the liver from the amino acids lysine and methionine. L-carnitine is concentrated in mammalian cardiac and skeletal muscle by an active membrane transport mechanism. In normal mammals, including dogs, plasma carnitine concentrations correlate closely with myocardial carnitine concentration. This close correlation is sometimes lost in canine DCM.

What does carnitine do in the heart?

The normal heart obtains approximately 60% of its total energy production from fatty acid oxidation [49]. L-carnitine plays an essential role in this process and likely also plays an important role in the regulation of glucose metabolism within the heart [50]. Like taurine, L-carnitine has also been proposed to play many other roles in the heart [51–53].

Free fatty acids in the cytosol are converted to their "reactive form" by combining with co-enzyme A (CoA) in a reaction catalyzed by fatty acyl CoA synthetase (thiokinase). B-oxidation of fatty acids occurs within the mitochondrial matrix. Therefore, fatty acids in the cytosol must be transported across the mitochondrial inner membrane, which is generally impermeable to bulky polar molecules, such as CoA. This is accomplished via the "carnitine shuttle." In the carnitine shuttle, the activated fatty acid reacts with carnitine to form a more permeable molecule. This reaction occurs on the outer surface of the inner mitochondrial membrane and is catalyzed by the enzyme carnitine acyltransferase I. This permeable (long-chain acyl-carnitine ester) molecule is transported across the inner mitochondrial membrane, where the long-chain acyl carnitine is converted back to free carnitine and long-chain fatty acids via the enzyme acyltransferase II.

Free carnitine within the mitochondrial inner matrix is also thought to assist in the transport of free acyl groups (R – C = O) across the inner mitochondrial membrane. By buffering the fluctuations in the acetyl CoA-to-free CoA ratio, carnitine may regulate the activity of pyruvate dehydrogenase, the key step in the funneling of pyruvate, the product of glycolysis, into the citric acid cycle. The reader will recall that the citric acid cycle is the final common pathway for the oxidation of fuel molecules: amino acids, fatty acids, and carbohydrates. Most fuel molecules enter the cycle as acetyl CoA via the reaction:

$$\text{Pyruvate} + \text{CoA} + \text{NAD}^+ \rightarrow \text{acetyl CoA} + \text{CO}_2 + \text{NADH}$$

The point of presenting this review in biochemistry is not to confuse or disinterest the reader but to provide a context for understanding why carnitine potentially plays a role in overall energy metabolism in cells. The interested reader is referred to textbooks of biochemistry [54] and general reviews on carnitine [52,55] for more detail on these reactions and mechanisms.

Does L-carnitine play a role in canine cardiac health management?

Biology

L-carnitine is not thought to be an essential nutrient in the diet of the dog. In normal dogs, synthesis in the liver is believed to be adequate. When the L-carnitine concentration in 50 commercial diets was tested in 1991, values determined ranged from 0.7% to 5% of that found in lean ground beef (3500 nmol/g) [56]. Mean plasma L-carnitine concentration increased significantly in laboratory dogs after 1 and 2 weeks of adding ground beef to the diet. Plasma L-carnitine concentration rose from a presupplement concentration of 26.2 ± 4.5 µmol/L to a postdietary supplement concentration of 55.9 ± 3.5 µmol/L after 1 week and 51.9 ± 8 µmol/L after 2 weeks.

L-carnitine deficiency

A variety of clinical signs have been reported in carnitine-deficient human beings, including encephalopathy, muscle weakness, recurrent infections, "failure to thrive," and CHF [57,58]. Carnitine deficiency has been associated with primary myocardial diseases in several species [59], including dogs [60–62]. More widespread studies have not been undertaken in dogs, however, because of the difficulty in thoroughly assessing carnitine status.

Deficiencies of carnitine are classified as either primary or secondary. Primary carnitine deficiencies may arise from genetic defects in synthesis, renal transport, intestinal absorption, or transmembrane uptake mechanisms. Excessive degradation of carnitine is also a possible cause [59]. In human beings, primary carnitine deficiencies have been reported to be associated with cardiomyopathy. These cardiomyopathies are typically not present at birth but usually take 3 to 4 years to develop, and L-carnitine therapy can prevent and reverse the cardiac dysfunction [59].

Secondary carnitine deficiencies are believed to be much more common in human beings and have multiple possible causes [59]. The incidence and genesis of carnitine deficiencies in dogs are unknown.

Currently, carnitine deficiency in the dog is classified descriptively as either plasma carnitine deficiency characterized by low concentrations of free plasma carnitine, systemic carnitine deficiency characterized by low concentrations of free plasma and tissue carnitine, or myopathic carnitine deficiency characterized by low free myocardial carnitine concentrations in the presence of normal and sometimes elevated plasma carnitine concentrations. Plasma carnitine deficiency alone is not a well-documented state and is included to account for the fact that in veterinary practice, plasma carnitine but not tissue carnitine sampling is often pursued.

Therefore, if only plasma carnitine is used to assess the carnitine status of a dog, if it is low, it can be helpful in making the diagnosis of carnitine deficiency. If plasma carnitine is normal, however, this does not rule out the possibility of the myopathic form of carnitine deficiency. Evaluating cardiac muscle carnitine concentrations requires a fluoroscopy-guided endomyocardial biopsy, which is not available in most private practice situations. For these reasons, the diagnosis and determination of the incidence of myopathic carnitine deficiency in asymptomatic dogs and dogs with cardiac disease remain elusive.

L-carnitine deficiency and association with myocardial disease states

Carnitine deficiency has been associated with DCM in dogs in a limited number of clinical reports [60,61,63]. L-carnitine deficiency was initially diagnosed in a family of Boxer dogs [60]. In this family, the sire, the dam, and two littermates had DCM at points in their lives. Only one had a low plasma L-carnitine concentration. This dog also had a low myocardial concentration, and after being treated with high-dose L-carnitine (220 mg/kg/d) orally, his shortening fraction increased from 18% to 28%. This dog's littermate had low myocardial and normal plasma L-carnitine concentrations. This dog similarly responded to administration of high-dose L-carnitine supplementation, increasing its shortening fraction from 2% to 24%. Interestingly, the latter dog experienced a decline in myocardial function after L-carnitine therapy was withdrawn. Both parents of these littermates had a normal plasma and low myocardial concentration. Unfortunately, both parents died soon after beginning L-carnitine supplementation.

This same group in collaboration with others reported the results of determining plasma and myocardial L-carnitine concentrations and subsequent treatment with L-carnitine, 150 mg/kg/d, orally in 18 Doberman Pinschers with DCM and heart failure [62]. Applicable conventional therapy was also given. In these dogs, myocardial carnitine deficiency was seen in 13 of 18 dogs, with plasma carnitine deficiency also present in 1 of 13 dogs. No differences in history, clinical signs, age, sex, severity of heart failure, or cardiac rhythm in dogs with and without myocardial carnitine deficiency were noted. Survival times were significantly longer in dogs with myocardial carnitine deficiency than in dogs with normal myocardial carnitine levels. All 5 dogs with normal myocardial carnitine levels died within 44 days (mean: 21 ± 14). Survival times reported in 11 of the 13 dogs with myocardial carnitine deficiency were less than 44 days (5 of 11 dogs), 60 to 100 days (2 of 11 dogs), 150 to 200 days (2 of 11 dogs), and greater than 365 days (2 of 11 dogs).

Another group presented a case report of two Boxer dogs with DCM [61]. One was treated with L-carnitine, 250 mg/kg, orally per day. The other was untreated. Myocardial concentration of L-carnitine was found to be low in the unsupplemented dog and elevated in the supplemented dog. Another recent report [64] describes a possible case of L-carnitine-responsive cardiomyopathy in a Boxer.

The only other available nonanecdotal data to add to this story are derived from the MUST study and ongoing work by Sanderson and his colleagues as described in the taurine section of this article and a prior review [6].

Interpretation of the available data

It is my impression that after the initial report of success in treating a few cases of DCM in Boxers with carnitine, large numbers of clinicians began treating dogs with DCM with L-carnitine. Now, years later, the general impression in the veterinary community is that the hope for success when treating any single dog with DCM with carnitine is low. When one considers the poor prognosis and lack of effective long-term therapy associated with this disease, however, it is not surprising that clinicians who have a strong need or desire to "do something" continue to grasp at any available options.

Carnitine, like taurine, is safe and relatively free of risk to "try" merely because there is little else to do. Unlike taurine, however, which is inexpensive, L-carnitine therapy can cost $1 to $3 per day depending on the size of the dog and dose chosen. This cost would not seem large if there were a reliable means of selecting which dogs are likely to respond favorably to therapy.

Clinical considerations

Conventional therapy

Independent of suspected or proven carnitine or taurine deficiency, patients with CHF or low-output heart failure require appropriate therapy with diuretics, ACE inhibitors, and digoxin in accordance with current standards of therapy. These therapies should be continued until patients supplemented with taurine or carnitine respond, clinically stabilize, and demonstrate significant echocardiographic improvement in myocardial function. In patients that respond to supplementation, weaning from conventional therapy should be gradual, beginning with removal of digoxin, then ACE inhibitors, and finally diuretics. Patients should be closely monitored throughout the process by the clinician and owner. The safety of the process is best ensured by instructing owners to count and log and report heart rate and respiratory rate at home, frequent communication between the veterinarian and client, and frequent rechecks with chest radiographic evaluation approximately 1 week after each change in medication.

Sample collection

To enable interpretation of the results, it is imperative that any samples collected be acquired before beginning supplementation with taurine or carnitine. Taurine and carnitine are best assessed in heparin anticoagulated plasma samples. A useful protocol follows:

1. "Wet" the surfaces of a 6-mL syringe by drawing up heparin, 1 mL, and allowing it to contact the entire interior barrel of the syringe by pulling back on the plunger with the syringe in an inverted position.
2. Empty the syringe of most of the heparin other than that which remains in the hub after ejecting the heparin back into the multidose vial from which it was drawn.
3. Change needles, and acquire 4 to 6 mL of blood from a vein.
4. Remove the needle, and slowly eject 1 mL of whole blood into a container for whole blood taurine analysis.
5. Eject the remaining volume into a tube, and centrifuge to separate the cells from the plasma.

6. Carefully harvest 1 to 2 mL of plasma from the tube, avoiding the buffy coat layer, and aliquot for shipping in one or two tubes for taurine or carnitine analysis. Consult your laboratory for the preferred method of storage and shipping.

Consult your laboratory for instructions on collection and preparation of tissue samples.

Normal values

Consult your laboratory. The following are guidelines based on current data from Keene and Sanderson (carnitine) and Kramer, Kittleson, and Sanderson (taurine).

Normal plasma and myocardial carnitine concentrations in dogs:

- Plasma carnitine (μmol/L): total (12–38), free (8–36), esterified (0–7)
- Myocardial carnitine (nmol/mg of noncollagenous protein): total (5–13), free (4–11), esterified (0–4)

Normal plasma and whole blood taurine concentrations in dogs (approximate[5]):

- Plasma taurine (nmol/mL): plasma (45–110), whole blood (>250)

Treatment considerations

Both taurine and carnitine are available at health food stores. To ensure the best results, it is wise to use a formulation from a known source. It is important to administer only the L-isomer of carnitine, because D-carnitine inactivates carnitine-containing enzyme systems and mammals have no endogenous ability to convert D-carnitine to L-carnitine. Neither D-carnitine nor the racemic mixture (D-L-carnitine) can be safely administered.

Both taurine and carnitine seem to be extremely safe, and the risk of therapy is minimal.

Taurine is quite inexpensive, but the financial cost of carnitine (approximately $80-$200 per month depending on the source) is substantial.

Recommended doses in dogs are as follows:

Carnitine
Large dogs (25–40 kg) receive 2 g (approximately 1 teaspoonful of the commercially available pure substance) mixed with food three times daily.
Small dogs (<25 kg) receive 1 g mixed with food three times daily.
Taurine
Large dogs (25–40 kg) receive 1 to 2 g orally (can be mixed with food) two to three times daily.

---

[5] Derived from combined observations at the University of California at Davis and University of Minnesota. The precise concentration at which disease susceptibility becomes a concern remains unclear.

Small dogs (<25 kg) receive 500 to 1000 mg mixed with food three times daily.

There is a wide variation in the literature regarding doses recommended for carnitine supplementation in dogs with DCM. The effective therapeutic dose may depend on the form of carnitine deficiency present, and a minimal effective dose has not been established yet.

In cases where it is elected to use L-carnitine, a suggested dose is 200 mg/kg administered orally three times daily. In the few cases where L-carnitine seemed effective, objective echocardiographic improvement was not observed for 3 to 4 months. Therefore, to fully evaluate whether carnitine supplementation is going to be beneficial in a dog with DCM, it is important to not only use a high enough dose but to use it for a long enough time during the trial period.

Summary

In this article, I presented my (admittedly biased) perspective of the current state of knowledge addressing the role of traditional and nontraditional therapeutics. The focus has been on the nontraditional therapeutics. Among these, the only ones I currently consider to have any documented value are taurine and, less commonly, L-carnitine. The role of taurine (and likely carnitine) remains limited to cases of documented deficiency. In the case of cats with taurine deficiency-induced myocardial failure, it is now clear that most cases are the result of formulation errors by owners and manufacturers. In dogs, it is less clear if the causes of taurine deficiencies represent manifestations of pathologic conditions or dietary formulations errors. Increasingly, it seems the latter may prove to be the case in most, if not all, circumstances.

Finally, I would like to reiterate the conclusions of the last time I addressed this topic (with coauthors Kittleson and Sanderson) in this publication. Remember that there is limited evidence to support the therapeutic recommendations you read or hear in most circumstances. The urge to do "something" for patients can be overwhelmingly attractive. Nevertheless, whether it is administration of drugs or prescribing nutraceuticals or prescription diets, strongly consider the source of the information urging you to prescribe, the strength of the evidence presented, the financial costs to the owner, and the potential risks and benefits to the patient.

References

[1] Pion PD, Kittleson MD, Rogers QR, Morris JG. Myocardial failure in cats associated with low plasma taurine: a reversible cardiomyopathy. Science 1987;237:764–8.
[2] Pion PD, Kittleson MD, Thomas WP, Skiles ML, Rogers QR. Clinical findings in cats with dilated cardiomyopathy and relationship of findings to taurine deficiency. J Am Vet Med Assoc 1992;201(2):267–74.

[3] Pion PD, Kittleson MD, Thomas WP, DeLellis LA, Rogers QR. Dilated cardiomyopathy in the cat: response to taurine supplementation. J Am Vet Med Assoc 1992;201:275–84.
[4] Pion PD, Kittleson MD, Skiles ML, Rogers QR, Morris JG. Dilated cardiomyopathy associated with taurine deficiency in the domestic cat: relationship to diet and myocardial taurine content. Adv Exp Med Biol 1992;315:63–73.
[5] Fox PR, Sturman JA. Myocardial taurine concentrations in cats with cardiac disease and in healthy cats fed taurine-modified diets. Am J Vet Res 1992;53(2):237–41.
[6] Pion PD, Sanderson SL, Kittleson MD. The effectiveness of taurine and levocarnitine in dogs with heart disease. Vet Clin North Am Small Anim Pract 1998;28(6):1495–514.
[7] Huxtable RJ. Physiological actions of taurine. Physiol Rev 1992;72(1):101–63.
[8] Sturman JA, Gargano AD, Messing JM, Imaki H. Feline maternal taurine deficiency: effect on mother and offspring. J Nutr 1986;116(4):655–67.
[9] Pion PD, Lewis J, Greene K, Rogers QR, Morris JG, Kittleson MD. Effect of meal-feeding and food deprivation on plasma and whole blood taurine concentrations in cats. J Nutr 1991;121(11 Suppl):S177–S178.
[10] Schuller-Levis G, Mehta PD, Rudelli R, Sturman J. Immunologic consequences of taurine deficiency in cats. J Leukoc Biol 1990;47(4):321–31.
[11] Huxtable RJ, Chubb J, Azari J. Physiological and experimental regulation of taurine content in the heart. Fed Proc 1980;39(9):2685–90.
[12] Hayes KC, Carey RE, Schmidt SY. Retinal degeneration associated with taurine deficiency in the cat. Science 1975;188(4191):949–51.
[13] Huxtable RJ. From heart to hypothesis: a mechanism for the calcium modulatory actions of taurine. Adv Exp Med Biol 1987;217:371–87.
[14] Takihara K, Azuma J, Awata N, Ohta H, Hamaguchi T, Sawamura A, et al. Beneficial effect of taurine in rabbits with chronic congestive heart failure. Am Heart J 1986;112(6):1278–84.
[15] Azuma J, Sawamura A, Awata N, Ohta H, Hamaguchi T, Harada H, et al. Therapeutic effect of taurine in congestive heart failure: a double-blind crossover trial. Clin Cardiol 1985;8(5):276–82.
[16] Schaffer SW, Seyed-Mozaffari M, Kramer J, Tan BH. Effect of taurine depletion and treatment on cardiac contractility and metabolism. Prog Clin Biol Res 1985;179:167–75.
[17] Morris JH, Rogers QR. The metabolic basis for the taurine requirement of cats. Adv Exp Med Biol 1992;315:33–44.
[18] Rabin B, Nicolosi RJ, Hayes KC. Dietary influences on bile acid conjugation in the cat. J Nutr 1976;106:1241–6.
[19] Kramer GA, Kittleson MD, Fox PR, et al. Plasma taurine concentrations in normal dogs and in dogs with heart disease. J Vet Intern Med 1995;9(4):253–8.
[20] Jacobsen JG, Thomas LL, Smith LH Jr. Properties and distribution of mammalian L-cysteine sulfinate carboxylases. Biochem Biophys Acta 1964;85:103–16.
[21] Haslewood GAD. The biological significance of chemical differences in bile salts. Biol Rev 1964;39:537–74.
[22] Kittleson MD, Keene B, Pion PD, et al. Results of the Multicenter Spaniel Trial (MUST): taurine- and carnitine-responsive dilated cardiomyopathy in American Cocker Spaniels with decreased plasma taurine concentration. J Vet Intern Med 1997;11(4):204–11.
[23] Kittleson MD, Pion PD, DeLellis LA, Tobias AH. Dilated cardiomyopathy in American cocker spaniels—taurine deficiency and preliminary results of response to supplementation. Presented at the American College of Veterinary Internal Medicine Scientific Proceedings, New Orleans, 1991.
[24] Hamaguchi T, Azuma J, Schaffer S. Interaction of taurine with methionine: inhibition of myocardial phospholipid methyltransferase. J Cardiovasc Pharmacol 1991;18(2):224–30.
[25] Lake N. Loss of cardiac myofibrils: mechanism of contractile deficits induced by taurine deficiency. Am J Physiol 1993;264(4 Part 2):H1323–26.

[26] Steele DS, Smith GL, Miller DJ. The effects of taurine on Ca2+ uptake by the sarcoplasmic reticulum and Ca2+ sensitivity of chemically skinned rat heart. J Physiol (Lond) 1990;422:499–511.
[27] Gentile S, Bologna E, Terracina D, Angelico M. Taurine-induced diuresis and natriuresis in cirrhotic patients with ascites. Life Sci 1994;54(21):1585–93.
[28] Sisson DD, Knight KH, Helinski C, Fox PR, Bond BR, Harpster NK, et al. Plasma taurine concentrations and M-mode echocardiographic measures in healthy cats and in cats with dilated cardiomyopathy. J Vet Intern Med 1991;5:232–8.
[29] Moise NS, Pacioretty LM, Kallfelz FA, Stipanuk MH, King JM, Gilmour RF. Dietary taurine deficiency and dilated cardiomyopathy in the fox. Am Heart J 1991;121:541–7.
[30] Liu S-K. Congestive heart failure in the cat. J Am Vet Med Assoc 1970;156(9):1319–30.
[31] Harpster, N.K., Acquired heart disease in the cat. In: Proceedings of the 40th Annual Meeting of the American Animal Hospital Association. Denver (CO): American Animal Hospital Association; 1973. p. 118–25.
[32] Liu SK. Pathology of feline heart disease. Vet Clin North Am Small Anim Pract 1977;7(2):323–39.
[33] Liu SK, Tilley LP. Animal models of myocardial diseases. Yale J Biol Med 1980;53:191–211.
[34] Van Vleet JF, Ferrans VJ, Weirich WE. Pathologic alterations in hypertrophic and congestive cardiomyopathy of cats. Am J Vet Res 1980;41:2037–48.
[35] Lord PF, Wood A, Tilley LP, Liu SK. Radiographic and hemodynamic evaluation of cardiomyopathy and thromboembolism in the cat. J Am Vet Med Assoc 1974;164(2):154–65.
[36] Lawler DF, Templeton AJ, Monti KL. Evidence for genetic involvement in feline dilated cardiomyopathy. J Vet Intern Med 1993;7(6):383–7.
[37] Hickman MA, Bruss ML, Morris JG, Rogers QR. Dietary protein source (soybean vs. casein) and taurine status affect kinetics of the enterohepatic circulation of taurocholic acid in cats. J Nutr 1992;122(4):1019–28.
[38] Hickman MA, Rogers QR, Morris JG. Taurine balance is different in cats fed purified and commercial diets. J Nutr 1992;122(3):553–9.
[39] Hickman MA, Rogers QR, Morris JG. Effect of processing on fate of dietary [14C] taurine in cats. J Nutr 1990;120(9):995–1000.
[40] Gavaghan BJ, Kittleson MD. Dilated cardiomyopathy in an American Cocker Spaniel with taurine deficiency. Aust Vet J 1997;75(12):862–8.
[41] Freeman LM, Michel KE, Brown DJ, Kaplan PM, Stamoulis ME, Rosenthal SL, et al. Idiopathic dilated cardiomyopathy in Dalmatians: nine cases (1990–1995). J Am Vet Med Assoc 1996;209(9):1592–6.
[42] Sanderson SL, Osborne CA, Lulich JP, Bartges JW. Evaluation of urinary carnitine and taurine excretion in 5 cystinuric dogs with carnitine and taurine deficiency. J Vet Intern Med 2001;15(2):94–100.
[43] Sanderson SL, Gross KL, Ogburn PN, Calvert C, et al. Effects of dietary fat and L-carnitine on plasma and whole blood taurine concentrations and cardiac function in healthy dogs fed protein-restricted diets. Am J Vet Res 2001;62(10):1616–23.
[44] Kim SW, Rogers QR, Morris JG. Dietary antibiotics decrease taurine loss in cats fed a canned heat-processed diet. J Nutr 1996;126(2):509–15.
[45] Torres CL, Backus RC, Fascetti AJ, Rogers QR. Taurine status in normal dogs fed a commercial diet associated with taurine deficiency and dilated cardiomyopathy. J Anim Physiol Anim Nutr (Berl) 2003;87(9–10):9–10.
[46] Stratton-Phelps M, Backus RC, Rogers QR, Fascetti AJ. Dietary rice bran decreases plasma and whole-blood taurine in cats. J Nutr 2002;132(6 Suppl 2):1745S–7S.
[47] Backus RC, Cohen GL, Pion PD, Good KL, Rogers QR, Fascetti AJ. Taurine deficiency in Newfoundlands fed commercially available complete and balanced diets. J Am Vet Med Assoc 2003;223:1130–6.

[48] Fascetti AJ, Reed JR, Rogers QR, Backus RC. Taurine deficiency in dogs with dilated cardiomyopathy: 12 Cases (1997–2001). J Am Vet Med Assoc 2003;223:1137–41.

[49] Neely JR, Morgan HA. Relationship between carbohydrate metabolism and energy balance of heart muscle. Annu Rev Physiol 1974;36:413–59.

[50] Broderic TL, Panagakis G, DiDomenico D, Gamble J, Lopaschuk GD, Shug AL, et al. L-carnitine improvement of cardiac function is associated with a stimulation in glucose but not fatty acid metabolism in carnitine-deficient hearts. Cardiovasc Res 1995;30:815–20.

[51] Bremer J. Carnitine—metabolism and functions. Physiol Rev 1983;63(4):1420.

[52] Rebouche CJ, Paulson DJ. Carnitine metabolism and functions in humans. Annu Rev Nutr 1986;6:41–66.

[53] Arsenian MA. Carnitine and its derivatives in cardiovascular disease. Prog Cardiovasc Dis 1997;40:265–86.

[54] Mayes PA. Oxidation of fatty acids: ketogenesis. In: Murray RK, Granner DK, Mayes PA, Rodwell VW, editors. Harper's biochemistry. 24th edition. East Norwalk, CT: Appleton & Lange; 1996. p. 224–35.

[55] Leibovitz BE. Carnitine. Advanced Research Press Inc; 1987. 1–13.

[56] Keene BW, Mier HC, Meurs KM, Schmidt MJ, Shug AL. Dietary L-carnitine deficiency and plasma L-carnitine concentrations in dogs [abstract]. J Vet Intern Med 1991;5(2):134.

[57] Engel AG, Angelini C. Carnitine deficiency of human skeletal muscle associated with lipid storage myopathy: a new syndrome. Science 1973;179:899.

[58] Tripp ME, Katcher ML, Peters HA, et al. Systemic carnitine deficiency presenting as familial endocardial fibroelastosis: a treatable cardiomyopathy. N Engl J Med 1981; 305:385.

[59] Paulson DJ. Carnitine deficiency-induced cardiomyopathy. Mol Cell Biochem 1998;180: 33–41.

[60] Keene BW, Panciera DP, Atkins CE, et al. Myocardial L-carnitine deficiency in a family of dogs with dilated cardiomyopathy. J Am Vet Med Assoc 1991;198:647.

[61] Costa ND, Labuc RH. Case report: efficacy of oral carnitine therapy for dilated cardiomyopathy in boxer dogs. J Nutr 1994;124(Suppl):2687S–92S.

[62] Keene W, Kittleson MD, Rush JE, Pion PD, Atkins CE, DeLellis LD, et al. Myocardial carnitine deficiency associated with dilated cardiomyopathy in Doberman Pinschers [abstract]. J Vet Intern Med 1989;3(2):126.

[63] Sanderson S, Osborne C, Ogburn P, et al. Canine cystinuria associated with carnitinuria and carnitine deficiency [abstract]. J Vet Intern Med 1995;9:212.

[64] Frater JL. A possible case of L-carnitine-responsive cardiomyopathy in a Boxer. Aust Vet Pract 2002;32(2):55–9.

[65] Keene BW. Understanding the importance of carnitine, taurine, and other neutraceuticals in the cardiology patient. Proceedings of the American College of Veterinary Internal Medicine. 2002.

[66] Freeman LM. Nutritional therapy of heart disease. In: Waltham/OSU Symposium, Small Animal Cardiology. 2002.

[67] Safi AM, Samala CA, Stein RA. Role of nutraceutical agents in cardiovascular disease: an update—part I. Cardiovasc Rev Rep 2003;24(7):381–91.

[68] Keene BW, Panciera DP, Atkins CE, et al. Myocardial L-carnitine deficiency in a family of dogs with dilated cardiomyopathy. J Am Vet Med Assoc 1991;198:647.

[69] Freeman LM, Rush JE, Kehayias JJ, et al. Nutritional alterations and the effect of fish oil supplementation in dogs with heart failure. J Vet Int Med 1998;12:440–8.

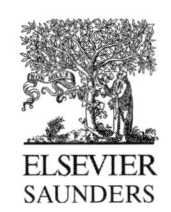

Vet Clin Small Anim
34 (2004) 217–228

THE VETERINARY
CLINICS
Small Animal Practice

Nutraceuticals, aging, and cognitive dysfunction

Elizabeth Head, PhD[a],*, Steven C. Zicker, PhD, DVM,[b]

[a]*Institute for Brain Aging and Dementia, University of California at Irvine, 1259 Gillespie NRF, Irvine, CA 92697-4540, USA*
[b]*Science and Technology Center, Hill's Pet Nutrition, Inc., P.O. Box 1658, Topeka, KS 66601-1658, USA*

Aging and cognitive dysfunction in dogs

Current estimates in the companion animal population suggest that there are more than 52 million senior and geriatric dogs over the age of 7 years [1]. Advanced age in dogs is frequently associated with severe behavioral and cognitive deficits. Deficits in learning and memory, which are measured using systematic and controlled laboratory testing procedures, have been observed [2–5]. In client-owned animals, behavioral signs such as disorientation, decreased social interaction, loss of prior housetraining, sleep disturbances, and decreased activity are reported [6]. Until recently, clinicians had regarded this constellation of behavioral observations to be indicative of senility associated with advanced age. It was also regarded in general as a progression of signs that had no plausible etiology and thus no viable intervention.

These authors have indicated that they have a relationship that, in the context of the subject of their presentation, could be perceived as an apparent conflict of interest. This pertains to relationships with food companies, pharmaceutical companies, or other corporations whose products or services are related to the subject matter of the presentation topic. The authors want it to be known that this article was written with integrity and that any perceived conflict of interest did not affect their research, information, or topic as described in this text. This work was supported by Grant No. AG12694 from the National Institutes of Aging, U.S. Department of the Army, Contract No. DAMD17-98-1-8622. The content of the information does not necessarily reflect the position or the policy of the government, and no official endorsement should be inferred. Hill's Pet Nutrition, Topeka, KS, provided additional funding.

* Corresponding author.
E-mail address: ehead@uci.edu (E. Head).

0195-5616/04/$ - see front matter © 2004 Elsevier Inc. All rights reserved.
doi:10.1016/j.cvsm.2003.09.007

Ruehl and collaborators [6,7], however, have proposed a terminology of canine cognitive dysfunction syndrome (CDS) to describe the behavioral deficits manifested in older dogs. Numerous studies using owner-based observational questionnaires have been performed to assess the prevalence of CDS in dogs. In a study of 26 pet owners, the most commonly reported complaints associated with older dogs included destructive behaviors, inappropriate urination or defecation, and excessive vocalization [6]. In other studies, approximately 18% (proprietary market research, 1999; pet owner sample size: 150; data on file, Pfizer Animal Health, New York, NY) to 75% (proprietary market research, 2001; pet owner sample size: 337; data on file, Hill's Pet Nutrition, Topeka, Kansas) of pet owners report that their senior dogs (7 years or older) exhibited at least one clinical symptom of CDS. Further, CDS might be a progressive disease; aged dogs that had impairments in one category were found within 12 to 18 months to have impairments in two or more categories [8,9].

Owner-evaluated, survey-based studies measure global brain dysfunction and might be insensitive to early and subtle changes in learning and memory associated with pathological aging in dogs. Surveys are also subjective, and the use of owners as untrained evaluators of behavioral traits is subject to large variation. An alternative method of classification involves the development of neuropsychological tests that provide quantitative and objective measures of cognitive function directly, without reliance on questionnaires [2,5]. These tests are labor-intensive, and (to date) they have only been performed in laboratory settings; however, they appear to be much more sensitive for identification of early cognitive impairment than the client-based behavioral questionnaires.

One well-developed method of testing takes place in a modified Wisconsin General Testing Apparatus (University of Toronto, Toronto, Canada), in which dogs are rewarded for making a correct response (Fig. 1).

Dogs are given access to a sliding tray that contains three recessed food wells that can be covered by objects to test visual learning and memory [5]. For example, an oddity discrimination task involves presenting dogs with a choice of responding to three objects, with one differing from the other two objects, which are identical. To perform this task accurately, the subject is required to learn that the odd object is associated with a food reward and to remember the general rule when tested at a later occasion. To distribute the sense of smell for the solution, an equal amount of food is placed in an inaccessible location of the nonrewarded objects.

Neuropsychological tests have been used to accomplish three objectives: (1) identify nonsubjective cognitive changes as a function of age in dogs, (2) characterize the neurobiological basis of age-dependent cognitive decline, and (3) screen potential interventions. As such, the populations of dogs tested to date display similar characteristics to those that are observed in the human population. It appears that there are old dogs that perform quite well for their age on these tests (successful agers), dogs that are mildly

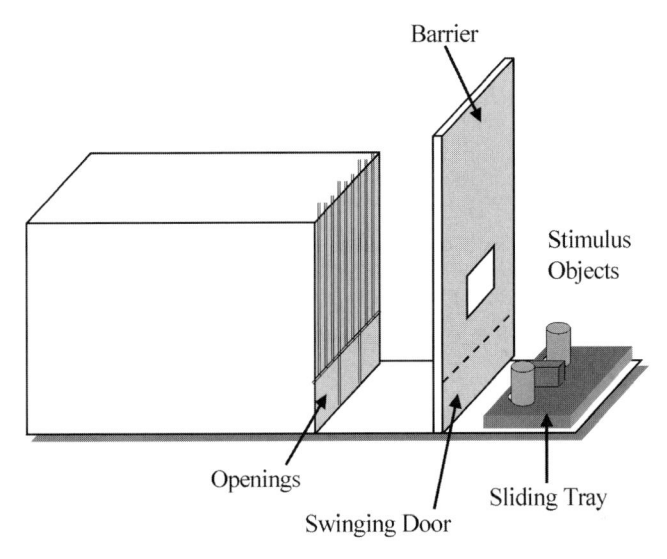

Fig. 1. Canine cognitive testing apparatus. Dogs are placed inside the test box with openings in the front. The swinging door is lifted and the sliding tray is pushed forward to present objects (stimuli) to the animal. Dogs move the objects aside to reach a food reward hidden in a recessed food well. In the task illustrated in the figure dogs are shown three objects, two of which are identical. The correct response is to select the block (*center*).

impaired (similar to age-associated memory impairments in humans), and dogs that are severely impaired (similar to dementia in humans).

The current terminology for classification of aged dogs based on cognitive and behavioral deficits might need refinement or revision as more research in this area is performed. With respect to measuring behavioral outcomes in dogs, the link between clinical measures of CDS and systematic laboratory cognitive tests is unknown, and it is not clear whether or not results from the laboratory translate directly into the clinic. It is important to make this distinction, because whether or not tests of learning and memory and the cognitive processing involved with laboratory-based tasks involve the same brain circuits that are compromised in CDS has yet to be established. Thus, it becomes difficult to classify a dog as having CDS based on the neuropsychological scores because no studies have been performed in which neuropsychological tests and in-home behavioral questionnaires have been done on the same group of dogs. Dogs that have the most severe cognitive deficits might be those that have the most noticed behavioral deficits, and therefore are truly dysfunctional. Alternatively, if there is no correlation between the behavioral deficits observed by owners and the cognitive deficits observed in the laboratory, it is possible that each evaluation is measuring different types of brain dysfunction. In either case, a full understanding of the correlates between these types of testing is needed to arrive at a logical classification terminology for this field of study.

Biological basis for cognitive dysfunction

A number of morphologic features of aging in the canine brain are similar to the hallmarks of human brain aging [10–12]. For example, cortical atrophy and ventricular widening occur with age in dogs and humans [13]. The aged canine brain also accumulates proteins within and around neurons with age that might be toxic [14–16]. One form of pathology, the accumulation of diffuse proteinaceous plaques, has received the most attention in dogs because it is thought to play a causative role in the development of Alzheimer's disease in humans [17]. Plaques contain a number of proteins, but the primary constituent is the β-amyloid peptide (Aβ), which has identical amino acid sequences in humans and dogs [18,19].

The extent of Aβ deposition in the canine brain is linked to the severity of cognitive deficits [20,21]. The extent and the location of Aβ are important. Aged dogs that are severely impaired on a reversal learning task, which measures the dog's ability to inhibit a previously learned behavior (sensitive to frontal lobe function), are the same dogs that show the most extensive prefrontal cortex Aβ pathology [22]; however, Aβ deposition does not account for all the variability in individual animal test scores, suggesting that other events occur that play a role in causing cognitive dysfunction. Because advancing age is one risk factor for the development of cognitive dysfunction in dogs, it is reasonable to examine other age-associated pathologies to determine if they also contribute to cognition dysfunction.

Reactive oxygen species and oxidative damage

Another candidate mechanism that might contribute to neuron dysfunction and the progressive accumulation of neuropathology is oxidative damage. In the brain, normal metabolic processes lead to the production of oxidants that accumulate over time and increase with age [23]. The free radical theory of aging was first proposed in 1956 by Denham Harman [24]. The theory postulates that excessive reactive oxygen species (ROS) produce cellular damage, and the cumulative inevitable response to that damage is age-dependent pathology in multiple tissues. It is now generally accepted that ROS are produced primarily as byproducts of mitochondrial aerobic respiration [25]. Accordingly, one interpretation of the free radical hypothesis of aging predicts that aging processes might be mitigated by appropriate reduction of excessive ROS. Recently, nutritional strategies based on dietary antioxidant intervention have been proposed and have gained some measure of credible proof [26]. The nutritional strategies reviewed in this discussion are to (1) enhance function of aged mitochondria, which results in decreased production of ROS, and (2) increase antioxidants in the antioxidant network system.

Reactive oxygen species

Oxidants, or ROS, are any atoms or molecules that contain one or more unpaired electrons. Most ROS are unstable because the unpaired electrons in the molecule thermodynamically seek other electrons with which they can pair, which results in ROS having a high potential for unregulated and nonspecific reactions. The increased potential for reactivity is not a problem in an isolated or inert system, but when ROS are introduced within the close confines of a complex functional matrix such as a mammalian cell, the potential for interaction, damage, and dysfunction is heightened.

Aerobic metabolism in mitochondria has been implicated in production of the majority (50–90%) of ROS generated, with the superoxide ion apparently being the ROS molecule of central interest. As mitochondria age or become dysfunctional from disease, a higher percentage of electrons are diverted to form superoxide, which might then undergo further uncontrolled reactions within the cell [23,27]. In addition to mitochondria, there are other sites and sources of metabolic generation of free radicals such as peroxisomes and neutrophil extrusion of oxidants to kill bacteria. Finally, exogenous influences such as ionizing radiation, pollutants (eg, ozone), and carcinogens might contribute to the production of free radicals in mammalian systems.

Antioxidant enzymes

A balance of superoxide production with detoxification appears to be important to cellular health and intracellular metabolic signals. Under normal conditions the cell has a variety of mechanisms to detoxify superoxide. As seen in Fig. 2, superoxide is normally converted to water by way of two consecutive enzymatic conversions. The first is the conversion of superoxide to hydrogen peroxide by Cu/Zn superoxide dismutase or Mn superoxide dismutase. The second is conversion of hydrogen peroxide to water by catalase or glutathione peroxidase (a selenoenzyme). If superoxide escapes these specific primary and redundant detoxification systems it can be detoxified by a less specific general free radical absorber such as vitamin E.

O_2^- —Nitric oxide→ **Peroxynitrite**

↓ → **Reduced Transition Metals**

H_2O_2 ⟶

↓   ↘

                          Hydroxyl radical
                                  ·OH⁻

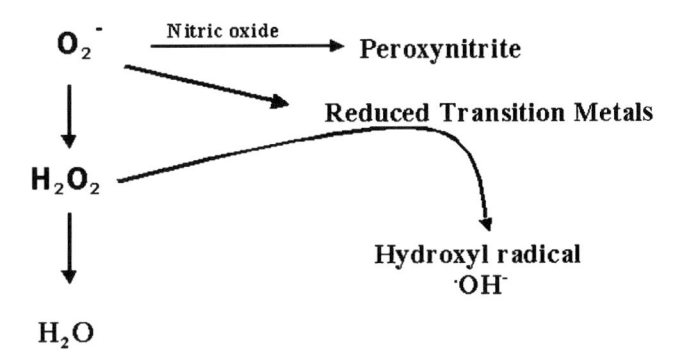

H_2O

Fig. 2. Potential pathways for superoxide metabolism.

Conversely, the superoxide can react with intracellular molecules to be converted to a more toxic molecule.

If superoxide is not detoxified because of impaired defense mechanisms, or if it is produced in excess of the detoxification systems, it is thermodynamically inclined to react with any molecule—biologic or not—within its sphere of influence. In the presence of nitric oxide, which by itself is an important biologic signaling molecule, superoxide can produce the toxic molecule peroxynitrite. In the presence of hydrogen peroxide and free transition metals such as iron or copper, superoxide is converted to the extremely toxic hydroxyl radical (Fig. 2).

Oxidative damage in the brains of aged dogs

Aging and the production of free radicals can lead to oxidative damage to proteins, lipids, and nucleotides that, in turn, can cause neuronal dysfunction and ultimately neuronal death. Several mechanisms are normally in place that balance the production of free radicals, but with age these protective mechanisms might begin to fail. For example, superoxide dismutase, an enzyme normally present in brains that converts reactive superoxide ions to hydrogen peroxide, is one step in a series of compensatory mechanisms to reduce dangerous free radicals, and this enzyme system appears to decline with age in canine brain [28].

The brains of aged dogs accumulate oxidative damage to proteins, which can be measured by the formation of carbonyl groups, nitrated tyrosine residues, or reduced glutamine synthetase activity [29]. These age-dependent modifications can potentially impair neuron function. The link between aging and oxidative damage suggests that the hypothesis that reducing oxidative damage in the brain might lead to improved cognitive function in aged dogs. One approach to reducing oxidative damage is through the use of compounds found in foods that might have specific functional effects in specific populations. Some sources refer to these substances as nutraceuticals, others as functional foods, and others as non-nutritive food-based compounds. Whatever the appropriate terminology, studies for testing these compounds are numerous and sometimes difficult to interpret.

Nutritional antioxidants

Antioxidants are substances that have the ability to scavenge ROS and reduce the overall number of oxidants in a system [23,30,31]. It has now been substantiated that antioxidants in biologic systems might act individually, but more likely in combination by way of a network of detoxification systems. For example, vitamin E can absorb an electron from ROS, but then the vitamin E is recycled by vitamin C, which is in turn recycled by glutathione, or lipoic acid, which is finally recycled by reduced NAD(P)H (Fig. 3). As evidenced by this system, there is a requirement for a complex mixture of antioxidants to achieve maximal effectiveness in vivo.

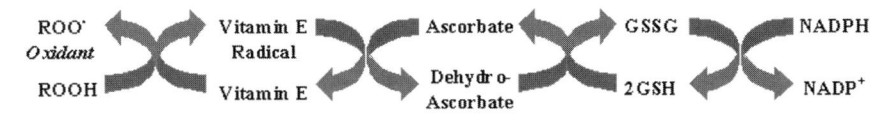

ROO˙ ⇌ Vitamin E ⇌ Ascorbate ⇌ GSSG ⇌ NADPH
Oxidant   Radical
ROOH ⇌ Vitamin E ⇌ Dehydro- ⇌ 2 GSH ⇌ NADP⁺
                   Ascorbate

Fig. 3. Possible network of antioxidants required to detoxify ROS.

A variety of antioxidant or antioxidant defense-associated molecules are derived from food sources. Vitamin E is found in high concentrations in nuts and oils, vitamin C is found in high concentrations in fruits, and β-carotene is found in certain vegetables. Trace minerals such as selenium, copper, zinc, and manganese, which are important to enzymes that specifically detoxify free radicals (Cu/Zn SOD) or help recycle antioxidants that detoxify free radicals (glutathione peroxidase), can be acquired from different food sources.

Recent research has shown that some molecules classified as mitochondrial cofactors (lipoic acid, l-carnitine) might also act to enhance the function of aged mitochondria such that less ROS are produced during aerobic respiration. It has been shown that chronic antioxidant damage to enzymes and cell membranes might reduce the capability of these molecules to bind mitochondrial enzyme cofactors, thus reducing their metabolic capacity [32]. Supplementation of foods with these mitochondrial cofactors increases their concentration within cells and restores binding to the enzymes that require them, which restores mitochondrial efficiency [32] and reduces oxidative damage to RNA [33].

Can antioxidants reduce cognitive impairments in aged dogs?

If brain aging in dogs and the progressive accumulation of oxidative damage causes cognitive dysfunction, the best test of the hypothesis is to reduce oxidative damage, which can hypothetically be accomplished through dietary enrichment with nutritional antioxidants (nutraceuticals). A longitudinal investigation of the effects of dietary intervention on cognitive function of beagle dogs is in progress. The experimental subjects are a group of 48 aged beagle dogs (10-13 years old) and 17 young dogs (3-5 years old). Each animal was assigned into one of two food groups using a counterbalanced design based on extensive baseline cognitive testing. No differences existed between the cognitive ability of the groups before dietary intervention. The test food group was fed an antioxidant/mitochondrial cofactor with dried fruit- and vegetable-fortified food, whereas the control group was maintained on an identical base food without the fortification that was nutrient adequate for senior dogs. Approximately 6 months after starting the dietary intervention, the dogs were tested on a series of oddity discrimination learning tasks [34].

As illustrated in Fig. 4, age and food effects were present, with old animals performing significantly worse than young dogs on all phases of the

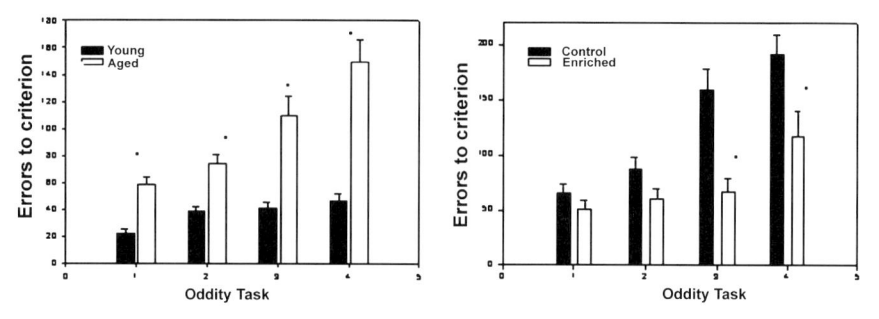

Fig. 4. Effect of age, food, and task difficulty on acquisition of an oddity discrimination learning task. The *left* panel compares the old animals on the test food with the old animals on the control food on four successive tasks. Overall, the number of errors made to achieve the criterion increased with each task from oddity task 1 to task 4. The *right* panel compares old and young dogs independent of food. There were highly significant differences on each of the tasks ($P < 0.05$).

test. With respect to food, old dogs fed the test food made significantly fewer errors on the more difficult tasks than old controls.

In addition to the laboratory testing, a behavioral field trial was performed to assess these categories of signs of cognitive dysfunction: (1) disorientation, (2) changes in sleep patterns, (3) changes in activity, (4) changes in interactions with others, and (5) loss of house training. Dogs more than 7 years old that exhibited signs in two or more of these categories were recruited for the study. Half of the dogs (n = 64) were fed a commercial dog food and the other half (n = 61) were fed a fortified food (Hill's Prescription Diet Canine b/d, Hill's Pet Nutrition). The ingredients included vitamins E and C, docosahexaenoic and eicosapentaenoic acids, lipoic acid, l-carnitine, and dried fruits and vegetables. At 60 days, the owners reported that dogs on the test food improved in all five categories, whereas owners of dogs on control food had improved in only two. Supplemented dogs improved in awareness of their surroundings, family and animal recognition and interaction, and enthusiasm in greeting. In addition, they circled less, soiled less in the house, and were more agile. Dogs on the control food and test food exhibited less aimless activity, vocalized less, and slept more regularly. Overall, the dogs on control food improved in 4 of 15 (27%) behaviors, whereas the experimental group improved in 13 of 15 (87%) behaviors. These findings support the hypothesis that reducing production of free radicals and neutralizing existing ones will improve the behavior of older dogs [35].

The most important aspect of this work is the discovery that cognitive performance can be improved by dietary manipulation. Furthermore, the effects of the dietary manipulation were relatively rapid. Antioxidants might therefore potentially act to prevent the development of these age-associated behaviors—and possibly even neuropathology—by counteracting oxidative stress.

Nutrition, aging, and cognitive dysfunction: potential pitfalls and caveats

A number of issues should be considered when interpreting the rapidly growing literature describing the use of antioxidants to improve cognitive dysfunction in aged animals. The three main issues are: (1) issues related to which compounds to use, the dosage range of the compound, the route of administration, when to begin use, and length of use; (2) issues related to biological outcome measures; and (3) behavioral outcome measures.

The selection of compounds, dosage range, length of administration, and route of administration vary considerably across species. The selection of specific compounds might depend on bioavailability. Supplementation with antioxidants might or might not increase absorption into tissues. Some antioxidants are absorbed more readily than others and might display species or meal variation differences in absorption. For example, vitamin E absorption has been shown to be highly variable based on timing of concurrent food intake [36]. Thus, different species might benefit from different types of antioxidant, but not all species might benefit from the same antioxidants. For example, canines cleave β-carotene in their intestine into vitamin A, but cats lack the metabolic enzymes to perform this function. Thus, the addition of carotenoids to these two species might have differential effects. Cats fed canthaxanthine displayed retinal pigmentation and regional vacuolization when fed a human equivalent dose of this antioxidant [37].

The dose of individual antioxidants might also vary as a function of species, and dose levels determined to be efficacious in rodents might not be translatable to other higher mammalian species because of intrinsic metabolic differences. Another important consideration is the metabolic changes with age of animals—many pharmaceuticals and likely nutraceuticals show different absorption, elimination, and toxicity profiles in older animals compared with younger animals. Route of administration is also important; single compound supplementation might not be as efficacious as multicompound administration within food, which is also true with amino acid nutrition.

To further complicate the issue, there is the question "when is the best time to begin antioxidant supplementation?" It is likely that young animals will not require nor respond to antioxidant interventions, which leaves the question "at what age would supplementation be prophylactic?" It is likely that the age at which benefits from nutraceuticals such as antioxidants are observed will vary in different species.

To critically evaluate the therapeutic potential for antioxidants and other nutraceuticals for the aging process, one must consider the outcome measures used to determine efficacy. A variety of new laboratory methods have been developed that purportedly measure the effects of ROS in biologic systems and, potentially, the results of an intervention. An increase in markers is presumed to be attributable to increased ROS being produced, thus more oxidative damage. A decrease is presumed to indicate less production of ROS and less cellular damage. Markers are specific for different biomolecules such as DNA, 8-oxodeoxyguanosine, lipids (alkenals, malondialdehyde [MDA], thiobarbituric acid-reactive substances [TBARS]), prostaglandins (isoprostanes), proteins (nitrotyrosine, protein carbonyls), and advanced glycation end products. The utility of these measures has been discussed in the literature but there currently is no consensus regarding their specific predictive usefulness for health outcomes. Further, less evidence is available indicating how systemic measures of oxidative damage reflect central nervous system damage. In addition, the methodology to perform these measures is sometimes complex and might be sensitive to sample preparation. Standard protocols are not available for all measures to be used across different laboratories. Nonetheless, some associations have been made between reduction of these markers of oxidative damage and improved health outcomes.

Behavioral outcome measures are even more vulnerable to a lack of standardized testing procedures and variability across laboratories. Behavioral studies are more limited because they are difficult to perform and the expense, length of time required for intervention, and ability to control the dietary intake of subjects is problematic. Nonetheless, behavioral studies are where the ultimate proof of efficacy must be shown on health outcomes. The study of animals that have shorter life spans than humans and potential for more dietary control (eg, dogs) is useful for developing nutritional strategies that might prove beneficial in determination of outcomes; however, translating results from studies of one species to must be done with caution because of issues related to doses and bioavailability.

Summary

Decline in cognitive function that accompanies aging in dogs might have a biological basis, and many of the disorders associated with aging in canines might be preventable through dietary modifications that incorporate specific nutraceuticals. Based on previous research and the results of laboratory and clinical studies, antioxidants might be one class of nutraceutical that benefits aged dogs. Brains of aged dogs accumulate oxidative damage to proteins and lipids, which can lead to dysfunction of neuronal cells. The production of free radicals and lack of increase in compensatory antioxidant enzymes might lead to detrimental modifications to important macromolecules within neurons. Reducing oxidative damage through food ingredients rich in a broad spectrum of antioxidants significantly improves, or slows the decline of, learning and memory in aged dogs; however, determining which compounds, combinations, dosage ranges, when to initiate intervention, and long-term effects constitute critical gaps in knowledge about this subject.

References

[1] AVM Association. U.S. Pet pwnership and demographics sourcebook. Schaumburg (IL): American Veterinary Medical Association; 1997.
[2] Adams B, Chan A, Callahan H, Siwak C, Tapp D, Ikeda-Douglas C, et al. Spatial learning and memory in the dog as a model of cognitive aging. Behav Brain Res 2000;108(1): 47–56.
[3] Chan AD, Nippak PM, Murphey H, Ikeda-Douglas CJ, Muggenburg B, Head E, et al. Visuospatial impairments in aged canines (Canis familiaris): the role of cognitive-behavioral flexibility. Behav Neurosci 2002;116(3):443–54.
[4] Head E, Mehta R, Hartley J, Kameka AM, Cummings BJ, Cotman CW, et al. Spatial learning and memory as a function of age in the dog. Behav Neurosci 1995;109:851–8.
[5] Milgram NW, Head E, Weiner E, Thomas E. Cognitive functions and aging in the dog: acquisition of nonspatial visual tasks. Behav Neurosci 1994;108:57–68.
[6] Ruehl WW, Bruyette DS, DePaoli A, Cotman CW, Head E, Milgram NW, et al. Canine cognitive dysfunction as a model for human age-related cognitive decline, dementia and Alzheimer's disease: clinical presentation, cognitive testing, pathology and response to l-deprenyl therapy. Prog Brain Res 1995;106:217–25.
[7] Ruchl WW, Neilson J, Hart B, Head E, Bruyette DS, Cummings BJ. Therapeutic actions of l-deprenyl in dogs: a model of human brain aging. In: Goldstein D, editor. Catecholamines: bridging basic science with clinical medicine, progress in brain research. New York: Elsevier; 1996. p. 217–25.
[8] Hart BL. Effect of gonadectomy on subsequent development of age-related cognitive impairment in dogs. J Am Vet Med Assoc 2001;219(1):51–6.
[9] Neilson JC, Hart BL, Cliff KD, Ruehl WW. Prevalence of behavioral changes associated with age-related cognitive impairment in dogs. J Am Vet Med Assoc 2001;218(11):1787–91.
[10] Cummings BJ, Head E, Ruehl WW, Milgram NW, Cotman CW. The canine as an animal model of human aging and dementia. Neurobiol Aging 1996;17:259–68.
[11] Head E, Milgram NW, Cotman CW. Neurobiological models of aging in the dog and other vertebrate species. In: Hof P, Mobbs CV, editors. Functional neurobiology of aging. San Diego: Academic Press; 2001. p. 457–68.
[12] Wisniewski HM, Wegiel J, Morys J, Bancher C, Soltysiak Z, Kim KS. Aged dogs: an animal model to study beta-protein amyloidogenesis. In: Maurer PRK, Beckman H, editors. Alzheimer's disease. Epidemiology, neuropathology, neurochemistry and clinics. New York: Springer-Verlag; 1990. p. 151–67.
[13] Su M-Y, Head E, Brooks WM, Wang Z, Muggenberg BA, Adam GE, et al. MR imaging of anatomic and vascular characteristics in a canine model of human aging. Neurobiol Aging 1998;19(5):479–85.
[14] Braunmuhl A. Kongophile angiopathie und senile plaques bei greisen hunden. Arch Psychiatr Nervenkr 1956;194:395–414 [in German].
[15] Lafora G. Neoformaciones dendriticas an las neuronas y alteraciones de la neuroglia en el perro senil. Trab del Lab de Investig Biol 1914;1 [in Spanish].
[16] Wisniewski HM, Johnson AB, Raine CS, Kay WJ, Terry RD. Senile plaques and cerebral amyloidosis in aged dogs. Lab Invest 1970;23:287–96.
[17] Selkoe DJ. Amyloid beta-protein and the genetics of Alzheimer's disease. J Biol Chem 1996;271:18295–8.
[18] Johnstone EM, Chaney MO, Norris FH, Pascual R, Little SP. Conservation of the sequence of the Alzheimer's disease amyloid peptide in dog, polar bear and five other mammals by cross-species polymerase chain reaction analysis. Brain Res Mol Brain Res 1991;10(4):299–305.
[19] Selkoe DJ, Bell DS, Podlisny MB, Price DL, Cork LC. Conservation of brain amyloid proteins in aged mammals and humans with Alzheimer's disease. Science 1987;235: 873–7.

[20] Colle M-A, Hauw J-J, Crespeau F, Uchiara T, Akiyama H, Checler F, et al. Vascular and parenchymal Aβ deposition in the aging dog: correlation with behavior. Neurobiol Aging 2000;21:695–704.
[21] Cummings BJ, Head E, Ruehl WW, Milgram NW, Cotman CW. Beta-amyloid accumulation correlates with cognitive dysfunction in the aged canine. Neurobiol Learn Mem 1996;66:11–23.
[22] Head E, Callahan H, Muggenburg BA, Cotman CW, Milgram NW. Visual-discrimination learning ability and beta-amyloid accumulation in the dog. Neurobiol Aging 1998;19(5):415–25.
[23] Ames BN, Shigenaga MK, Hagen TM. Oxidants, antioxidants, and the degenerative diseases of aging. Proc Natl Acad Sci USA 1993;90:7915–22.
[24] Harman D. Aging: a theory based on free radical and radiation chemistry. J Gerontol 1956;11:298–300.
[25] Beckman KB, Ames BN. The free radical theory of aging matures. Physiol Rev 1998;78(2):547–81.
[26] Joseph JA, Denisova N, Fisher D, Bickford P, Prior R, Cao G. Age-related neurodegeneration and oxidative stress: putative nutritional intervention. Neurol Clin 1998;16(3):747–55.
[27] Cottrell DA, Turnbull DM. Mitochondria and ageing. Curr Opin Clin Nutr Metab Care 2000;3(6):473–8.
[28] Kiatipattanasakul W, Nakamura S, Kuroki K, Nakayama H, Doi K. Immunohistochemical detection of anti-oxidative stress enzymes in the dog brain. Neuropathology 1997;17:307–12.
[29] Head E, Liu J, Hagen TM, Muggenburg BA, Milgram NW, Ames BN, et al. Oxidative damage increases with age in a canine model of human brain aging. J Neurochem 2002;82:375–81.
[30] De Ruvo C, Amodio R, Algeri S, Martelli N, Intelangelo A, D'Ancona GM, et al. Nutritional antioxidants as antidegenerative agents. Int J Dev Neurosci 2000;18(4–5):359–66.
[31] Haramaki N, Stewart DB, Aggarwal S, Ikeda H, Reznick AZ, Packer L. Networking antioxidants in the isolated rat heart are selectively depleted by ischemia-reperfusion. Free Radic Biol Med 1998;25(3):329–39.
[32] Liu J, Killilea DW, Ames BN. Age-associated mitochondrial oxidative decay: improvement of carnitine acetyltransferase substrate-binding affinity and activity in brain by feeding old rats acetyl-L-carnitine and/or R-alpha -lipoic acid. Proc Natl Acad Sci USA 2002;99(4):1876–81.
[33] Liu J, Head E, Gharib AM, Yuan W, Ingersoll RT, Hagen TM, et al. Memory loss in old rats is associated with brain mitochondrial decay and RNA/DNA oxidation: partial reversal by feeding acetyl-L-carnitine and/or R-alpha -lipoic acid. Proc Natl Acad Sci USA 2002;99(4):2356–61.
[34] Milgram, NW, Zicker SC, Head E, Muggenburg BA, Murphey H, Ikeda-Douglas C, et al. Dietary enrichment counteracts age-associated cognitive dysfunction in canines. Neurobiol Aging 2002;23:737–45.
[35] Dodd C, Zicker SC, Jewell DE, Lowry SR, Fritsch D, Toll PW. Effects of an investigational food on age related behavioral changes in dogs. In: Hill's European Symposium on Canine Brain Ageing. 2002. Barcelona, Spain.
[36] Leonard SW, Good C, Guggar E, Traber MG. Improved vitamin E bioavailability from a fortified breakfast cereal as compared with a vitamin E supplement. FASEB J 2002;16(4):A373–A374.
[37] Scallon LJ, Burke JM, Mieler WF, Kies JC, Aaberg TM. Canthaxanthine-induced retinal pigment epithelial changes in the cat. Curr Eye Res 1988;7(7):687–93.

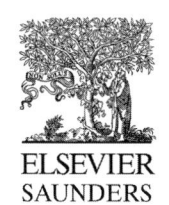

Modulation of immune response through nutraceutical interventions: implications for canine and feline health

Michael G. Hayek, PhD*, Stefan P. Massimino, MS, Michael A. Ceddia, PhD

The Iams Company Research and Development, PO Box 189, Lewisburg, OH 45338, USA

The interaction between nutrition and the immune response has been an area of intense research over the past four decades. A bidirectional interaction between nutrition, immune response, and infectious disease was suggested by Scrimshaw et al [1] in the 1950s. Subsequently, it was recognized that malnourished individuals were at risk for infection [2]. Follow-up studies have demonstrated that deficiencies of most micronutrients result in impaired host defense [3–6]. Conversely, others have demonstrated that the supplementation of certain nutrients beyond accepted requirements may improve certain indices of the immune response. This has led to a plethora of studies examining the influence of dietary components on the immune system.

Nutraceuticals, or functional foods and pharmafoods as they have also been referred to, is a relatively new word in this science of food and food extracts. A nutraceutical has been defined in many ways; however, for the purpose of this article, we shall define it as a food or naturally occurring food component thought to have a beneficial effect on health. The nutraceutical field is an extensive one and is becoming increasingly more difficult to define, because this terminology includes many natural remedies

---

These authors have indicated that they have a relationship that, in the context of the subject of their presentation, could be perceived as an apparent conflict of interest. This pertains to relationships with food companies, pharmaceutical companies, or other corporations whose products or services are related to the subject matter of the presentation topic. The authors want it to be known that this article was written with full integrity and that any perceived conflict of interest did not affect their research, information, or topic as described in this text.

* Corresponding author.
 E-mail address: hayek.mg@pg.com (M.G. Hayek).

0195-5616/04/$ - see front matter © 2004 Elsevier Inc. All rights reserved.
doi:10.1016/j.cvsm.2003.09.002

that have been known for centuries (eg, ginseng, green tea) as well as substances that have been extracted from natural products (eg, vitamin E).

Recently, many nutraceuticals and their respective effects on immunity have been studied. It is important to understand that although benefits are reported, not all nutraceuticals influence the immune system in the same ways. These range from no effect to modulating various parts of the immune system, including the nonspecific immune system, the specific immune system, cellular activity, and cytokine secretion. These differences become apparent as we review various nutraceuticals and their reported effects on health as determined by immune function modulation.

Immune system overview

The immune system is an interactive network of cells, proteins, and signaling agents designed to provide protection to the host from environmental pathogens, parasites, malignant cells, allergens, and toxins [7]. The immune system (Fig. 1) can be divided into two interactive parts: innate or antigen nonspecific and acquired or antigen specific [8,9]. Innate immunity consists of nonspecific barriers and cellular and chemical defense mechanisms. Nonspecific physical barriers, such as skin and mucous membranes, protect against the initial entry of pathogens, such as bacteria, viruses, and parasites. Once those barriers are overwhelmed, however, a functional immune system is required to mount a specific response to clear the infection and protect the individual. Cellular and chemical defenses rely heavily on detection of the difference between invading microorganisms (nonself) and what is considered "self" or part of the individual's body. When these pathogens are detected, enzymes that digest bacterial cell walls are activated and cells that recognize these invading microorganisms and destroy them are deployed. This response is nonspecific to the invading organism and does not require priming (no lag time), but it is slow and usually not sufficient to clear the pathogen once it has become established.

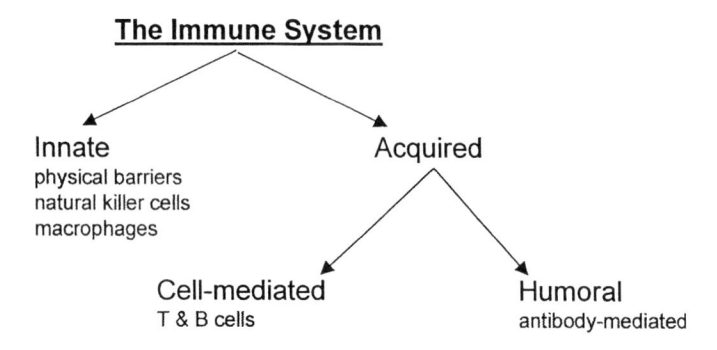

Fig. 1. Interactive arms of the immune system.

Rather, it serves to contain the infection until the next level of defense, known as acquired immunity, develops.

Acquired immunity can be further divided into humoral and cell-mediated immunity. Humoral immunity includes the production of antibodies (also referred to as immunoglobulins) from B cells. There are five different immunoglobulin isotypes (IgG, IgA, IgM, IgD, and IgE) consisting of different subclasses within these isotypes. These antibodies can work in concert with the complement system to rid the body of invading antigens [7,10].

The cellular portion of the immune system includes the interaction of bone marrow–derived macrophages and B cells as well as thymus-derived T cells. T cells can be further divided into subsets based on cell surface protein expression [10–12]. These subsets include the (CD4+) or T helper (Th) cells and the (CD8+) or T-cytotoxic/suppresser cells. Th cells can be further classified based on the cytokines that they produce. Th_1 cells secrete interleukin (IL)-2, interferon (INF)-γ, tumor necrosis factor (TNF), and IL-12 and are important in bacterial responses, whereas Th_2 cells secrete IL-4, IL-10, and IL-13 and are important in parasite infections [13]. CD8+ cells may either play a role as a killer cell that assists in a response to a viral antigen and cancer or as a suppresser role to regulate the immune response. Another set of cells that play an important role are the natural killer (NK) cells. NK cells can help to rid the host of tumor cells and viruses in the body. A summary of these cells and functions is presented in Table 1.

Cells of the immune system use hormone-like substances to communicate intracellularly. These protein mediators have been classified by different names based on their cellular origin. Lymphocyte-derived mediators that are capable of regulating the growth and mobility of leukocytes were collectively called lymphokines [14]. It was then discovered that non-lymphoid cells can also produce these lymphokines; thus, the term *cytokine* was suggested [15]. Another term used to describe most immune mediators is *interleukin*, a word that refers to their basic property of serving as communication vehicles between different cells [16].

To evaluate the impact of nutraceuticals, one must conduct experiments on the immune system. A variety of tests have been developed to assess

Table 1
Various cells of the immune system

Cell type	Function
Macrophage	Phagocytosis and antigen presentation to T cells
B cells	Antibody production
T helper-1 cells (CD4+)	Activation of B cells (bacterial response)
T helper-2 cells (CD4+)	Activation of B cells (parasite response)
T cytotoxic/suppresser cells (CD8+)	Regulation of cellular-mediated immunity, viral clearance
Natural killer cells	Attack tumor-or virus-containing cells

immunologic status or function. These include in vivo tests, such as delayed-type hypersensitivity, titer response to vaccine, antibody response to a protein challenge, and circulating lymphocyte concentrations. In vitro tests include response of lymphocytes to mitogen compounds, cytokine production, phagocytic function (particle uptake and bacterial killing), NK cell activity, and cytotoxic T-cell activity. No single test or group of tests is perfect for evaluating immunologic assessment; however, a combination of in vitro and in vivo indices should provide a useful indication of immune status within an individual.

Dietary modulation of the immune response

Interactions between nutrition and immunity have been well documented (the reader is referred to an article by Gershwin et al [17] for a review). Diets deficient in protein, energy, minerals, vitamins, and essential fatty acids have long been known to impair immunity. More recently, supplementation of minerals greater than the minimum required levels has been reported to be successful in improving health and immune function in a wide range of species. Initial research in this area focused on altering the intake of required dietary nutrients. A summary of some of the research conducted with vitamins and mineral is presented in Tables 2 and 3.

Currently, studies have focused on dietary components that are not traditionally recognized as nutritional requirements of mammals. Some of these compounds may be derived from foods or food ingredients. Some examples of these are garlic, grape seed extracts, green tea, and isoflavones. Other compounds are derived from herbs and botanicals that are not typically consumed as part of the diet. A summary of the reported effects of various nutraceuticals on the immune system is presented in Table 4.

There are several interesting points that should be considered when evaluating these interactions. Inspection of the results demonstrates that the various nutraceuticals interact with various parts of the immune system. Therefore, it should be noted that although two compounds are reported to enhance the immune response, they might have quite different mechanisms of action. Another important aspect to note is that certain compounds have mixed reports on their effect on the immune system. For instance, several reports demonstrated that echinacea was beneficial for antibody response and NK cell activity [70,71], whereas others have reported a lack of effect with a concern that it may be immunosuppressive under certain conditions [69].

Differential effects of a nutraceutical may be a result of the concentration used in the studies. Zimecki et al [115] demonstrated various in vitro effects of lactoferrin at different concentrations on lymphocyte proliferation. A positive effect of lactoferrin on proliferation was observed at low concentrations, and a reduction in proliferation was observed when lactoferrin was present at higher concentrations.

Table 2
Vitamins demonstrated to have immunoenhancing properties greater than recognized required intakes

Vitamin	Species	Effect
Thiamin	Human	Increases neutrophil motility [18]
Vitamin B6	Human	Increases lymphocyte proliferation in elederly subjects [19]
	Human	Maintenance of immune function in the elderly [20]
Vitamin C	Human	Increases neutrophil motility and lymphocyte proliferation [21]
	Human	Increases lymphocyte proliferation and DTH [22]
	Human	Increases lymphocyte proliferation and DTH [23]
	Human	Increases serum IgG, IgM, and complement in elderly women [24]
	Human	Reduces severity of viral infections [25,26]
Vitamin E	Rodent	Increases T-cell mitogenesis [27]
	Rodent	Increases Th cell function [28]
	Rodent	Increases B-cell mitogenesis [27]
	Rodent	Increases antibody titer [29]
	Rodent	Increases plaque-forming cells [27]
	Rodent	Increases IL-2 production [30]
	Rodent	Increases delayed-type hypersensitivity [30]
	Rodent	Increases NK cell activity [31]
	Rodent	Decreases live influenza pulmonary titers [32]
	Chicken	Increases antibody titer [33]
	Chicken	Increases plaque-forming cells [29]
	Calves	Increases lymphocyte proliferation [34]
	Pigs	Increases lymphocyte proliferation [35]
	Sheep	Increases antibody titer [36]
	Human	Increases polymorphonuclear cell phagocytosis [37]
	Human	Increases T-cell mitogenesis [38]
	Human	Increases IL-2 production [38]
	Human	Increases DTH [38]
β-Carotene	Rodent	Increases IL-2 receptor expression [39]
	Rodent	Increases proliferation of cytotoxic T cells [40]
	Cattle	Increases lymphocyte proliferation [41,42]
	Pigs	Increases lymphocyte proliferation [42]
	Human	Increases percent Th cells, NK cells, and IL-2 receptor [43]
	Human	Increases NK cell activity [44]
	Human	Increases DTH response [44]
	Human	Increases Th cell number [45]

Abbreviations: DTH, delayed type hypersensitivity; IL, interleukin; NK, natural killer; Th, T helper.

Lastly, one should consider potential interactions with other treatment regimens. This can be seen with research on β-glucan. Several studies reported that β-glucan can stimulate macrophage number and cytokine production [102,103]. Toxic effects have been reported in mice provided with β-glucan in conjunction with the nonsteroidal anti-inflammatory drug indomethacin, however [119,120]. It was suggested that this may have been the result of maladjustment of the cytokine network by β-glucan [120].

Table 3
Minerals demonstrated to have immunoenhancing properties greater than recognized required intakes

Mineral	Species	Effect
Zinc	Rodent	Increases T-cell and macrophage function resistance to *Candida albicans* and virus infection [46]
	Human	Increases circulating T cells, DTH, antibody titer response [47]
Selenium	Sheep	Increases T-cell mitogen response [48]
	Rodent	Increases NK cell activity [49]
	Rodent	Increases T-cell mitogen response [51]
	Rodent	Increases expression of IL-2 receptors [52]
	Human	Increases NK cell activity [50]
Chromium	Cattle	Increases antibody production [53–58]
	Cattle	Increases T-cell mitogen response [55,56]

Abbreviations: DTH, delayed type hypersensitivity; IL, interleukin; NK, natural killer.

In summary, there is a strong potential for modulating the immune response by various nutraceuticals. It is important to understand the mechanism of action for the nutraceutical of interest and to be sure that the concentration of interest has been demonstrated to produce the desired effect on the species of interest.

Potential application for dogs and cats

There are various conditions in the life of dogs and cats in which the immune response is not functioning at peak performance. By understanding the mechanism for the immune dysregulation at these times, it may be possible to design nutritional interventions that can aid the immune response. The effects of nutritional interventions on immune function have been examined in the immune status in cats, puppies, and senior dogs as well as in dogs undergoing intense exercise.

When puppies are born, they emerge from a sterile environment (the uterus) and become exposed to a hostile environment filled with pathogenic microorganisms. Unfortunately, their immune systems are not fully developed at birth and require significant time to become fully functional. As a result, newborn puppies are especially vulnerable to infection in the first few weeks of life and require immune assistance to survive. This assistance is provided by the bitch by means of transfer of antibodies through the colostrum and milk, which immediately confers some level of immune protection for the newborn. This transfer of immunity from dam to newborn is important for the newborn's survival.

The immune system then requires time to develop to its fully functional capacity. The distribution of immune cell types and their responses have been reported to change as puppies and kittens grow and develop [121]. T-cell populations are significantly smaller and their proliferation response to

Table 4
Nutraceutical compounds that have been demonstrated to interact with the immune system

Nutraceutical	Species	Effect
L-arginine	Human	Modulates immune cell phenotypes [57]
	Rodent	Activates macrophage activity [58]
	Murine	Increases NK cell activity [59]
L-cysteine	In vitro	Glutathione precursor, potentiates H_2O_2-induced killing of Escherichia coli [60]
L-glutamine	Murine	Enhances T-cell responsiveness [61]
	Human	Modulates cytokine secretion [62]
	In vitro	Enhances is lymphocyte proliferation and cytokine production [63,64]
N-acetyl-L-cysteine	Human	Glutathione precursor [65]
	Human, in vitro	Antioxidant activity [65,66]
	Human	Modulates cytokine secretion [67]
Selenomethionine	Murine	Component of glutathione peroxidase, inhibits IL-10 secretion [68]
Echinacea	Rodent	No effects reported [69]
	Rodent	Increases antigen-specific immunoglobulin production [70]
	Human	Enhances is killer cell cytotoxicity [71]
Garlic	Murine	Augments macrophage and T-cell functions [72]
	Murine	Inhibits tumor growth [73]
	Murine	Decreased antigen-specific ear swelling in rodents [73]
	Canine	No effect [74]
Genistein	Murine	Suppresses cell-mediated immunity [75]
	Murine	Increases host resistance to tumor incidence [76]
Ginkgo biloba	Human	Dilates blood vessels [77]
	In vitro	Potent free radical scavenger [78]
	In vitro	Inhibits neutrophil function [79]
Ginseng	Rodent	Activation of a Th-1–type cellular immunity [80]
	Rodent	Enhances bacterial clearance and decreases lung pathology in rats [81,82]
Goldenseal	Rodent	Increases antigen-specific immunoglobulin production [70]
Grape seed extract	In vitro	Cytotoxic effects against some cancer cells [83]
	Rodent	Increases the resistance against oxidative stress [84]
Green tea	Murine	Ameliorates tumor-related immune dysfunction [85,86]
Maitake mushroom (Grifola frondosa)	Murine	Enhances the antigen-specific antibody response [87]
	Murine	Anti tumor activity [88]
Pine bark extract (Pycnogenol)	Murine	Enhances IL-2 production by mitogen-stimulated splenocytes [89]
	Murine	Reduces elevated levels of IL-6 and IL-10 [90]
	In vitro	Enhances macrophage TNFα production [91]

(continued on the next page)

Table 4 (*continued*)

Nutraceutical	Species	Effect
Quercetin	In vitro	Antitumor properties [92]
	In vitro	Inhibits platelet function [93]
	In vitro	Reduces oxidative stress–induced cell membrane damage [94]
Reishi mushroom (Ganoderma lucidum)	Human	Anti-inflammatory [95]
Resveratrol	Human	Modulates cytokine activity and both CTL and NK cell cytotoxic activity [96]
Spirulina	Chicken	Enhances humoral and cell-mediated immune functions [97]
	Human	Activates the innate immune system [98]
	Murine	Enhances antibody production during allergic reaction [99]
	Cats	Enhances macrophage phagocytic function [100]
	Chicken	Enhances macrophage phagocytic function [101]
β-1,3-glucan	In vitro	Stimulates cytokine release from macrophages [102]
	Murine	Increases macrophage number [103]
Soy isoflavones	Murine	Increases nonspecific and humoral immunity [104]
α-Lipoic acid	In vitro	Increases T-cell glutathione levels [105]
Blue green algae	Chicken	Increases humoral and cell-mediated immunity [101]
	Human	Increases immune cell translocation and activity [106]
Conjugated linoleic acid (CLA)	Murine	Decreases tumorigenesis [107]
	Murine, porcine	Modulates immune cell phenotypes and enhances cytotoxicity [108–110]
Lactoferrin	Murine	Supports health and function of GIT [111]
	Murine	Reduces systemic and intestinal inflammation [112]
	Murine	Promotes healthy gut bacteria [112]
	Murine	Enhances delayed-type hypersensitivity reaction [113]
	Murine	Protective in septic shock model [114]
	In vitro	Dose-dependent effect on lymphocyte proliferation [115]
	Human	Dose-dependent effect [116]
		Decreases IL-6 and TNFα production [117]
Melatonin	Murine	Increases nonspecific immune cell populations [117]
Phytoserol (β-sitosterol)	Rodent	Anti-inflammatory and antipyretic activity [118]

Abbreviations: CTL, cytotoxic T-lymphocyte; DTH, delayed type hypersensitivity; GIT, gastrointestinal tract; IL, interleukin; NK, natural killer; Th, T helper.

stimulation is less in puppies compared with adult dogs. After 16 weeks of age, puppies have been reported to possess a lymphocyte population similar to that of healthy adult dogs.

Unfortunately, puppy deaths do occur during growth and development, specifically in utero, at birth, immediately after birth, and immediately after weaning. Losses during this postweaning period typically occur as a result of infection caused by dysregulation or a compromised immune system.

Therefore, a stronger immune system as early as possible can help puppies to grow and develop into healthy adult dogs. A recently conducted study [122] showed that puppies receiving a diet from weaning (6 weeks of age) supplemented with the antioxidants vitamin E, β-carotene, and lutein had higher levels of T- and B-cell activation at 14 and 22 weeks of age compared with their age-matched controls (fed a diet with standard vitamin E levels and no added lutein or β-carotene).

Puppies that were fed an antioxidant-supplemented diet produced higher antibody levels to specific vaccines, such as distemper, parvovirus, and parainfluenza. To summarize, puppies fed diets formulated with antioxidant nutrients (ie, β-carotene, lutein, vitamin E) possess increased immune systems, which decreases the likelihood of infections and death. During this vulnerable period, puppies are at a higher risk for developing disease. Previous research in adult dogs as well as in other species shows that nutritional supplementation can influence immune function. Dietary supplementation with antioxidants can improve cell-mediated (T- and B-cell response) and humoral immune function (antibody production), which enhances the responses necessary to protect animals against infections and disease.

Exercise and immunity

Sporting dogs generally have a higher level of exercise incorporated into their daily routine than nonsporting dogs. The interaction between exercise and immune function has only recently been demonstrated to exist. It has been observed that certain types of exercise modulate the immune system. Nutritional interventions may aid this modulation.

NK cells are part of the innate immune system; as such, they act as the first barrier of defense against pathogens that breach the body's physical barriers. These cells are involved in the early response to viral infection and tumor growth. NK cell cytotoxic activity increases acutely and proportionately with exercise intensity and then returns to resting levels soon after exercise ceases [123,124]. It continues to decline and remains below resting levels for up to 6 hours after intense and prolonged exercise, however [125].

Neutrophils, which are also known as polymorphonuclear leukocytes, represent 50% to 60% of the total circulating leukocytes. Once an inflammatory response is initiated, neutrophils are the first cells to be recruited to sites of infection or injury. Their targets include bacteria, fungi, protozoa, viruses, virally infected cells, and tumor cells. Studies have suggested that although acute exercise stimulates neutrophil function, prolonged periods of intense exercise are associated with downregulation of neutrophil function [126].

Macrophages are a first line of defense against pathogens and malignancies by nature of their phagocytic, cytotoxic, and intercellular killing capacities. Ceddia and Woods [127] demonstrated that exhaustive exercise suppressed macrophage function for up to 24 hours after exercise. This suppression in macrophage function was caused by the inability of macrophages to degrade pathogens [128].

Lymphocytes are also influenced by exercise. Lymphocyte stimulation has been reported to be particularly sensitive to exercise-induced changes. Brief moderate exercise has little effect (it may actually slightly stimulate lymphocyte activation), but intense or prolonged exercise suppresses the proliferative response for up to 3 hours [125,129].

The effect of intensive exercise on oxidative stress was examined in sled dogs. Several studies [130–132] have examined the levels of oxidative stress markers released in the blood of sled dogs during a 3-day exercise bout (racing 15–20 miles per day for 3 days). During this exercise period, the authors noted increases in serum uric acid, isoprostane levels [131], and serum 7,8-dihydro-8-oxo-2′deoxyguanosine and an increase in the lag time of in vitro oxidation of lipoprotein particles [132]. These findings indicate an increase in free radical production as a result of the exercise regimen.

As a result of the increase in oxidative stress noted in the sled dog, it was of interest to determine if there is an effect on the immune system similar to that reported in other species [133]. In this study, 62 trained sled dogs were randomized to either a sedentary group (n = 22), an exercised group (n = 21), or an exercised plus supplemental antioxidants group (n = 19). All dogs were fed a commercially available diet containing 35% protein, 30.8% fat, 23.1% carbohydrates, and a ω-6–to–ω-3 fatty acid ratio of 5.9:1. Antioxidant supplementation consisted of one biscuit per day containing β-carotene, 21.6 mg, and lutein, 18.4 mg, as well as α-tocopherol, 400 IU, in the form of a soft-gel capsule.

Similar to observations in other species, several immune indices were altered as a result of the 3-day exercise session. The proportion of blood neutrophils was increased, whereas the proportions of lymphocytes, eosinophils, and monocytes were decreased. Also, a decrease in lymphocyte activity and alterations in the proportions of T cells and B cells were noted. Lastly, exercise resulted in an increase in the blood levels of acute-phase proteins, indicating that the exercise resulted in a generalized inflammatory response. Supplementation with antioxidants resulted in normalization of the acute-phase proteins as well in as the proportions of certain T cells and B cells. These data demonstrate that supplementation with antioxidants results in alleviation of some of the effects of exercise on the immune response.

Aging and immunity

The dysregulation in immune function is a well-documented consequence of aging. This can lead to an increased incidence of morbidity (illness) and mortality (death). Cell-mediated immunity is clearly the component of the immune system most adversely affected with advancing age, primarily T cells (the reader is referred to an article by Pawelec et al [134] for a review). Age-related T-cell immunity dysfunction has been implicated as the cause of many chronic degenerative diseases in elderly human beings, including arthritis, cancer, autoimmune diseases, and increased susceptibility to infectious diseases. There are many theories that have been put forth to try and explain the mechanism(s) responsible for this decline, but no one theory can fully account for all the changes observed. Among all the theories to date, the free radical theory of aging is particularly interesting because it is based on a premise that a single common process modifiable by genetics and environmental factors is responsible for the aging and death of all living things. Proposed by Harmon [135] in 1956, this theory postulates that aging is caused by free radical reactions and accumulation of reactive oxygen byproducts. As explained previously in this article, free radical production and accumulation can have several damaging effects on various cells, including those of the immune system. Therefore, much research with aging animals has been done looking at dietary antioxidants as a means of reducing free radical reactions and accumulation.

Senior dogs have been reported to show a decreased immune system response compared with younger dogs. Older dogs also differ in the makeup of their immune system compared with younger dogs. Based on these observations, the aging process results in a dysregulation of the immune response in dogs similar to that seen in other species. This dysregulation may be corrected with nutritional interventions. This was observed in a recently conducted study [136] which reported benefits from feeding senior dogs a diet supplemented with β-carotene. In this study β-carotene supplementation reversed the age-associated decline in T-cell population numbers and T-cell proliferation activity.

Although the interaction of vitamin E and the immune response has been well documented in a variety of species, there were no data in the literature with regard to the domestic cat. A recently conducted study [137] attempted to determine this interaction. In this study, 38 cats (19 young cats and 19 old cats) were fed a baseline diet for a 60-day period that contained a basal level of vitamin E (60-IU/kg diet). Half the young and old cats were then switched to diets (in a step-up fashion) that contained supplemental levels of vitamin E (250-IU/kg and 500-IU/kg diets) for 60-day feeding periods, respectively. Immune function was assessed at the end of each 60-day feeding period, with the other half of the cats maintained on the baseline diet as controls throughout the course of the study. In agreement with previous canine studies, old cats exhibited a marked decrease in proliferation to T-cell mitogens compared with their younger counterparts. There was, however, no age difference seen in B-cell response. When the old cats were fed the 250-IU/kg vitamin E diet, T- and B-cell proliferation was higher than in their age-matched controls. No effect was seen on young cats. When old cats received the 500-IU/kg vitamin E diet, the concanavalin A–stimulated T-cell response was lower versus that in age-matched controls. Taken together with the canine data, these studies demonstrate that the age-associated decline in the immune response can be mitigated through specific nutritional interventions.

Summary

Mounting research demonstrates that certain nutraceutical compounds interact with the immune system. These interactions may be positive or negative depending on the compound or dose administered to the individual. Understanding the mechanisms by which these compounds work should provide opportunities to design nutritional interventions to bolster the health of dogs and cats.

References

[1] Schrimshaw NS, Taylor CE, Gordon JE. Interaction of nutrition and infection. Am J Med Sci 1959;237:367–403.
[2] Chandra RK. Immunocompetence in undernutrition. J Pediatr 1972;81:1194–200.
[3] Keush GT, Wilson CS, Waksal SD. Nutrition, host defenses and lymphoid system. Arch Host Def Mech 1983;2:275–359.
[4] Chandra S, Chandra RK. Nutrition and immune response outcome. Prog Food Nutr Soc 1986;10:1–65.
[5] Beisel WR. Single nutrients and immunity. Am J Clin Nutr 1982;35(2 Suppl):417–68.
[6] Hwang D. Essential fatty acids and immune response. FASEB J 1989;3:2052–61.
[7] Chandra RK. Basic immunology and its application to nutritional problems. In: Forse RA, Bell S, Blackburn GL, Kabbash LG, editors. Diet, nutrition and immunity. Boca Raton: CRC Press; 1994. p. 1–8.
[8] Brostoff J, Scanding GK, Male D, Roitt IM. Clinical immunology. London: Grower Medical Publishing; 1991.
[9] Chandra RK. Primary and secondary immunodeficiency disorders. Edinburgh: Churchill Livingstone; 1983.
[10] Cruse JM, Lewis RE. Illustrated dictionary of immunology. Boca Raton: CRC Press; 1995.
[11] Nossal GJ. Current concepts: immunology. The basic components of the immune system. N Engl J Med 1987;316(21):1320–5.
[12] Goodman JW. The immune response. In: Stites DP, Terr AI, editors. Basic and clinical immunology. East Norwalk, CT: Appleton & Lange; 1991. p. 34–44.
[13] Scott P, Kaufmann HE. The role of T-cell subsets and cytokines in the regulation of infection. Immunol Today 1991;12:346–8.
[14] Dumonde DC, Wolstencroft RA, Panayi GS, Matthew M, Morley J, Howson WT. Lymphokines: non-antibody mediators of cellular immunity generated by lymphocyte activation. Nature 1969;224:38–42.
[15] Anonymous. Current state of studies of mediators of cellular immunity: a progress report. Cell Immunol 1977;33:233–44.
[16] Meydani SN. Dietary modulation of cytokine production and biological functions. Nutr Rev 1990;48:361–9.
[17] Gershwin ME, German BJ, Keen CL, editors. Nutrition and immunology; principles and practice. Totowa, NJ: Humana Press; 2000.
[18] Jones PT, Anderson R. Oxidative inhibition of polymorphonuclear leukocyte motility mediated by the peroxidase/H_2O_2/halide system: studies on the reversible nature of the inhibition and mechanism of protection of migratory responsiveness by ascorbate, levamisole, thiamine and cysteine. Int J Immunopharmacol 1983;5(5):377–89.

[19] Talbott MC, Miller LT, Kervliet NI. Pyridoxine supplementation: effect on lymphocyte response in elderly persons. Am J Clin Nutr 1987;46:659–64.
[20] Meydani SN, Ribaya-Mercado JD, Russell RM, Sahyoun N, Morrow RD, Gershoff SN. Vitamin B6 deficiency impairs interleukin-2 production and lymphocyte proliferation in elderly adults. Am J Clin Nutr 1991;53:1275–80.
[21] Anderson R, Oosthuizen R, Maritz R, Theron A, Van Rensburg AJ. The effects of increasing weekly doses of ascorbate on certain cellular and humoral immune functions in normal volunteers. Am J Clin Nutr 1980;33(1):71–6.
[22] Kennes B, Dumont I, Brohee D, Hubert C, Neve P. Effect of vitamin C supplements on cell-mediated immunity in old people. Gerontology 1983;29(5):305–10.
[23] Panush RS, Delafuente JC, Katz P, Johnson J. Modulation of certain immunologic responses by vitamin C. III. Potentiation of in vitro and in vivo lymphocyte responses. Int J Vitam Nutr Res Suppl 1982;23:35–47.
[24] Ziemlanski S, Wartanowicz M, Klos A, Raczka A, Klos M. The effect of ascorbic acid and alpha-tocopherol supplementation on serum proteins and immunoglobulin concentration in elderly. Nutr Res Int 1986;2:1–5.
[25] Siegel BV. Vitamin C and the immune response in health and disease. In: Klurfeld DM, editor. Nutrition and immunity. New York: Plenum Press; 1993. p. 167–96.
[26] Anderson R, Smith MJ, Joon GK, Van Standen AM. Vitamin E and cellular immune functions. Ann NY Acad Sci 1990;587:34–48.
[27] Corwin LM, Schloss J. Influence of vitamin E on the mitogenic response of murine lymphocytes. J Nutr 1980;110:916–23.
[28] Tanaka J, Fuyiwara H, Torisu M. Vitamin E and immune response: enhancement of T-helper activity by dietary supplementation of vitamin E in mice. Immunology 1979;38: 727–34.
[29] Tengerdy RP, Heinzerling RH, Methias MM. Effect of vitamin E on disease resistance and immune response. In: de Dune C, Hayaishi O, editors. Tocopherol, oxygen and biomembranes. Amsterdam: Elsevier/North-Holland Biomedical Press; 1978. p. 191–200.
[30] Meydani SN, Meydani M, Verdon CP, Shapiro AC, Blumberg JB, Hayes KC. Vitamin E supplementation suppresses prostaglandin E2 synthesis and enhances the immune response of aged mice. Mech Ageing Dev 1986;34:191–201.
[31] Moriguchi S, Kobayashi N, Kishino Y. High dietary intakes of vitamin E and cellular immune functions in rats. J Nutr 1990;120:1096–102.
[32] Hayek MG, Taylor SF, Bender BS, Han SN, Meydani M, Smith DE, et al. Vitamin E supplementation decreases lung virus titers in mice infected with influenza. J Infect Dis 1997;176:273–6.
[33] Tengerdy RP, Lactera NG. Vitamin E adjuvant formulations in mice. Vaccine 1991;9: 204–6.
[34] Reddy PG, Morill JL, Minocha HC, Morill MB, Dayton AB, Frey RA. Effects of supplemental vitamin E on the immune system of calves. J Dairy Sci 1985;69:164–71.
[35] Larsen HJ, Tollersrud S. Effect of dietary vitamin E and selenium on the phytohemagglutin response in pig lymphocytes. Am J Vet Sci 1981;31:301–5.
[36] Afzal M, Tengerdy RP, Ellis RP, Kimberling CV, Morris CJ. Protection of rams against epididymitis by a B. Ovis-vitamin E vaccine. Vet Immunol Immunopathol 1984;7:293–304.
[37] Baehner RL, Boxer LA, Allen JM, Davis J. Autooxidation as a basis for altered function of polymorphonuclear leukocytes. Blood 1977;50:327–35.
[38] Meydani SN, Barklund MP, Liu S, Meydani M, Miller RA, Cannon JG, et al. Vitamin E supplementation enhances cell-mediated immunity in healthy elderly subjects. Am J Clin Nutr 1990;52(3):557–63.
[39] Prabhala RH, Maxey V, Hicks MJ, Watson RR. Enhancement of the expression of activation markers on human peripheral blood mononuclear cells by in vitro culture with retinoids and carotenoids. J Leukoc Biol 1989;45(3):249–54.

[40] Seifter E, Rettura G, Padawer J, Levenson SM. Moloney murine sarcoma virus tumors in CBA/J mice: chemopreventive and chemotherapeutic actions of supplemental beta-carotene. J Natl Cancer Inst 1982;68(5):835–40.
[41] Daniel LR, Chew BP, Tanaka TS, Tjoelker LW. In vitro effects of β-carotene and vitamin A on peripartum bovine peripheral blood mononuclear cell proliferation. J Dairy Sci 1991;74:911–5.
[42] Michal JJ, Heiman LR, Wong TS, Chew BP. Modulatory effects of dietary β-carotene on blood and mammary leukocyte function in periparturient dairy cows. J Dairy Sci 1994;77:1408–21.
[43] Watson RR, Prabhala RH, Pleiza PM, Alberts DS. Effect of beta-carotene on lymphocyte subpopulations in elderly humans: evidence for a dose response relationship. Am J Clin Nutr 1991;53:90–9.
[44] Santos MS, Meydani SN, Leka L, Wu D, Fotouhi N, Meydani M, et al. Natural killer cell activity in elderly men is enhanced by beta-carotene supplementation. Am J Clin Nutr 1996;64(5):772–7.
[45] Alexander M, Newmark H, Miller R. Oral beta-carotene can increase number of OKT4+ cells in human blood. Immunol Lett 1985;9:221–4.
[46] Singh KP, Zaidi SI, Raisuddin S, Saxena AK, Murthy RC, Ray PK. Effect of zinc on immune functions and host resistance against infection and tumor challenge. Immunopharmacol Immunotoxicol 1992;14(4):813–40.
[47] Duchateau J, Delepesse G, Vrijens R, Collet H. Beneficial effects of oral zinc supplementation on the immune response of old people. Am J Med 1981;70:1001–4.
[48] Larson HJ. Effect of selenium on lymphocyte responses to mitogens. Res Vet Sci 1988;45:11–5.
[49] Talcott PA, Exon JH, Koller LD. Attraction of natural killer cell-mediated cytotoxicity in rats treated with selenium, diethylnitrosamine and ethylnitrosourea. Cancer Lett 1984;23:313–9.
[50] Kiremidjian-Schumacher L, Roy M, Wishe HI, Cohen MW, Stotzky G. Supplementation with selenium and human immune cell functions. II. Effect on cytotoxic lymphocytes and natural killer cells. Biol Trace Elem Res 1994;41(1–2):115–27.
[51] Kiremidjian-Schumacher L, Roy M, Wishe HI, Cohen MW, Stotzky G. Selenium and immune cell functions. I. Effect of lymphocyte proliferation and production of interleukin 1 and interleukin 2. Proc of Soc Exp Biol and Med 1990;193:136–42.
[52] Roy M, Kiremidjian-Schumacher L, Wishe HI, Cohen MW, Stotzky G. Effect of selenium on the expression of high affinity interleukin 2 receptors. Proc of Soc Exp Biol and Med 1992;200:36–43.
[53] Burton JL, Mallard BA, Mowat DN. Effects of supplemental chromium on immune responses of peripaturient and early lactation cows. J Anim Sci 1993;71:1532–9.
[54] Burton JL, Malard BA, Mowat DN. Effects of supplemental chromium on responses of newly weaned beef calves to IBR/PI3 vaccination. Can J Vet Res 1994;58:148–51.
[55] Chang X, Mowat DN. Supplemental chromium for stressed and growing feeder calves. J Anim Sci 1992;70:559–65.
[56] Kegley EB, Spears JW. Immune response, glucose metabolism, and performance of stressed feeder calves fed inorganic and organic chromium. J Anim Sci 1995;73:2721–6.
[57] Baligan M, Giardina A, Giovannini G, Laghi MG, Ambrosioni G. L-arginine immunity. Study of pediatric subjects. Minerva Pediatr 1997;49(11):537–42.
[58] Angele MK, Smail N, Ayala A, Cioffi WG, Bland KI, Chaudry IH. L-arginine: a unique amino acid for restoring the depressed macrophage functions after trauma-hemorrhage. J Trauma 1999;46(1):34–41.
[59] Lieberman MD, Nishioka K, Redmond HP, Daly JM. Enhancement of interleukin-2 immunotherapy with L-arginine. Ann Surg 1992;215(2):157–65.
[60] Berglin EH, Edlund MB, Nyberg GK, Carlsson J. Potentiation by L-cysteine of the bactericidal effect of hydrogen peroxide in Escherichia coli. J Bacteriol 1982;152(1):81–8.

[61] Kew S, Wells SM, Yaqoob P, Wallace FA, Miles EA, Calder PC. Dietary glutamine enhances murine T-lymphocyte responsiveness. J Nutr 1999;129(8):1524–31.
[62] Yaqoob P, Calder PC. Cytokine production by human peripheral blood mononuclear cells: differential sensitivity to glutamine availability. Cytokine 1998;10(10):790–4.
[63] Yaqoob P, Calder PC. Glutamine requirement of proliferating T lymphocytes. Nutrition 1997;13(7–8):646–51.
[64] Wells SM, Kew S, Yaqoob P, Wallace FA, Calder PC. Dietary glutamine enhances cytokine production by murine macrophages. Nutrition 1999;15(11–12):881–4.
[65] De Vries N, De Flora S. N-acetyl-L-cysteine. J Cell Biochem Suppl 1993;17F:270–7.
[66] Aruoma OI, Halliwell B, Hoey BM, Butler J. The antioxidant action of N-acetylcysteine: its reaction with hydrogen peroxide, hydroxyl radical, superoxide, and hypochlorous acid. Free Radic Biol Med 1989;6(6):593–7.
[67] Baier JE, Neumann HA, Moeller T, Kissler M, Borchardt D, Ricken D. Radiation protection through cytokine release by N-acetylcysteine. Strahlenther Onkol 1996;172(2):91–8.
[68] Rafferty TS, Walker C, Hunter JA, Beckett GJ, McKenzie RC. Inhibition of ultraviolet B radiation-induced interleukin 10 expression in murine keratinocytes by selenium compounds. Br J Dermatol 2002;146(3):485–9.
[69] South EH, Exon JH. Multiple immune functions in rats fed Echinacea extracts. Immunopharmacol Immunotoxicol 2001;23(3):411–21.
[70] Rehman J, Dillow JM, Carter SM, Chou J, Le B, Maisel AS. Increased production of antigen-specific immunoglobulins G and M following in vivo treatment with the medicinal plants Echinacea angustifolia and Hydrastis canadensis. Immunol Lett 1999;68(2–3):391–5.
[71] See DM, Broumand N, Sahl L, Tilles JG. In vitro effects of echinacea and ginseng on natural killer and antibody-dependent cell cytotoxicity in healthy subjects and chronic fatigue syndrome or acquired immunodeficiency syndrome patients. Immunopharmacology 1997;35(3):229–35.
[72] Lau BH, Yamasaki T, Gridley DS. Garlic compounds modulate macrophage and T-lymphocyte functions. Mol Biother 1991;3(2):103–7.
[73] Kyo E, Uda N, Kasuga S, Itakura Y. Immunomodulatory effects of aged garlic extract. J Nutr 2001;131(3 Suppl):1075S–9S.
[74] Turek JJ, Massimino SP, Boebel KP, Hayek MG. Investigation of garlic as an immunomodulator in canines. In: Reinhart GA, Carey DP, editors. Recent advances in canine and feline nutrition, vol. 3. 2000 Iams Nutrition Symposium Proceedings. Wilmington: Orange Frazer Press; 2000. p. 573–82.
[75] Yellayi S, Zakroczymski MA, Selvaraj V, Valli VE, Ghanta V, Helferich WG, et al. The phytoestrogen genistein suppresses cell-mediated immunity in mice. J Endocrinol 2003;176(2):267–74.
[76] Guo TL, McCay JA, Zhang LX, Brown RD, You L, Karrow NA, et al. Genistein modulates immune responses and increases host resistance to B16F10 tumor in adult female B6C3F1 mice. J Nutr 2001;131:3251–8.
[77] Mehlsen J, Drabaek H, Wiinberg N, Winther K. Effects of a Ginkgo biloba extract on forearm haemodynamics in healthy volunteers. Clin Physiol Funct Imaging 2002;22:375–8.
[78] Pincemail J, Dupuis M, Nasr C, Hans P, Haag-Berrurier M, Anton R, et al. Superoxide anion scavenging effect and superoxide dismutase activity of Ginkgo biloba extract. Experientia 1989;45(8):708–12.
[79] Pincemail J, Thirion A, Dupuis M, Braquet P, Drieu K, Deby C. Ginkgo biloba extract inhibits oxygen species production generated by phorbol myristate acetate stimulated human leukocytes. Experientia 1987;43(2):181–4.
[80] Song Z, Kharazmi A, Wu H, Faber V, Moser C, Krogh HK, et al. Effects of ginseng treatment on neutrophil chemiluminescence and immunoglobulin G subclasses in a rat

model of chronic Pseudomonas aeruginosa pneumonia. Clin Diagn Lab Immunol 1998;5(6):882–7.
[81] Song ZJ, Johansen HK, Faber V, Hoiby N. Ginseng treatment enhances bacterial clearance and decreases lung pathology in athymic rats with chronic P. aeruginosa pneumonia. APMIS 1997;105(6):438–44.
[82] Song Z, Wu H, Mathee K, Hoiby N, Kharazmi A. Gerimax ginseng regulates both humoral and cellular immunity during chronic Pseudomonas aeruginosa lung infection. J Altern Complement Med 2002;8(4):459–66.
[83] Ye X, Krohn RL, Liu W, Joshi SS, Kuszynski CA, McGinn TR, et al. The cytotoxic effects of a novel IH636 grape seed proanthocyanidin extract on cultured human cancer cells. Mol Cell Biochem 1999;196:99–108.
[84] Koga T, Moro K, Nakamori K, Yamakoshi J, Hosoyama H, Kataoka S, et al. Increase of antioxidative potential of rat plasma by oral administration of proanthocyanidin-rich extract from grape seeds. J Agric Food Chem 1999;47:1892–7.
[85] Zhu M, Gong Y, Yang Z, Ge G, Han C, Chen J. Green tea and its major components ameliorate immune dysfunction in mice bearing Lewis lung carcinoma and treated with the carcinogen NNK. Nutr Cancer 1999;35(1):64–72.
[86] Zhu M, Gong Y, Yang Z. Protective effect of tea on immune function in mice. Zhonghua Yu Fang Yi Xue Za Zhi 1998;32(5):270–4.
[87] Suzuki I, Itani T, Ohno N, Oikawa S, Sato K, Miyazaki T, et al. Effect of a polysaccharide fraction from Grifola frondosa on immune response in mice. J Pharmacobiodyn 1985;8(3):217–26.
[88] Adachi K, Nanba H, Kuroda H. Potentiation of host-mediated anti-tumor activity in mice by beta-glucan obtained from Grifola frondosa (maitake). Chem Pharm Bull (Tokyo) 1987;35(1):262–70.
[89] Cheshier JE, Ardestani-Kaboudanian S, Liang B, Araghiniknam M, Chung S, et al. Immunomodulation by pycnogenol in retrovirus-infected or ethanol-fed mice. Life Sci 1996;58(5 PL):87–96.
[90] Miodini P, Fioravanti L, Di Fronzo G, Cappelletti V. The two phyto-oestrogens genistein and quercetin exert different effects on oestrogen receptor function. Br J Cancer 1999;80(8):1150–5.
[91] Park YC, Rimbach G, Saliou C, Valacchi G, Packer L. Activity of monomeric, dimeric, and trimeric flavonoids on NO production, TNF-alpha secretion, and NF-kappaB-dependent gene expression in RAW 264.7 macrophages. FEBS Lett 2000;465(2–3):93–7.
[92] Pignatelli P, Pulcinelli FM, Celestini A, Lenti L, Ghiselli A, Gazzaniga PP, et al. The flavonoids quercetin and catechin synergistically inhibit platelet function by antagonizing the intracellular production of hydrogen peroxide. Am J Clin Nutr 2000;72(5):1150–5.
[93] Ferrali M, Signorini C, Caciotti B, Sugherini L, Ciccoli L, Giachetti D, et al. Protection against oxidative damage of erythrocyte membrane by the flavonoid quercetin and its relation to iron chelating activity. FEBS Lett 1997;416(2):123–9.
[94] Stavinoha W, Satsangi N, Weintraub S. Study of the anti-inflammatory efficacy of Ganoderma lucidum. In: Kim BK, Kim YS, editors. Recent advances in Ganoderma lucidum research, Seoul: The Pharmaceutical Society of Korea; 1995. p. 3–7.
[95] Stavinoha W, Satsangi N, Weintraub S. Study of the antiinflammatory efficacy of *Ganoderma lucidum*. In: Kim B-K, Kim Y, editors. Recent advances in *Ganoderma lucidum* research. Seoul, Korea: The Pharmaceutical Society of Korea; 1995. p. 3–7.
[96] Falchetti R, Fuggetta MP, Lanzilli G, Tricarico M, Ravagnan G. Effects of resveratrol on human immune cell function. Life Sci 2001;70(1):81–96.
[97] Qureshi MA, Garlich JD, Kidd MT. Dietary Spirulina platensis enhances humoral and cell-mediated immune functions in chickens. Immunopharmacol Immunotoxicol 1996;18(3):465–76.
[98] Hirahashi T, Matsumoto M, Hazeki K, Saeki Y, Ui M, Seya T. Activation of the human innate immune system by Spirulina: augmentation of interferon production and NK

cytotoxicity by oral administration of hot water extract of Spirulina platensis. Int Immunopharmacol 2002;2(4):423–34.
[99] Hayashi O, Hirahashi T, Katoh T, Miyajima H, Hirano T, Okuwaki Y. Class specific influence of dietary Spirulina platensis on antibody production in mice. J Nutr Sci Vitaminol (Tokyo) 1998;44(6):841–51.
[100] Qureshi MA, Ali RA. Spirulina platensis exposure enhances macrophage phagocytic function in cats. Immunopharmacol Immunotoxicol 1996;18(3):457–63.
[101] Al-Batshan HA, Al-Mufarrej SI, Al-Homaidan AA, Qureshi MA. Enhancement of chicken macrophage phagocytic function and nitrite production by dietary Spirulina platensis. Immunopharmacol Immunotoxicol 2001;23(2):281–9.
[102] Olson EJ, Standing JE, Griego-Harper N, Hoffman OA, Limper AH. Fungal beta-glucan interacts with vitronectin and stimulates tumor necrosis factor alpha release from macrophages. Infect Immun 1996;64(9):3548–54.
[103] Burgaleta C, Golde DW. Effect of glucan on granulopoiesis and macrophage genesis in mice. Cancer Res 1977;37(6):1739–42.
[104] Zhang R, Li Y, Wang W. Enhancement of immune function in mice fed high doses of soy daidzein. Nutr Cancer 1997;29(1):24–8.
[105] Han D, Tritschler HJ, Packer L. Alpha-lipoic acid increases intracellular glutathione in a human T-lymphocyte Jurkat cell line. Biochem Biophys Res Commun 1995;207(1): 258–64.
[106] Jensen GS, Ginsberg DI, Huerta P, Citton M, Drapeau C. Consumption of Aphanizomenon flos-aquae has rapid effects on the circulation and function of immune cells in humans. J Am Nutraceutical Assoc 2000;2(3):50–8.
[107] Belury MA. Inhibition of carcinogenesis by conjugated linoleic acid: potential mechanisms of action. J Nutr 2002;132(10):2995–8.
[108] Wong MW, Chew BP, Wong TS, Hosick HL, Boylston TD, Shultz TD. Effects of dietary conjugated linoleic acid on lymphocyte function and growth of mammary tumors in mice. Anticancer Res 1997;17:987–93.
[109] Bassaganya-Riera J, Hontecillas R, Zimmerman DR, Wannemuehler MJ. Dietary conjugated linoleic acid modulates phenotype and effector functions of porcine CD8(+) lymphocytes. J Nutr 2001;131(9):2370–7.
[110] Hayek MG, Han SN, Wu D, Watkins BA, Meydani M, Dorsey JL, et al. Dietary conjugated linoleic acid influences the immune response of young and old C57BL/6NCrlBR mice. J Nutr 1999;129(1):32–8.
[111] Kruzel ML, Harari Y, Chen CY, Castro GA. Lactoferrin protects gut mucosal integrity during endotoxemia induced by lipopolysaccharide in mice. Inflammation 2000;24(1): 33–44.
[112] Kruzel ML, Harari Y, Chen CY, Castro GA. The gut. A key metabolic organ protected by lactoferrin during experimental systemic inflammation in mice. Adv Exp Med Biol 1998;443:167–73.
[113] Zimecki M, Kruzel ML. Systemic or local co-administration of lactoferrin with sensitizing dose of antigen enhances delayed type hypersensitivity in mice. Immunol Lett 2000;74(3):183–8.
[114] Kruzel ML, Harari Y, Mailman D, Actor JK, Zimecki M. Differential effects of prophylactic, concurrent and therapeutic lactoferrin treatment on LPS-induced inflammatory responses in mice. Clin Exp Immunol 2002;130(1):25–31.
[115] Zimecki M, Stepniak D, Szynol A, Kruzel ML. Lactoferrin regulates proliferative response of human peripheral blood mononuclear cells to phytohemagglutinin and mixed lymphocyte reaction. Arch Immunol Ther Exp (Warsz) 2001;49(2):147–54.
[116] Zimecki M, Spiegel K, Wlaszczyk A, Kubler A, Kruzel ML. Lactoferrin increases the output of neutrophil precursors and attenuates the spontaneous production of TNF-alpha and IL-6 by peripheral blood cells. Arch Immunol Ther Exp (Warsz) 1999;47(2):113–8.

[117] Currier NL, Sun LZ, Miller SC. Exogenous melatonin: quantitative enhancement in vivo of cells mediating non-specific immunity. J Neuroimmunol 2000;104(2):101–8.
[118] Gupta MB, Nath R, Srivastava N, Shanker K, Kishor K, Bharguva KP. Anti-inflammatory and antipyretic activities of B-sitosterol. Planta Med 1980;39:157–63.
[119] Takahashi H, Ohno N, Adachi Y, Yadomae T. Association of immunological disorders in lethal side effect of NSAIDs on beta-glucan-administered mice. FEMS Immunol Med Microbiol 2001;31(1):1–14.
[120] Yoshioka S, Ohno N, Miura T, Adachi Y, Yadomae T. Immunotoxicity of soluble beta-glucans induced by indomethacin treatment. FEMS Immunol Med Microbiol 1998;21(3):171–9.
[121] Bortnick SJ, Orandle MS, Papadi GP, Johnson CM. Lymphocyte subsets in neonatal and juvenile cats: comparison of blood and lymphoid tissues. Lab Anim Sci 1999;49(4):395–400.
[122] Massimino SP, Daristotle L, Ceddia MA, Hayek MG. The influence of diet on the puppy's developing immune system. In: Canine reproduction and neonatal health. Tufts Animal Expo, Boston, 2001. p. 15–9.
[123] Nielsen HB, Secher NH, Christensen NJ, Pedersen BK. Lymphocytes and NK cell activity during repeated bouts of maximal exercise. Am J Physiol 1996;271(1):R222–7.
[124] Nieman DC, Miller AR, Henson DA, Warren BJ, Gusewitch G, Johnson RL, et al. Effects of high- vs moderate-intensity exercise on natural killer cell activity. Med Sci Sports Exerc 1993;25(10):1126–34.
[125] Nieman DC, Simandle S, Henson DA, Warren BJ, Suttles J, Davis JM, et al. Lymphocyte proliferative response to 2.5 hours of running. Int J Sports Med 1995;16(6):404–9.
[126] Pyne DB, Baker MS, Fricker PA, McDonald WA, Telford RD, Weidemann MJ. Effects of an intensive 12-wk training program by elite swimmers on neutrophil oxidative activity. Med Sci Sports Exerc 1995;27(4):536–42.
[127] Ceddia MA, Woods JA. Exercise suppresses macrophage antigen presentation. J Appl Physiol 1999;87(6):2253–8.
[128] Ceddia MA, Voss EW, Woods JA. Intracellular mechanisms responsible for exercise-induced suppression of macrophage antigen presentation. J Appl Physiol 2000;88:804–10.
[129] Mitchell JB, Paquet AJ, Pizza FX, Starling RD, Holtz RW, Grandjean PW. The effect of moderate aerobic training on lymphocyte proliferation. Int J Sports Med 1996;17(5):384–9.
[130] Hinchcliff KW, Reinhart GA, DiSilvestro R, Reynolds A, Blostein-Fujii A, Swenson RA. Oxidant stress in sled dogs subjected to repetitive endurance exercise. Am J Vet Res 2000a;61:512–7.
[131] Hinchcliff KW, Piercy RJ, Baskin CR, DiSilvestro RA, Reinhart GA, Hayek MG, et al. Oxidant stress, oxidative damage and antioxidants: review and studies in Alaskan sled dogs. In: Reinhart GA, Carey DP, editors. Recent advances in canine and feline nutrition, vol. 3. 2000 Iams nutrition symposium proceedings. Wilmington: Orange Frazer Press; 2000. p. 517–30.
[132] Baskin CR, Hinchcliff KW, DiSilvestro RA, Reinhart GA, Hayek MG, Chew BP, et al. Effects of dietary supplementation on oxidative damage and resistance to oxidative damage during prolonged exercise in sled dogs. Am J Vet Res 2000;61:886–91.
[133] Chew BP, Park JS, Kim HW, Wong TS, Cerveny C, Park HJ, et al. Effects of heavy exercise and the role of dietary antioxidants in immune response in the Alaska sled dog. In: Reinhart GA, Carey DP, editors. Recent advances in canine and feline nutrition, vol. 3. 2000 Iams nutrition symposium proceedings. Wilmington: Orange Frazer Press; 2000. p. 531–9.
[134] Pawelec G, Wagner W, Adibzadeh M, Engel A. T cell immunosenescence in vitro and in vivo. Exp Gerontol 1999;34:419–29.

[135] Harmon D. Aging: a theory based on free radical and radiation therapy. J Gerontol 1956;11:298–300.
[136] Kearns RJ, Loos KM, Chew BP, Massimino SP, Burr JR, Hayek MG. The effect of age and dietary β-carotene on immunological parameters in the dog. In: Reinhart GA, Carey DP, editors. Recent advances in canine and feline nutrition, vol. 3. 2000 Iams nutrition symposium proceedings. Wilmington: Orange Frazer Press; 2000. p. 389–401.
[137] Hayek MG, Massimino SP, Burr JR, Kearns RJ. Dietary vitamin E improves immune function in cats. In: Reinhart GA, Carey DP, editors. Recent advances in canine and feline nutrition, vol. 3. 2000 Iams nutrition symposium proceedings. Wilmington: Orange Frazer Press; 2000. p. 555–63.

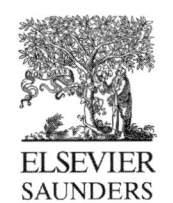

The use of nutraceuticals in cancer therapy

Philip Roudebush, DVM[a],*, Deborah J. Davenport, DVM, MS[a], Bruce J. Novotny, DVM[b]

[a]*Technical Information Services, Hill's Pet Nutrition, Inc. Hill's Science and Technology Center, PO Box 1658, Topeka, KS 66601, USA*
[b]*Helios Communications, LLC, 5826 Park Circle, Shawnee, KS 66216, USA*

Few diseases evoke as much emotion as cancer. Most pet owners have had or will have a personal experience with cancer either in themselves, a family member, or a close personal friend. Furthermore, the popular press is filled with articles about cancer prevention and the promise of therapeutic breakthroughs, including the use of functional foods and nutraceuticals. Thus, pet owners have a heightened awareness of human cancer, and this suggests that veterinarians and veterinary health care teams should approach pets with cancer and their owners in a positive, compassionate, and knowledgeable manner. Pet owners are also able to understand the importance of nutrition in animals with cancer and how proper feeding and use of functional foods or nutraceuticals can enhance the quality and length of life in pets with cancer.

Human patients with cancer commonly use unconventional and complementary therapy, including nutraceuticals [1–4]. In one study, investigators found that only 7% of human cancer patients used unconventional medical therapies when they were asked routine questions by physicians [1]. Extended questioning revealed that 40% of cancer patients were actually using herbal supplements, megavitamins, or other nonherbal preparations, however [1]. In another study, more than half of human patients with colorectal cancer took nutritional supplements. In this study, most patients took more than one type of supplement [2]. Vitamins, calcium,

---

These authors have indicated that they have a relationship that, in the context of the subject of their presentation, could be perceived as an apparent conflict of interest. This pertains to relationships with food companies, pharmaceutical companies, or other corporations whose products or services are related to the subject matter of the presentation topic. The authors want it to be known that this article was written with full integrity and that any perceived conflict of interest did not affect their research, information, or topic as described in this text.

* Corresponding author.
E-mail address: phil_roudebush@hillspet.com (P. Roudebush).

and botanical supplements were used most often [2]. A third study revealed that 80% of adult human cancer patients used vitamin supplements (multivitamins, vitamin C, or vitamin E) and that 54% used herbal products, including green tea, echinacea, shark cartilage, grape seed extract, and milk thistle [4]. The high prevalence of nutraceutical use among human cancer patients further suggests that nutraceutical use in pets with cancer is probably common.

This article focuses on the use of functional foods and nutraceuticals for complementary therapy in pets with cancer. Functional foods are usually defined as any modified food or food ingredient that may provide a health benefit beyond the traditional nutrients it contains. The broad topic of nutrients and foods for prevention of cancer is beyond the scope of this article and is covered in other sources.

Metabolic alterations in patients with cancer

Metabolic alterations have been identified in human and canine patients with cancer. In human beings, these alterations have been associated with cachexia, decreased response to therapy, decreased remission rates, and increased mortality.

Alterations in carbohydrate metabolism

Carbohydrate metabolism is dramatically altered in dogs with cancer. Altered metabolism occurs because tumors preferentially metabolize glucose (carbohydrates) for energy, forming lactate (lactic acid) as an end product. Dogs with cancer must then expend energy to convert lactate back to glucose, resulting in a net energy gain by the tumor and net loss by the animal. Consequently, dogs with cancer lose energy to the tumor and have elevated blood lactate and insulin levels (ie, laboratory evidence of altered carbohydrate metabolism). Studies to delineate carbohydrate metabolism in cats with cancer have not been published. Research has documented that dogs with lymphoma and a wide variety of other malignant diseases have significant alterations in carbohydrate metabolism, including the following [5–10]:

- Dogs with a wide variety of malignant conditions have elevated resting insulin and lactate levels compared with levels in dogs without cancer. The mechanisms for elevated blood lactic acid levels in dogs and people with a wide variety of malignancies remain uncertain, but increased rates of anaerobic glycolysis have been documented in people with cancer and lactic acidosis. Tumor cells have also been hypothesized to be the source of the increased lactic acid. Neoplastic cells may use embryonic forms of key enzymes of anaerobic metabolism, such as hexokinase, 6-phosphofructokinase, and pyruvate kinase, which are less subject to host feedback mechanisms. It is likely, although still

conjectural, that inflammatory cytokine-mediated increases in host tissue glycolysis are responsible for increased production of lactic acid in many, if not all, tissues in the body. Futile cycles resulting from elevated Cori cycle activity of lactic acid interconversion with glucose may increase the daily energy needs of human patients with cancer cachexia by approximately 20%.
- Insulin and lactate levels in dogs with cancer increase above baseline values in response to intravenous glucose and food tolerance tests compared with levels in control dogs. Elevated blood insulin concentrations have been reported in dogs, laboratory animals, and people with cancer. Results of studies in human beings and laboratory animals with cancer cachexia provide ample evidence of decreased postreceptor insulin responsiveness resulting in part from increased serum concentrations of free fatty acids and lipoproteins as well as other insulin-antagonistic metabolic defects.
- Elevated lactate and glucose levels do not improve for a period of time after dogs with cancer are rendered free of disease with chemotherapy and surgery, suggesting that the malignancy causes fundamental changes in metabolism that persist after clinical evidence of cancer is eliminated.
- Elevated lactate levels cause inefficient conversion of lactate back to glucose, resulting in a net energy loss to the patient.
- Administration of lactate- or glucose-containing fluids increases lactate levels in dogs with lymphoma, suggesting that these types of fluids should not be used routinely in animals with cancer unless specifically indicated.
- Increased levels of key glycolytic and glucose transport enzymes are found in canine cancer tissue compared with normal tissues [10].
- Alterations in metabolic factors are hypothesized to reduce the quality of life for animals with cancer.

Alterations in protein metabolism

Human patients with cancer and weight loss have decreased body muscle mass, decreased skeletal protein synthesis, and altered nitrogen balance [11]. These patients concurrently have increased skeletal muscle protein breakdown, liver protein synthesis, and whole-body protein synthesis to support tumor growth. The reprioritization of liver protein synthesis is commonly known as the acute-phase reactant response [12]. The presence of an acute-phase protein response is strongly associated with reduced survival in human patients with several different forms of cancer. If protein intake does not keep pace with use, an imbalance occurs that alters immune response, gastrointestinal function, and wound healing.

Increased expression of the ubiquitin-proteasome proteolytic pathway is a major cause of skeletal muscle loss in patients with cancer [11–14].

Accelerated proteolysis via the ubiquitin-proteasome pathway is the principle cause of muscle wasting induced by cancer, fasting, metabolic acidosis, disuse, denervation, diabetes, sepsis, burns, hyperthyroidism, and glucocorticoid excess [14]. Multiple systems control this pathway, including cytokines, hormones, nutrients, and tumor-derived proteolysis-inducing factor (PIF). Studies in many muscle-wasting rodent models and in human cancer patients have detected serum PIF. Loss of skeletal muscle mass correlates with the presence of PIF.

Cytokines, such as tumor necrosis factor-α (TNFα), are also involved in protein catabolism. TNFα does not induce muscle protein catabolism directly but rather adversely affects important factors that replenish wasted muscle [11,12].

In one study, cancer-bearing dogs had significantly lower plasma concentrations of threonine, glutamine, glycine, valine, cystine, and arginine and significantly higher concentrations of isoleucine and phenylalanine than did normal control dogs [15]. Alterations in plasma amino acid profiles did not normalize after tumors were removed surgically. This finding suggests that cancer induces long-lasting changes in canine protein metabolism and may involve mechanisms similar to those described previously.

Alterations in fat metabolism

Adipose tissue catabolism is the second major feature of cachexia in various chronic diseases, including cancer [11–13]. A decrease in fat synthesis or an increase in lipolysis can deplete fat stores. A lipid-mobilizing factor (LMF) has been isolated from a cachexia-inducing murine tumor and from the urine of human patients with cancer and weight loss [11–13]. LMF acts directly on adipose tissue, causing the release of free fatty acids and glycerol by increasing levels of cyclic AMP in a manner similar to that of the natural lipolytic hormones [12]. Studies in animal models suggest that production of LMF by tumors may account for loss of body fat, especially when combined with decreased food intake.

Several cytokines alter lipid metabolism. TNFα is the major cytokine implicated in the catabolism of adipose tissue during cachexia. TNFα inhibits lipoprotein lipase, decreases insulin receptor activity, and inhibits glucose transporter activity [13]. All these actions indirectly stimulate lipolysis by TNFα. Altered lipid profiles in dogs with lymphoma suggest that similar changes may occur in pets with cancer [16]. Studies to delineate fat metabolism in cats with cancer have not been published.

In addition, some tumor cells have a limited ability to use fat to meet energy needs versus soluble carbohydrates and protein [17]. This finding led to the hypothesis that foods relatively high in fat may benefit animals with cancer compared with foods relatively high in carbohydrates. The type of fat in the food also seems to be important. High levels of ω-3 fatty acids have many clinical benefits, including reduced tumorigenesis, tumor growth, and metastasis, as well as altered eicosanoid synthesis and anticatabolic effects [18–20]. Practical use of these findings in animals with cancer is explored in the next section.

The ideal nutritional profile for patients with cancer

The ideal nutritional profile for animals with cancer is not definitively known; however, information that exists in a number of species is being used to support cancer patients today. Alterations in carbohydrate, protein, and fat metabolism precede obvious clinical disease and cachexia in dogs with cancer. These metabolic alterations may persist in animals with clinical remission or apparent recovery from their cancer. Until research results dictate differently, pathophysiologic and therapeutic principles for cats with cancer should follow those of people and dogs with cancer.

Key nutritional factors in animals with cancer include soluble carbohydrate, fiber, protein, arginine, fat, and ω-3 fatty acids (Table 1). These key nutritional factors should be considered in the nutritional management of every patient with cancer. Efficacy of other nutraceuticals, including antioxidant vitamins, trace minerals, glutamine, protease inhibitors (Bowman-Birk inhibitor [BBI]), garlic, tea polyphenols, vitamin A, and shark cartilage, has not been substantiated in clinical trials in pets with cancer. Their potential use is discussed elsewhere in this article.

Soluble carbohydrate and fiber

Most dogs and cats do not have a requirement for soluble carbohydrates and fiber in their diet. Pet food manufacturers and homemade recipes use ingredients containing soluble carbohydrates because they are well used as energy sources and they have unique properties that aid in manufacturing and cooking processes. Soluble carbohydrates may be poorly used by animals with cancer, however, because the soluble carbohydrates may enhance insulin and contribute to increased lactate production. Thus, soluble carbohydrates should be minimized in the dry matter content of foods (see Table 1).

Soluble (fermentable) and insoluble (poorly fermentable) fiber sources are important to help maintain intestinal health, especially in animals undergoing chemotherapy, radiation therapy, or surgery. Increased dietary fiber may help to prevent and treat abnormal stool quality (eg, soft stools, diarrhea) encountered when changing from a high-carbohydrate commercial dry food to a high-fat commercial or homemade food. Crude fiber levels greater than 2.5% dry matter are recommended.

Protein and arginine

Dietary protein should be highly digestible and exceed levels normally used for maintenance of adult animals (see Table 1), because patients with

Table 1
Key nutritional factors for dogs and cats with cancer and levels in selected commercial foods[a]

	Protein	Soluble carbohydrate	Fat	Omega-3 fatty acids	Arginine	Crude fiber
Recommended levels for dogs with cancer:	30–45	<25	25–40	>5	>2.5	>2.5
Recommended levels for cats with cancer:	40–50	<25	25–40	2–3	>2.5	>2.5
Products						
Hill's Prescription Diet Canine n/d, moist	38.0	19.9	33.2	7.3	2.95	2.7
Hill's Prescription Diet Canine/Feline a/d, moist	45.7	14.7	30.5	2.6	2.1	1.3
Hill's Prescription Diet Feline p/d, moist	47.6	12.2	32	0.41	2.7	0.7
Hill's Science Diet Feline Adult Seafood Recipe, moist	45.1	20.1	25.4	0.82	2.8	2.5
Iams Eukanuba Maximum Calorie/Canine & Feline, moist	43.3	7.6	41.1	0.78	2.6	1.6
Iams Eukanuba Maximum Calorie/Canine, dry	40.1	22.7	29	0.9	na	2.3
Iams Eukanuba Maximum Calorie/Feline, dry	44.2	19.1	29.6	0.93	na	1.4
Purina CV Feline Formula, moist	42.5	23.1	26.8	na	na	1.0
Purina DM Feline Formula, dry	59.3	12.9	17.5	0.44	na	1.3
Purina DM Feline Formula, moist	56.9	8.1	23.8	0.88	na	3.7
Select Care Feline Development Formula, moist	48.0	12.1	32.2	na	na	1.4
Dry grocery brand dog foods (average)[b]	25.3	52.2	12.3	<1	<2	3.1
Dry specialty brand dog foods (average)[b]	28.1	45.1	16.3	<1	<2	3.3
Moist grocery brand dog foods (average)[b]	41.2	19.9	27.1	<1	<2	1.8
Dry grocery brand cat foods (average)[b]	34.8	43.9	12.3	<1	<2	2.2
Dry specialty brand cat foods (average)[b]	35.3	37.4	18.5	<1	<2	2.4
Moist grocery brand cat foods (average)[b]	51.2	9.7	26.6	<1	<2	1.5

Abbreviation: na, information not available from manufacturer.

[a] Nutrients expressed on a percent dry matter basis. Values obtained from manufacturers' published information.
[b] *Data from* Debraekeleer J. Nutrient profiles of commercial dog and cat foods (Appendix L). In: Hand MS, Thatcher CD, Remillard RL, Roudebush P, editors. Small animal clinical nutrition, 4th edition. Topeka (KS): Mark Morris Institute; 2000. p. 1073–83.

cancer have altered protein metabolism and may suffer loss of lean muscle mass (cachexia). Protein levels should be highly bioavailable and moderate in an amount of 30% to 45% dry matter in foods for dogs with cancer and 40% to 50% dry matter in foods for cats with cancer.

Arginine is an essential amino acid that may have specific therapeutic value in animals with cancer. Adding arginine to parenteral solutions decreases tumor growth and metastatic rates in rodent cancer models [21,22]. Increased dietary arginine in conjunction with increased dietary ω-3 fatty acid intake improves clinical signs, quality of life, and survival time in dogs treated for cancer. In a group of dogs receiving chemotherapy for lymphoma, consumption of food supplemented with arginine and ω-3 fatty acids elevated plasma arginine and fatty acid concentrations [23]. Plasma levels of arginine and ω-3 fatty acids were positively correlated with survival time; however, it is unclear if the arginine had an independent effect [23]. Similarly, in dogs undergoing radiation therapy for nasal tumors and fed food supplemented with arginine and ω-3 fatty acids, elevated plasma levels of arginine and ω-3 fatty acids were positively correlated with quality of life and negatively correlated with inflammatory mediators and mucositis in irradiated areas [24]. The exact mechanisms whereby arginine benefits patients with cancer are unknown but may include modulating the immune system or altering neuroendocrine responses. The minimum effective level of dietary arginine for animals with cancer is unknown; however, the positive correlation between plasma arginine concentrations and survival in dogs with lymphoma receiving chemotherapy suggests that it is appropriate to provide more than 2.5% arginine on a dry matter basis. Cats should receive foods with similar levels until research discloses a more effective level.

Glutamine

Like arginine, glutamine seems to have great potential benefits for pets with cancer. For many years, glutamine was considered a nonessential amino acid; however, numerous studies have demonstrated that endogenous glutamine storage and synthesis may not be adequate to meet the body's needs in certain situations, such as critical illness, trauma, sepsis, and cancer [25]. Glutamine levels in plasma and skeletal muscle are decreased in tumor-bearing animals [26].

Glutamine has many important biochemical roles and is a preferred energy fuel for cells with rapid turnover, such as lymphocytes, enterocytes, and malignant cells. There has been considerable interest in giving supplemental glutamine to patients with cancer, because glutamine deficiency may contribute to cancer cachexia and poor immune response. Glutamine supplementation is a concern for cancer patients because glutamine may potentially enhance tumor growth. Studies have shown that glutamine supplementation does not enhance DNA content in tumors, indicating that supplemented glutamine can be used by nontumor tissues, such as muscle, lymphocytes, and the gut mucosa. Studies using rodent cancer models and clinical trials in human patients with cancer have shown that glutamine supplementation (1) stabilizes weight loss, (2) improves protein metabolism, (3) improves systemic immune response, and (4) improves gut-barrier function (less bacterial translocation) during radiochemotherapy [25,26]. One study revealed that feeding a glutamine-supplemented and amino acid–based purified food was unable to preserve intestinal function in a methotrexate-induced enteritis model in cats, however [27]. Additional studies are needed to determine optimal glutamine intake for pets with cancer. Supplementation of pet foods with L-glutamine is difficult, because the amino acid is unstable when heated or cooked. Glutamine is best supplied by high-quality and high-protein pet foods.

Protease inhibitors

Certain protease inhibitors are effective at preventing or suppressing carcinogen-induced transformation in vitro and carcinogenesis in animal model systems [28]. One protease inhibitor, the soybean-derived BBI, is particularly effective in suppressing malignant transformation in vitro and carcinogenesis and metastases in vivo without toxicity. BBI has been investigated most closely for control of leukoplakia in the oral cavity, a surrogate marker of head and neck cancer development in people. One study was performed using a feline model of methotrexate-induced enteritis to determine the impact of foods containing intact soybean protein, casein, or crystalline amino acids on intestinal structure and function [29]. This study revealed an association between feeding a soybean protein-based food and improved intestinal integrity (ie, less villous atrophy). These findings might be the result of a greater secretogogue effect of soybean protein-based foods, which stimulate trophic gut hormones, such as cholecystokinin. Further studies are needed to determine the role for soybean protein, BBI, and protease inhibitors in the routine management of pets with cancer.

Fat and ω-3 fatty acids

Some tumor cells have difficulty in using lipids as a fuel source, although host tissues continue to oxidize lipids for energy. As mentioned previously, this finding led to the hypothesis that foods moderately high in fat may benefit animals with cancer compared with foods relatively high in carbohydrates. Pets in North America receive most of their nutrient intake from commercial dry pet foods. These foods are usually high in soluble carbohydrate (25%–60%) and relatively low in fat (7%–25%). These characteristics likely make most commercial dry foods less optimal for nutritional management of animals with cancer. Table 1 compares recommended levels of soluble carbohydrate, protein, and fat for animals with cancer with nutrient levels in typical commercial pet foods and selected therapeutic foods.

The ω-3 fatty acids, especially those found in certain types of fish and fish oil (eicosapentaenoic acid [EPA] and docosahexaenoic acid [DHA]), are probably the most important nutraceuticals to consider for animals with cancer. Several human epidemiologic studies have suggested that consumption of fish or higher levels of ω-3 fatty acids is beneficial. Fish consumption protects against colorectal cancer in women and prostate cancer in men [30,31]. Higher ω-3 fatty acid concentrations in adipose tissue are associated with a reduced risk of breast cancer in women [32]. The recommendation for feeding high levels of ω-3 fatty acids, such as EPA and DHA, to pets with cancer is based on (1) in vitro cell culture studies, (2) extensive studies in rodent models using several different types of cancer, (3) clinical trials in human patients with severe forms of cancer, and (4) clinical trials in dogs treated for lymphoma and nasal tumors. Table 2 summarizes the metabolic basis for the use of ω-3 fatty acids for patients with cancer and lists results of in vitro and laboratory animal studies. These findings are discussed below. Results of human and canine clinical trials using ω-3 fatty acid supplements or enriched foods are discussed in the next section.

Fish oil and EPA/DHA supplementation inhibits lipolysis and muscle protein degradation associated with cachexia in various animal models. EPA inhibits LMF as discussed previously, which presumably explains the ability of EPA to preserve fat stores in patients with cancer [11–13,18]. EPA also inhibits PIF and thus helps to limit muscle protein degradation mediated by the ubiquitin-proteasome proteolysis pathway [12,13]. EPA significantly reduces protein degradation and tumor-induced lipolysis in rodent models of cancer [20]. Thus, EPA plays a key role in helping to reverse tumor-induced catabolic effects [11,12,20].

Matrix metalloproteinases (MMPs) are a family of zinc-dependent enzymes that play a key role in degrading basement membrane components and extracellular matrix. MMP activity is detectable in canine and feline neoplastic tissue and serum of tumor-bearing animals [33,34]. MMP activity is higher in tumor tissue than in unaffected stromal tissue, indicating that MMP may be involved in the pathogenesis of tumor growth and metastasis [33,34]. The ω-3 fatty acids can modulate MMP activity and may influence tumor growth and metastasis via this mechanism [19].

Several hundred studies using laboratory animal cancer models or in vitro cell cultures have evaluated the effects of fish oil or EPA/DHA on various facets of tumorigenesis, tumor growth, metastasis, and cancer therapy [18,19]. Findings include the following:

- EPA/DHA administration reduces cancerous transformation of irradiated fibroblasts and inhibits proliferation and metabolism in various cancer cell lines.

Table 2
Mechanisms and beneficial effects of omega-3 fatty acid supplementation in patients with cancer

Mechanisms and Effects	Species	Type of study
Reduced cancerous transformation of cells	Mouse	Irradiated fibroblasts
Inhibited growth of aberrant cells	Rat	Colon crypt cell biopsies
Inhibited proliferation and metabolism of cancer cells	Human being	Colon cancer cell culture
Increased radiation sensitivity of cancer cells	Rat	Brain tumor cell culture
Inhibited growth of primary tumors	Rat, mouse	Models of mammary, colon, prostate, lung and liver cancer
Inhibited growth of metastatic tumors	Mouse	Models of mammary and lung cancer
Decreased cytokine production	Rat	Mammary cancer model
	Human being	Clinical study of pancreatic cancer
Enhanced effects of chemotherapeutic agents on cancer cells	Human being	Cancer cell culture
	Mouse, rat	Models of mammary cancer
	Human being	Clinical study of breast cancer
Reduced blood vascular area in solid tumors	Mouse	Model of mammary cancer
Inhibited catabolic mediators	Mouse	Models of mammary and colon cancer
	Human being	Clinical study of pancreatic cancer
Reduced acute-phase proteins	Human being	Clinical study of pancreatic cancer
Reversed or stabilized weight loss	Human being	Clinical study of pancreatic cancer
Improved metabolic abnormalities	Dog	Clinical study of lymphoma
Reduced radiation damage to normal tissues	Dog	Clinical study of nasal tumors
Increased survival time when used with chemotherapy	Dog	Clinical study of lymphoma
Increased disease free interval when used with chemotherapy	Dog	Clinical study of lymphoma
Increased quality of life	Human being	Clinical study of pancreatic cancer
Increased quality of life when used with chemotherapy	Dog	Clinical study of lymphoma

- EPA/DHA supplementation inhibits growth of aberrant colon crypt cells, which are biomarkers for colon cancer.
- Oxidation products of ω-3 fatty acids promote apoptosis (programmed cell death) of tumor cells.
- Fish oil supplementation results in EPA/DHA incorporation into cell membranes of malignant cells.
- Fish oil or EPA/DHA supplementation inhibits growth of colon, liver, lung, prostate, and mammary tumors in rodent cancer models.

- Fish oil or EPA/DHA supplementation inhibits metastasis of colon and mammary tumors in rodent cancer models.
- Fish oil or EPA/DHA supplementation regulates the expression or activity of MMPs.
- Fish oil or EPA/DHA supplementation modulates the secretion of cytokines and eicosanoids, such as TNFα, interleukin (IL)-1, IL-6, and prostaglandin E_2, that have catabolic effects or impair immune responsiveness.
- Fish oil or EPA/DHA supplementation enhances the antitumor effects of certain cancer chemotherapeutic agents.
- Fish oil or EPA/DHA supplementation enhances the response of tumors to ionizing radiation.
- Fish oil supplementation reduces the blood vascular area in solid tumors.

Taken together, these extensive findings suggest a role for providing high levels of ω-3 fatty acids in the diet of pets with cancer. Table 1 compares recommended levels of fat and total ω-3 fatty acids for animals with cancer with nutrient levels in typical commercial pet foods and selected therapeutic foods. Clinical trials in people and well-controlled randomized clinical trials in dogs have further validated the benefits of using high levels of dietary ω-3 fatty acids in patients with cancer.

Clinical studies using ω-3 fatty acids in patients with cancer

Human clinical trials with fish oil or EPA/DHA supplementation have focused on patients with severe forms of cancer that carry a poor prognosis and have significant morbidity associated with pronounced cachexia. Fish oil or EPA/DHA supplementation in human patients with unresectable pancreatic cancer reverses weight loss, normalizes energy expenditure, reduces cytokine production, decreases production of catabolic mediators, and reduces or stabilizes production of acute-phase proteins [35–42]. As mentioned previously, the presence of an acute-phase protein response is strongly associated with reduced survival in patients with cancer, thus demonstrating a beneficial response to ω-3 fatty acid supplementation. Other clinical studies have shown that (1) fish oil supplementation modulates the immune response and prolongs survival of human patients with solid tumors [43], (2) EPA supplementation improves cell-mediated immune function in human patients with esophageal cancer [44], and (3) ω-3 fatty acid levels are higher in adipose tissue of women responding to chemotherapy for breast cancer [45].

Several well-controlled clinical trials have evaluated the use of a moderate-fat, low-carbohydrate, arginine- and fish oil–supplemented food (Prescription Diet Canine n/d; Hill's Pet Nutrition, Inc., Topeka, Kansas) in normal dogs and dogs undergoing chemotherapy for lymphoma or radiation therapy for nasal tumors. In normal dogs, food supplemented with high levels of fish oil elevated serum concentrations of EPA and DHA within 1 week. Furthermore, these elevated concentrations persisted for several weeks after dietary supplementation was discontinued [46].

One controlled randomized study evaluated the effects of Prescription Diet Canine n/d in decreasing or eliminating the metabolic alterations seen in dogs with stage IIIa and IVa lymphoma treated concurrently with doxorubicin chemotherapy [47]. Dogs fed the fish oil– and arginine-supplemented food had the following changes: (1) higher serum concentrations of EPA, DHA, and arginine; (2) lower serum glucose, lactate, and insulin values for intravenous glucose and food tolerance tests; and (3) more normal serum IL-6 and acute-phase protein concentrations. This study was followed by two controlled randomized trials in dogs with histologically confirmed high-grade stage IIIa or IVa lymphoblastic lymphoma [23,48]. Dogs fed the fish oil– and arginine-supplemented food had higher serum levels of ω-3 fatty acids and arginine compared with levels in dogs fed the unsupplemented control food. Higher serum levels of EPA and DHA were associated with lesser plasma lactic acid responses to intravenous glucose and food tolerance testing. Increasing ω-3 fatty acid levels were significantly associated with a longer disease-free interval, longer survival time, and improved quality of life for dogs fed the supplemented food (Table 3).

Moderate ω-3 fatty acid–supplemented foods do not seem to affect the pharmacokinetics of doxorubicin [49]. This finding suggests that the beneficial effects of ω-3 fatty acids are probably not related to altered drug metabolism or excretion in animals undergoing chemotherapy.

A separate controlled and randomized clinical trial evaluated the effect of fish oil and arginine supplementation on the acute effects of radiation injury in dogs with nasal tumors [24]. Dogs fed the supplemented food had higher serum concentrations of EPA, DHA, and arginine compared with values from control dogs. Higher serum levels of EPA and DHA were associated with lower plasma lactic acid concentrations, lower tissue concentrations of inflammatory mediators, improved performance scores, and a lesser degree of histologic damage to normal tissues from radiation therapy.

Together, these clinical studies suggest that feeding a moderate-fat and low-carbohydrate food supplemented with arginine and high levels of ω-3 fatty acids (1) is associated with an increase in the survival time of dogs undergoing single-agent cancer chemotherapy; (2) increases the survival time of a subset of dogs undergoing single-agent cancer chemotherapy by more than 30% compared with the survival time of similar dogs consuming an unsupplemented food; (3) reduces the severity of some acute phases of radiation therapy, thereby improving the quality of life for dogs with cancer; (4) suppresses the clinical signs of cancer for longer intervals (ie, longer periods of remission); and (5) counteracts select persistent metabolic changes found in canine cancer patients. Although clinical trials with functional foods have been performed for only a limited number of cancer types, the underlying metabolic abnormalities caused by cancer have been documented in dogs with many different types of tumors [8,9]. These

Table 3
Survival times of dogs with lymphoma receiving chemotherapy and a control or experimental food

Treatment	Median survival time (days)
None (historical)	30
Doxorubicin alone (historical)	230[a]
Control food plus doxorubicin[b]	275[c]
Canine n/d plus doxorubicin[d]	354[c]
Multidrug protocol[e]	397[e]

[a] *Data from* Postorino NC, Susaneck SJ, Withrow SJ, et al. Single-agent therapy with Adriamycin for canine lymphosarcoma. J Am Anim Hosp Assoc 1989;25:221–5.

[b] Control food was identical to Canine n/d except soybean oil replaced menhaden fish oil and arginine was not added.

[c] *Data from* Ogilvie GK, Fettman MJ, Mallinckrodt CH, Walton JA, Hansen RA, et al. Effect of fish oil, arginine and doxorubicin chemotherapy on remission and survival time for dogs with lymphoma. Cancer 2000;88:1916–28.

[d] Prescription Diet Canine n/d, Hill's Pet Nutrition, Inc., Topeka, KS.

[e] *Data from* Garrett LD, Thamm DH, Chun R, Dudley R, Vail DM. Evaluation of a 6-month chemotherapy protocol with no maintenance therapy for dogs with lymphoma. J Vet Intern Med 2002;16:704–9.

findings may suggest that similar clinical responses would be expected in animals with a wide range of cancer types; however, additional studies need to be performed to document this hypothesis.

In general, dietary supplementation with high levels of fish oil is safe for dogs. Potential adverse effects include poor wound healing, coagulopathies (eg, platelet dysfunction), gastrointestinal upset (eg, soft stools, diarrhea), pancreatitis, fishy breath odor, and nutrient interactions (eg, the vitamin E requirement increases with the amount of polyunsaturated fatty acids, including ω-3 fatty acids, in the food). Hemograms and serum biochemical profiles are not adversely affected by fish oil–supplemented foods in dogs with lymphoma and hemangiosarcoma [50]. Enrichment with ω-3 fatty acids also seems not to significantly alter wound healing [51]. High levels of dietary ω-3 fatty acids can potentially alter platelet function; however, studies in normal dogs and dogs with cancer have not shown such effects [52,53]. The same may not be true for cats. One study failed to detect significant changes in platelet aggregation or mucosal bleeding time in normal cats supplemented with purified EPA and DHA [54]; however, two other studies revealed decreased platelet aggregation and increased toenail or mucosal bleeding time in normal cats fed ω-3 fatty acid–enriched foods [55,56]. Because of the potential for serious bleeding problems, cats with cancer should be given foods with lower levels of fish oil or ω-3 fatty acids than those levels recommended for dogs with cancer (see Table 1).

Clinical experience suggests that approximately 10% of dogs with cancer develop soft stools or diarrhea when initially fed a high-fat canned dog food in conjunction with other cancer therapy. Of these dogs, about half adjust to the dietary change and develop normal stool consistency. The other half (about 5% of total cases) continue to have stool consistency issues that pet owners find unacceptable. Abnormal stool quality can be minimized or managed by gradually changing from commercial dry foods to higher fat canned foods over 10 to 14 days, adding dietary fiber or high-fiber foods to make up 5% to 10% of the total food intake, or using intestinal antibiotics as needed to control secondary clostridial enterocolitis.

Additional dietary fiber options include (1) adding psyllium husk fiber (Metamucil; Proctor & Gamble, Cincinnati, OH), 1 teaspoon per 5 to 10 kg of body weight with each meal; (2) adding a high-fiber cereal (Post 100% Bran cereal, Kraft Foods, Rye Brook, NY [28% fiber], Kellogg All-Bran cereal, Kellogg, Battle Creek, MI [50% fiber], or General Mills Fiber One cereal, General Mills, Minneapolis, MN [43% fiber]) by mixing cereal, 0.5 to 1 cup, per can of food; or (3) replacing approximately 10% of the total daily calories with higher fiber foods (Prescription Diet Canine r/d or Canine w/d dry foods; Hill's Pet Nutrition, Inc.) by mixing the dry product with the canned food at each meal. Foods with high levels of fat should also be used with caution in dogs at risk for pancreatitis.

In general, the use of commercial therapeutic foods formulated to aid in the nutritional management of dogs with cancer (Canine n/d, Hills Pet Nutrition, Inc.) is preferable to supplementing typical pet foods with fish oil and arginine. To achieve levels of ω-3 fatty acids found in Canine n/d, typical pet foods need to be supplemented with 12 to 20 fish oil capsules per day for a 10-kg dog. Use of an appropriate therapeutic food is more economic and increases pet owner compliance compared with administering multiple daily supplements.

Other nutraceuticals of interest in patients with cancer

Antioxidant vitamins

As mentioned earlier, many human cancer patients use vitamin supplements as complementary therapy, usually without the recommendation or knowledge of their physician [1–4]. Owners of pets with cancer may also commonly provide vitamin supplementation; however, this assumption has not been studied specifically. The need for vitamin E in the diet is markedly influenced by the composition of the food. The vitamin E requirement increases with increasing levels of polyunsaturated fatty acids (including ω-3 fatty acids), oxidizing agents, and trace minerals and decreases with increasing levels of fat-soluble vitamins, sulfur-containing amino acids, and selenium. Manufacturers of many specialty brand pet foods have increased levels of antioxidant vitamins, such as vitamins E and C, because they seem to improve immune function and reduce cell damage in normal animals. The role of antioxidant vitamins in animals with cancer is more complex, however.

At present, two opposing hypotheses exist regarding the use of antioxidant nutrients for patients with cancer [57]. One hypothesis suggests that supplementation with high doses of multiple micronutrients, including high-dose dietary antioxidants (eg, vitamins C and E, carotenoids, selenium), may improve the efficacy of cancer therapy by improving immune function, increasing tumor response to radiation or chemotherapy, decreasing toxicity to normal cells, and helping to reverse metabolic changes contributing to cachexia. The other hypothesis suggests that dietary antioxidants should not be used because they may protect cancer cells against damage by chemotherapy or radiation therapy. The second hypothesis is based on evidence that dietary fish oil inhibits tumor growth by increasing lipid peroxidation within cancer cells and that the beneficial effects of fish oil supplementation can be blocked by concurrent administration of vitamin E. Each of these hypotheses is derived from results obtained from hundreds of different studies and experimental designs.

Additional studies are needed to determine optimal antioxidant nutrient intake for pets with cancer. At the present time, megadose vitamin therapy does not seem to be indicated if the animal is fed a complete and balanced commercial food. The levels of vitamin E and other antioxidant nutrients should be appropriate for the level of polyunsaturated fatty acids, trace minerals, and oxidants in the food.

Trace minerals

Serum zinc, chromium, and iron concentrations are lower in dogs with lymphoma and osteosarcoma than levels in normal dogs [58]. The clinical significance of these abnormalities is unknown, however, especially because serum levels may or may not correlate with tissue levels of trace minerals. Additional studies are needed to determine optimal trace mineral intake for pets with cancer. At the present time, trace mineral supplementation does not seem to be indicated if the animal is fed a complete and balanced commercial food; however, trace mineral supplementation is essential if the owner feeds a home-prepared food.

Garlic

Epidemiologic studies suggest that garlic consumption has a preventive effect in human stomach and colorectal cancers [59]. Animal and in vitro studies provide further evidence that active ingredients in garlic and other allium vegetables (eg, onions, leeks, chives) have an anticarcinogenic effect. The positive effect seems to be related to the presence of oil- and water-soluble organosulfur compounds, primarily allyl derivatives like allicin [60,61]. The exact cancer-preventive mechanisms and effects are not clear; however, organosulfur compounds (1) modulate the activity of several enzymes that detoxify carcinogens, (2) deplete intracellular glutathione levels transiently in cancer cells, (3) depress cell division and induce apoptosis, (4) regulate nuclear factors involved in immune function and inflammation, (5) affect eicosanoid metabolism and cells that produce these metabolites, (6) regulate fatty acid metabolism, (7) inhibit platelet function by interfering with thromboxane synthesis, and (8) inhibit oxidative reactions [60–62]. Whether garlic powder and tablets possess similar levels of active compounds as fresh garlic preparations is subject to debate [62].

Preliminary studies of garlic powder inclusion in a complete and balanced dry dog food failed to show significant immunomodulatory effects in normal dogs [63]. Garlic extract oxidizes erythrocyte membranes and hemoglobin in dogs, inducing hemolysis associated with the appearance of eccentrocytes and Heinz bodies [64]. Routine use of garlic extracts in pets with cancer is discouraged because of the potential for toxicity and lack of clear evidence of efficacy.

Tea polyphenols

Several animal studies have demonstrated an anticarcinogenic effect of polyphenols, including flavones, flavonols, isoflavones, and catechins [65]. Extracts derived from the tea plant (*Camellia sinensis*) contain many polyphenolic compounds, which account for up to 30% of the dry weight of green tea leaves. Most of the polyphenols in green tea are flavonols, commonly known as catechins. In addition, caffeine, theobromine, theophylline, and phenolic acids like gallic acid are present as minor constituents of green tea. Black tea also contains several polyphenols, such as bisflavanals, theaflavins, and thearubigens.

Oral consumption or topical application of green tea or its polyphenolic constituents protects mice against tumor development induced by chemicals or ultraviolet radiation [66]. Polyphenols isolated from green tea or water extract of green tea afford protection against chemically induced carcinogenesis in several different organ systems in other animal models [66]. In addition, green tea modulates and increases the efficacy of cancer chemotherapeutic drugs in animal models [66]. The following mechanisms may be associated with the biologic effects of tea polyphenols: (1) inhibiting enzymes, such as cytochrome P450, which are involved in the bioactivation of carcinogens; (2) inducing apoptosis in cancer cells but not normal cells; (3) inhibiting growth of cancer cells by arresting the cell cycle; (4) inhibiting cell proliferation and tumor progression by binding to epidermal growth factor receptors; (5) modifying inflammation and carcinogenesis by inhibiting nitric oxide production; (6) inhibiting tumor promotion by decreasing activator protein; and (7) inhibiting angiogenesis through suppression of IL-8.

Green tea extracts are found in a few commercial pet foods and are available as supplements. Tea polyphenols may have relevance for cancer prevention and chemotherapy in the future if the results summarized here can be verified in pets.

Vitamin A

Retinol, retinal, and retinoic acid are three natural compounds that have vitamin A activity in mammals. Food sources include retinyl esters (vitamin A palmitate) in animal tissues and carotenoids (β-carotene) in vegetables. The term *retinoids* refers to the entire group of naturally occurring and synthetic vitamin A derivatives. The general functions of vitamin A include growth promotion, differentiation and maintenance of epithelial tissues, and maintenance of normal reproductive and visual functions. Retinoic acid affects differentiation and proliferation of epithelial cells by binding to and activating specific cell nuclear receptors that can modify rates of gene transcription.

In the last 25 years, many synthetic retinoids have been developed to offer better therapeutic responses and less toxicity than naturally occurring vitamin A compounds. These are classified as drugs rather than as nutraceuticals. Isotretinoin (Accutane; Roche Pharmaceuticals, Nutley, New Jersey) has been the synthetic retinoid used most commonly by veterinary dermatologists for cutaneous neoplastic disorders, such as epitheliotropic lymphoma (cutaneous T-cell lymphoma) and multiple keratoacanthomas [67]. Isotretinoin has been ineffective for the treatment of preneoplastic and squamous cell carcinoma lesions in cats, however [68].

Shark cartilage

The discovery that angiogenesis (ie, blood vessel growth and development) is a key condition for growth and metastasis of tumors has brought about a new approach for treating cancer using nutraceuticals and drugs that inhibit formation of new blood vessels [69]. Inhibition of tumoral angiogenesis may slow tumor growth and metastasis. Initially, cartilage was considered as a possible natural source of antiangiogenic compounds because of its avascular nature. The use of crude shark cartilage extracts for the treatment of cancer in people remains controversial, however, because of unsatisfactory patient outcomes in clinical trials [69] and lack of data that correlate bioavailability of shark cartilage with therapeutic effects [70]. At this point, there is no clear evidence that shark cartilage benefits pets with cancer.

More recently, antiangiogenic compounds have been extracted and purified from cartilage (Neovastat; Aeterna Laboratories, Quebec City, Quebec, Canada). These compounds are considered drugs rather than nutraceutical ingredients. Components of Neovastat seem to prevent angiogenesis in tumors by (1) preventing binding of vascular endothelial growth factor, (2) inhibiting MMP activity, (3) inducing endothelial cell–specific apoptosis, and (4) increasing levels of angiostatin at the tumor site [71]. Multiple human clinical trials are underway using this angiogenesis inhibitor in several different types of cancer, and results are expected within the next few years.

Results of these clinical trials may offer new therapeutic options in the future for pets with cancer.

References

[1] Metz JM, Jones H, Devine P, Hahn S, Glatstein E. Cancer patients use unconventional medical therapies far more frequently than standard history and physical examination suggest. Cancer J 2000;7:149–54.
[2] Sandler RS, Halabi S, Kaplan EB, Baron JA, Paskett E, Petrelli NJ. Use of vitamins, minerals, and nutritional supplements by participants in a chemoprevention trial. Cancer 2001;91:1040–5.
[3] Ernst E. Complementary therapies in palliative cancer care. Cancer 2001;91:2181–5.
[4] Bernstein BJ, Grasso T. Prevalence of complementary and alternative medicine use in cancer patients. Oncology (Huntingt) 2001;15:1267–72.
[5] Vail DM, Ogilvie GK, Wheeler SL, Fettman MJ, Johnston SD, Hegstad RL. Alterations in carbohydrate metabolism in canine lymphoma. J Vet Intern Med 1990;4:8–11.
[6] Vail DM, Ogilvie GK, Fettman MJ, Wheeler SL. Exacerbations of hyperlactemia by infusion of lactated Ringer's solution in dogs with lymphoma. J Vet Intern Med 1990;4:228–32.
[7] Ogilvie GK, Vail DM, Wheeler SL, Fettman MJ, Salman MD, Johnston SD, et al. Effects of chemotherapy and remission on carbohydrate metabolism in dogs with lymphosarcoma. Cancer 1992;69:233–8.
[8] Ogilvie GK, Walters L, Salman MD, Fettman MJ, Johnston SD, Hegstad RL. Alterations in carbohydrate metabolism in dogs with non-hematopoietic malignancies. Am J Vet Res 1997;56:277–81.
[9] Mazzaferro EM, Hackett TB, Stein TP, Ogilvie GK, Wingfield WE, Walton J, et al. Metabolic alterations in dogs with osteosarcoma. Am J Vet Res 2001;62:1234–9.
[10] Arai T, Ogino T, Gunji M, Washizu T, Komori S, Washizu M. Changes in glucose transport activities in mammary adenocarcinoma of dogs. Res Vet Sci 1997;62:85–6.
[11] Costelli P, Baccino FM. Cancer cachexia: from experimental models to patient management. Curr Opin Clin Nutr Metab Care 2000;3:177–81.
[12] Inui A. Cancer anorexia-cachexia syndrome: current issues in research and management. CA Cancer J Clin 2002;52:72–91.
[13] Langhans W. Peripheral mechanisms involved with catabolism. Curr Opin Clin Nutr Metab Care 2002;5:419–26.
[14] Jagoe RT, Goldberg AL. What do we really know about the ubiquitin-proteasome pathway in muscle atrophy? Curr Opin Clin Nutr Metab Care 2001;4:183–90.
[15] Ogilvie GK, Vail DM, Wheeler SL. Alterations in fat and protein metabolism in dogs with cancer [abstract]. In: Proceedings of Veterinary Cancer Society. Estes Park, CO, 1988. Veterinary Cancer Society. p. 31.
[16] Ogilvie GK, Ford RD, Vail DM, Walters DM, Salman SD, Babineau C, et al. Alterations in lipoprotein profiles in dogs with lymphoma. J Vet Intern Med 1994;8:62–6.
[17] Hansell DT, Davies JW, Shenkin A, Burns HJ. The oxidation of body fuel stores in cancer patients. Ann Surg 1986;204:637–42.
[18] Bougnoux P. n-3 Polyunsaturated fatty acids and cancer. Curr Opin Clin Nutr Metab Care 1999;2:121–6.
[19] Zhou J-R, Blackburn GL. Dietary lipid modulation of immune response in tumorigenesis. In: Heber D, Blackburn GL, Go VLW, editors. Nutritional oncology. San Diego: Academic Press; 1999. p. 195–213.
[20] Ross JA, Moses AGW, Fearon KCH. The anti-catabolic effects of n-3 fatty acids. Curr Opin Clin Nutr Metab Care 1999;2:219–26.
[21] Ye SL, Istan NW, Driscoll DF, Bristrian BR. Tumor and host response to arginine and branched chain amino acid-enriched total parenteral nutrition. Cancer 1992;69:261–70.

[22] Tachibana K, Mukai K, Hiraoka I, Moriguchi S, Takama S, Kishino Y. Evaluation of the effect of arginine-enriched amino acid solution on tumor growth. J Parenter Enteral Nutr 1985;9:428–34.
[23] Ogilvie GK, Fettman MJ, Mallinkrodt CH, Walton JA, Hansen RA, Davenport DJ, et al. Effect of fish oil, arginine, and doxorubicin chemotherapy on remission and survival time for dogs with lymphoma. Cancer 2000;88:1916–28.
[24] Anderson CR, Ogilvie GK, Fettman MJ, LaRue SM, Powers BE, Hansen RA, et al. Effect of fish oil and arginine on acute effects of radiation injury in dogs with nasal tumors: a double-blind randomized study [abstract]. In: Proceedings of Veterinary Cancer Society and American College of Veterinary Radiology. Chicago, 1997. Veterinary Cancer Society. p. 33–4.
[25] Neu J, DeMarco V, Li N. Glutamine: clinical applications and mechanisms of action. Curr Opin Clin Nutr Metab Care 2002;5:69–75.
[26] Yoshida S, Karibara A, Ishibashi N, Shirouzu K. Glutamine supplementation in cancer patients. Nutrition 2001;17:766–8.
[27] Marks SL, Cook AK, Reader R, Kass PH, Theon AP, Greve C, et al. Effects of glutamine supplementation of an amino acid-based purified diet on intestinal integrity in cats with methotrexate-induced enteritis. Am J Vet Res 1999;60:755–63.
[28] Kennedy AR. The Bowman-Birk inhibitor from soybeans as an anticarcinogenic agent. Am J Clin Nutr 1998;68(Suppl):1406S–12S.
[29] Marks SL, Cook AK, Griffey S, Kass PH, Rogers QR. Dietary modulation of methotrexate-induced enteritis in cats. Am J Vet Res 1997;58:989–96.
[30] Mishina T, Watanabe H, Araki H, Nakao M. Epidemiological study of prostatic cancer by matched-pair analysis. Prostate 1998;6:423–36.
[31] Kato I, Akhmedkhanov A, Koenig K, Toniolo PG, Shore RE, Riboli E. Prospective study of diet and female colorectal cancer: the New York University Women's Health Group. Nutr Cancer 1997;28:276–81.
[32] Simonsen N, van't Veer P, Strain JJ, Martin-Moreno JM, Huttunen JK, Navajas JF, et al. Adipose tissue omega-3 and omega-6 fatty acid content and breast cancer in the EURAMIC study. Am J Epidemiol 1998;147:342–52.
[33] Lana SE, Ogilvie GK, Hansen RA, Powers RE, Dernell WS, Withrow SJ. Identification of matrix metalloproteinases in canine neoplastic tissue. Am J Vet Res 2000;61:111–4.
[34] Jankowski MK, Ogilvie GK, Lana SE, Fettman MJ, Hansen RA, Powers BE, et al. Matrix metalloproteinase activity in tumor, stromal tissue and serum from cats with malignancies. J Vet Intern Med 2002;16:105–8.
[35] Barber MD, Ross JA, Fearon KC. Changes in nutritional, functional and inflammatory markers in advanced pancreatic cancer. Nutr Cancer 1999;35:106–10.
[36] Barber MD, Ross JA, Voss AC, Tisdale MK, Fearon KC. The effect of an oral nutritional supplement enriched with fish oil on weight-loss in patients with pancreatic cancer. Br J Cancer 1999;81:80–6.
[37] Barber MD. Cancer cachexia and its treatment with fish-oil-enriched nutritional supplementation. Nutrition 2001;17:751–5.
[38] Barber MD, McMillan DC, Preston T, Ross JA, Fearon KC. Metabolic response to feeding in weight-losing pancreatic cancer patients and its modulation by a fish-oil-enriched nutritional supplement. Clin Sci (Lond) 2000;98:389–99.
[39] Barber MD, Ross JA, Preston T, Shenkin A, Fearon KC. Fish oil-enriched nutritional supplement attenuates progression of an acute-phase response in weight-losing patients with advanced pancreatic cancer. J Nutr 1999;129:1120–5.
[40] Barber MD, Fearon KC, Tisdale MJ, McMillan DC, Ross JA. Effects of a fish oil-enriched nutritional supplement on metabolic mediators in patients with pancreatic cancer cachexia. Nutr Cancer 2001;40:118–24.
[41] Wigmore SJ, Fearon KC, Maingay JP, Ross JA. Down-regulation of the acute-phase response in patients with pancreatic cancer cachexia receiving oral eicosapentaenoic acid is mediated via suppression of interleukin-6. Clin Sci (Lond) 1997;92:215–21.

[42] Wigmore SJ, Barber MD, Ross JA, Tisdale MJ, Fearon KC. Effects of oral eicosapentaenoic acid on weight loss in patients with pancreatic cancer. Nutr Cancer 2000;36: 177–84.
[43] Gogos CA, Ginopoulos P, Salsa B, Apostolidou E, Zoumbos NC, Kalfarentzos F. Dietary omega-3 polyunsaturated fatty acids plus vitamin E restore immunodeficiency and prolong survival for severely ill patients with generalized malignancy: a randomized control trial. Cancer 1998;82:395–402.
[44] Takagi K, Yamamori H, Furukawa K, Miyazaki M, Tashiro T. Perioperative supplementation of EPA reduces immunosuppression induced by postoperative chemoradiation therapy in patients with esophageal cancer. Nutrition 2001;17:478–9.
[45] Bougnoux P, Germain E, Chajes V, Hubert B, Lhuillery C, Le Floch O, et al. Cytotoxic drug efficacy correlates with adipose tissue docosahexaenoic acid level in locally advanced breast carcinoma. Br J Cancer 1999;79:1765–9.
[46] Hansen RA, Ogilvie GK, Davenport DJ, Gross KL, Walton JA, Richardson KL, et al. Duration of effects of dietary fish oil supplementation on serum eicosapentaenoic acid and docosahexaenoic acid concentrations in dogs. Am J Vet Res 1998;59:864–8.
[47] Ogilvie GK, Salman MD, Fettman MJ, Davenport D, Gross K, Hansen RA, et al. Omega-3 fatty acids improve hyperlactatemia and hyperinsulinemia [abstract]. In: Proceedings of the Veterinary Cancer Society. Tucson, AZ, 1995. Veterinary Cancer Society. p. 17–8.
[48] Ogilvie GK, Fettman MJ, Mallinckrodt CH, Walton JA, Hansen RA, Davenport DJ, et al. Effect of fish oil, arginine and doxorubicin chemotherapy on remission and survival time in dogs with lymphoma: a double blind, randomized placebo controlled study [abstract]. In: Proceedings of American College of Veterinary Internal Medicine Annual Meeting. Seattle, WA, 2000. American College of Veterinary Internal Medicine. p. 766.
[49] Selting KA, Ogilvie GK, Gustafson DL, Long M, Lana SM, Hansen RS, et al. Effect of n-3 fatty acids on the pharmacokinetics of doxorubicin [abstract]. In: Proceedings of the Veterinary Cancer Society. Baton Rouge, LA, 2001. Veterinary Cancer Society. p. 24.
[50] Walton JA, Ogilvie GK, Fettman MJ, Wells ML, Hansen RA, Richardson KL, et al. Effect of a fish oil supplemented diet and doxorubicin on hemograms and biochemical profiles from dogs with lymphoma and hemangiosarcoma: a double blind, randomized, placebo controlled study [abstract]. In: Proceedings of the Veterinary Cancer Society. Pacific Grove, CA, 2000. Veterinary Cancer Society. p. 101.
[51] Scardino MS, Swaim SF, Sartin EA, Hoffman CE, Ogilvie GK, Hansen RA, et al. The effects of omega-3 fatty acid enrichment on wound healing. Vet Dermatol 1999;10:283–90.
[52] Myers NC, Gross KL, Armstead EA, Davenport DJ. The effect of dietary n-6:n-3 fatty acid ratio on hemostatic parameters and platelet aggregation in the dog [abstract]. In: Proceedings of the American College of Veterinary Internal Medicine Annual Meeting. San Antonio, TX, 1996. American College of Veterinary Internal Medicine. p. 753.
[53] McNiel EA, Ogilvie GK, Mallinckrodt C, Richardson K, Fettman MJ. Platelet function in dogs treated for lymphoma and hemangiosarcoma and supplemented with dietary n-3 fatty acids. J Vet Intern Med 1999;13:574–80.
[54] Bright JM, Sullivan PS, Melton SL, Schneider JF, McDonald TP. The effects of n-3 fatty acid supplementation on bleeding time, plasma fatty acid composition and in vitro platelet aggregation in cats. J Vet Intern Med 1994;8:247–52.
[55] Sullivan P, Bright J. Role of n-3 fatty acid supplementation for the prevention of thrombosis in cats with cardiovascular disease [abstract]. In: Proceedings of the American College of Veterinary Internal Medicine Annual Meeting. Lake Buena Vista, FL, 1995. American College of Veterinary Internal Medicine. p. 482–3.
[56] Saker KE, Eddy AL, Thatcher CD, Kalnitsky J. Manipulation of dietary (n-6) and (n-3) fatty acids alters platelet function in cats. J Nutr 1998;128(12 Suppl):2645S–7S.
[57] Prasad KN, Cole WC, Kumaar B, Che Prasad K. Pros and cons of antioxidant use during radiation therapy. Cancer Treat Rev 2002;28:79–91.

[58] Kazmierski KJ, Ogilvie GK, Fettman MJ, Lana SE, Walton JA, Hansen RA, et al. Serum zinc, chromium and iron concentrations in dogs with lymphoma and osteosarcoma. J Vet Intern Med 2001;15:585–8.
[59] Fleischauer AT, Arab L. Garlic and cancer: a critical review of the epidemiologic literature. J Nutr 2001;131(Suppl):1032S–40S.
[60] Knowles LM, Milner JA. Possible mechanisms by which allyl sulfides suppress neoplastic cell proliferation. J Nutr 2001;131(Suppl):1061S–6S.
[61] Pinto JT, Rivlin RS. Antiproliferative effects of allium derivatives from garlic. J Nutr 2001; 131(Suppl):1058S–60S.
[62] Hirsch K, Danilenko M, Giat K, Miron T, Rabinkov A, Wilchek M, et al. Effect of purified allicin, the major ingredient of freshly crushed garlic, on cancer cell proliferation. Nutr Cancer 2000;38:245–54.
[63] Turek JJ, Massimino SP, Boebel KP, Hayek MG. Investigation of garlic as an immunomodulator in canines. In: Reinhart GA, Carey DP, editors. Recent advances in canine and feline nutrition, vol 3. Wilmington: Orange Frazer Press; 2000. p. 573–82.
[64] Lee K-W, Yamato O, Tajima M, Kuraoka M, Omae S, Maede Y. Hematologic changes associated with the appearance of eccentrocytes after intragastric administration of garlic extract in dogs. Am J Vet Res 2000;61:1446–50.
[65] Yang CS, Landau JM, Huang M-T, Newmark HL. Inhibition of carcinogenesis by dietary polyphenolic compounds. Annu Rev Nutr 2001;21:381–406.
[66] Ahmad N, Mukhtar H. Green tea polyphenols and cancer: biologic mechanisms and practical implications. Nutr Rev 1999;57:78–83.
[67] Scott DW, Miller WH, Griffin CE. Synthetic retinoids. In: Small animal dermatology. 6th edition. Philadelphia: WB Saunders; 2001. p. 241–3.
[68] Evans AG, Madewell BR, Stannard AA. A trial of 13-cis-retinoic acid for treatment of squamous cell carcinoma and preneoplastic lesions of the head in cats. Am J Vet Res 1985; 46:2553–7.
[69] Gonzalez RP, Leyva A, Moraes MO. Shark cartilage as source of antiangiogenic compounds: from basic to clinical research. Biol Pharm Bull 2001;24:1097–101.
[70] Miller DR, Anderson GT, Stark JJ, Granick JL, Richardson D. Phase I/II trial of the safety and efficacy of shark cartilage in the treatment of advanced cancer. J Clin Oncol 1998;16:3649–55.
[71] Falardeau P, Champagne P, Poyet P, Hariton C, Dupont E. Neovastat, a naturally occurring multifunctional antiangiogenic drug, in phase III clinical trials. Semin Oncol 2001;28:620–5.

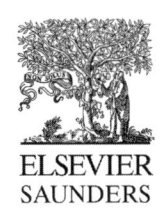

Use of nutraceuticals and chondroprotectants in osteoarthritic dogs and cats

Brian S. Beale, DVM

Gulf Coast Veterinary Specialists, 1111 West Loop South, Suite 160, Houston, TX 77027, USA

Chondroprotectants and nutraceuticals have become an attractive adjunctive or alternative treatment for cats and dogs suffering from osteoarthritis (OA). OA, also commonly referred to as degenerative joint disease (DJD), is characterized by varying amounts of joint pain and dysfunction depending on the severity and course of disease. Clinical signs might initially be limited to behavioral changes, occasional stiffness, difficulty rising, or reluctance to exercise. As the condition progresses, clinical signs such as lameness, loss of joint range of motion, and muscle atrophy become readily identifiable. Clinical signs might be exacerbated by exercise, long periods of rest or recumbancy, and weather changes (particularly cold weather). Some pets show signs of a restricted, stiff gait rather than obvious lameness. This presentation is seen commonly in cats and dogs that have mild DJD or those that have multiple joints with degenerative changes. Pets might also have a history of previous joint trauma (intra-articular fracture, ligamentous injury, dislocation, and so forth), osteochondral disease (osteochondrosis, ununited anconeal process, fragmented coronoid process), or congenital deformity (patellar luxation, hip dysplasia). OA might be more frequently diagnosed in cats today because of more critical observation and greater diagnostic effort. The osteoarthritic patient can be managed satisfactorily in most situations with a combination of optimization of body condition, exercise modification, anti-inflammatory therapy, and use of chondroprotectants agents. Chondroprotectants are available as oral nutraceuticals and injectable pharmaceuticals. Presently, recommendations cannot be made regarding which chondroprotectant is best for each dog and cat afflicted with osteoarthritis. Head-to-head comparisons of these products

E-mail address: drbeale@gcvs.com (B.S. Beale).

have not been made, and it is not known when the different mediators of OA play an important role. Mediators of pain and degradation (prostaglandins, free radicals, metalloproteinases, serine proteases, and so forth) might change during the course of disease. It would be ideal to know what the predominant mediators were in an individual animal suffering from OA to select the best product to treat that individual patient. The best current recommendation is to use products that have well-designed experimental and clinical research evaluating efficacy and safety and products that are manufactured under the high quality standards practiced by the pharmaceutical industry.

Chondroprotectants and nutraceuticals: definition

The term chondroprotectant is applied to various compounds that are proposed to have a positive effect on the health and metabolism of chondrocytes and synoviocytes. This definition is quite broad and thus has been used to label a wide variety of veterinary products that differ considerably in their structure, function, and degree of purity. Other terms have been used to describe these types of products, including slow-acting, disease-modifying osteoarthritic agents (SADMOA), structure/disease-modifying anti-OA drug, and symptomatic slow-acting drug for OA [1–6]. Because of the great variation in nomenclature and molecular structure of these compounds, care should be taken when attempting to compare one chondroprotectant agent to another. When applicable, it is always preferable to use generic compound names rather than trade names or broad descriptive terms (eg, chondroprotectant, SADMOA, and so forth) when discussing the effects or comparing the merits of these agents. Nevertheless, the term chondroprotectant is used in this article to help bridge the information presented here with that reported elsewhere previously.

Chondroprotective agents are purported to have three primary effects:

1. Support or enhance metabolism of chondrocyte and synoviocyte (anabolic)
2. Inhibit degradative enzymes within synovial fluid and cartilage matrix (catabolic)
3. Inhibit formation of thrombi in small blood vessels supplying the joint (antithrombotic)

Many types of compounds have been purported to have chondroprotective effects, including glycosaminoglycans (GAGs), amino sugars, structural proteins, enzymes, minerals, preparations of whole tissue, and semisynthetic compounds [1,2]. These compounds are available in oral and injectable forms. Most oral chondroprotectants are classified as dietary supplements. A subset of oral chondroprotectant agents is designated as nutraceuticals. A veterinary nutraceutical has been defined by the North American Veterinary Nutraceutical Council as a nondrug substance that is produced in a purified or extracted form and administered orally to provide compounds required for normal body structure and function with the intent of improving health and well-being [3]. Injectable chondroprotectants are drugs including glycosaminoglycan polysulfate ester, pentosan polysulphate, and hyaluronic acid.

Regulation of chondroprotectants

In the United States, dietary supplements for humans are regulated under the Dietary Supplements Health and Education Act (DSHEA). This law was enacted to permit consumer freedom to make purchasing decisions regarding supplements. Such products must be safe, but no premarketing approval is required (as is required for pharmaceuticals).

DSHEA does not apply to veterinary dietary supplements. Strict interpretation of the Food, Drug, and Cosmetic Act classifies oral veterinary compounds as foods, food additives, or pharmaceuticals. The same dietary supplements legally sold under DSHEA for human use are therefore technically unapproved veterinary pharmaceuticals when sold for animal use; however, to date the CVM has exercised regulatory discretion in the removal of veterinary dietary supplements from the market. Provided that the product is safe, poses no risk to the human food supply, and does not claim to treat, cure, prevent, or mitigate a disease, veterinary dietary supplements have not been forced to withdrawal from the market.

Chondroprotective agents administered by routes other than oral (eg, topical or injectable) are considered to be drugs and fall under the regulation of the Food and Drug Administration.

Manufacturing and quality control of chondroprotectants

The manufacturing process of chondroprotectant products varies widely. Manufacturers should apply high-quality standards similar to those practiced by the pharmaceutical industry (good manufacturing practice). The raw materials and finished product should be tested for purity and consistency by validated analytical methods to ensure the label accuracy of the product reaching the consumer. Problems with truth-in-labeling and quality control of oral chondroprotectant products have been documented [7,8]. The consumer cannot always be assured that the ingredients listed on the container are actually present in the product at the claimed concentration or purity. Presently, the results of clinical and experimental research on one product cannot be extrapolated to another similar product because of inconsistencies in manufacturing and quality control standards. Until regulation of these products improves, it is probably best to heed the recommendation found in the Arthritis Foundation's Guide to Alternative Therapies: when a supplement has been studied with good results, find out which brand was used in the study, and buy that brand.

Chondroprotectants and nutraceuticals: mechanism of action

The mechanism of action of many of these products is unknown or unproven, but some products have been substantiated with experimental and clinical trials. Dietary supplements and nutraceuticals cannot be sold under the premise of being a treatment for a medical condition, and these products cannot be marketed with the intent to diagnose, treat, cure, or prevent disease. Instead, they must be marketed as nutrients necessary for supporting or improving normal structure and function of the joint. Chondroprotective agents presumably influence cartilage metabolism by providing substrate and upregulating chondrocytes. They also appear to inhibit degradative enzymes, including metalloproteinases, serine proteases, and free radicals. Some of these products inhibit the formation of microthrombi in the periarticular vasculature, thus supporting a normal blood supply to the joint tissues. The mechanism of action of specific products, if known, is discussed in the appropriate section of this article.

The normal joint: structure and function

Diarthrodial joints are composed of a joint capsule, synovial fluid, articular cartilage, and subchondral bone. Normal joint function requires normal structure and function of these tissues. The joint capsule is composed of an outer fibrous capsule and an inner synovial membrane. The integrity of the joint capsule is important for normal gliding function, production of hyaluronic acid, and defense mechanisms. Synovial fluid is as ultrafiltrate of plasma containing the glycosaminoglycan hyaluronic acid. Synovial fluid functions include lubrication, protection (through its viscoelastic properties and participation in defense mechanisms), provision of nutrients, and removal of metabolic waste products from the cartilage. Articular cartilage is composed of hyaline cartilage. This type of cartilage has special viscoelastic properties that allow it to function at low levels of friction, which is needed to withstand the long-term forces experienced by the joint over a lifetime. Cartilage is a living tissue composed of chondrocytes embedded in an extracellular matrix composed of water, collagen, and proteoglycans. Proteoglycans are composed of small proteins, a hyaluronic acid backbone, and GAGs (keratin sulfate and chondroitin sulfate [CS]). GAGs are long chains of disaccharides. Glucosamine, a hexosamine sugar, is a precursor for the disaccharide units of GAG. GAGs play an important role in maintaining the proper concentration of water in the cartilage, which is essential for normal viscoelastic function. Chondrocytes are metabolically active cells producing collagen and proteoglycans needed for the cartilage matrix. These cells have little mitotic ability; they are not replaced when they die. Thus, it is imperative to support the health of chondrocytes. The subchondral bone plays an important role in dissipating concussive forces to the joint. This cushioning effect protects the overlying articular cartilage by decreasing the load on the cartilage and chondrocyte. As OA progresses, the subchondral bone can become more dense, causing increased loads to be placed on the cartilage, leading to damage. Disruption of any of these components can lead to suboptimal performance, pain, and progression of osteoarthritis.

Pathophysiology of osteoarthritis

OA is characterized by a low-grade inflammatory process that leads to progressive changes in the structure and function of the joint. Joint capsular thickening and inflammation leads to pain, decreased range of motion, and decreased function. Synovial fluid alterations cause pain, a change in joint biomechanics, and a reduction in the protective mechanisms of the joint. Loss of articular cartilage leads to pain and loss of function and establishes a mechanism for perpetuating low-grade inflammation and progressive OA. Increased density of the subchondral bone affects the joint indirectly by increasing the amount of force placed on the articular cartilage.

The two broad classes of OA are primary (idiopathic) and secondary. Primary OA is often referred to as wear-and-tear joint disease owing to its insidious onset, which is thought to be caused by long-term use combined with aging. Primary OA is not associated with an identifiable predisposing cause, but this might be because of clinicians' inability to detect subtle abnormalities. Secondary OA, identified more commonly, results from an initiating cause such as joint instability, trauma, osteochondral defects, or joint incongruity.

OA is characterized by changes in the structural components of articular cartilage. The initial change involves the loss of proteoglycans from the extracellular matrix caused by increased destruction and decreased production. The breakdown and loss of collagen and chondrocytes occur as the disease progresses, leading to irreversible change.

An understanding of the pathogenesis of OA is essential to develop a rational approach to management of the condition. Although OA is usually categorized as a noninflammatory joint disease, low-grade inflammation plays an important role in its pathogenesis. Inflammation of the synovial membrane leads to extravasation of inflammatory cells, primarily mononuclear cells, from synovial capillaries to synovial fluid. Leukocytes and synoviocytes release a variety of inflammatory mediators including prostaglandins, leukotrienes, neutral metalloproteinases, serine proteases, oxygen-derived free radicals, lysosomal enzymes (proteases, glycosidases, collagenases), oncoproteins, interleukins, tumor necrosis factor (TNF), and other cytokines. The neutral metalloproteinase stromelysin is thought to be the primary factor responsible for proteoglycan degradation in degenerative cartilage. Collagenase also plays a role in the long-term destruction of cartilage in osteoarthritis. The severity of the inflammatory process appears to be enhanced compared with human counterparts, especially when observing dogs that have cranial cruciate disease (Fig. 1).

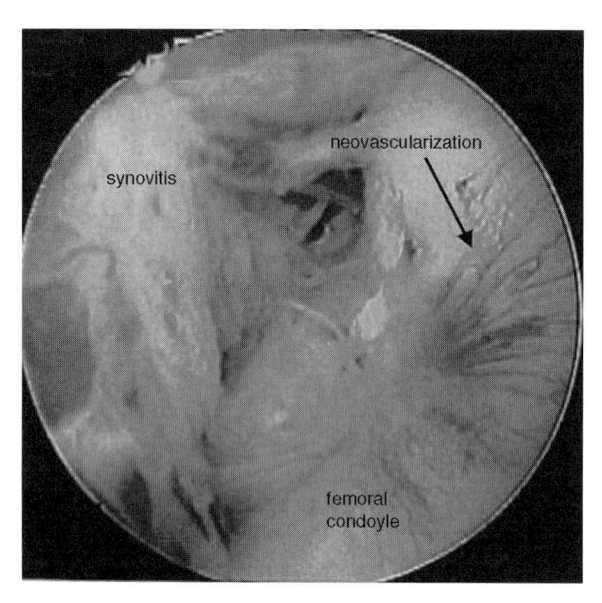

Fig. 1. Inflammation associated with OA in dogs can be progressive and severe. This dog suffered a partial tear of the cranial cruciate ligament and has been clinically lame for approximately 1 year.

Treatment of osteoarthritis

Treatment of OA might include weight loss, exercise modification, physical therapy, pharmacologic therapy, or surgery. In cases of secondary OA, the underlying cause must be identified and eliminated (if possible) to minimize the progression and long-term effects of OA, which might imply removal of an osteochondral fragment or stabilization of a stifle after rupture of a cranial cruciate ligament. Weight loss, when indicated, lessens clinical signs of OA because of decreased forces being placed on abnormal joint surfaces. Weight reduction before surgery reduces postoperative stress placed on the surgical repair. Decreased body weight has been found to be an important factor in lessening the prevalence and severity of OA in dogs that have hip dysplasia [9]. Enforced rest and restricted activity provide an opportunity for transient episodes of inflammation to resolve and decrease stress placed on the repair. Pharmacologic management of OA includes a wide variety of pharmaceuticals, most of which have gained popularity based on use in humans. Consideration should be given to drugs that inhibit the release or activity of prostaglandins, leukotrienes, neutral metalloproteases (stromelysin, collagenase), serine proteases, oncoproteins, interleukins, and TNF. Nonsteroidal anti-inflammatory drugs (NSAIDs) and glucocorticoid drugs are common examples. Other drugs such as chondroprotective agents not only inhibit mediators of inflammation within the joint but also might stimulate metabolic activity of synoviocytes and chondrocytes. Such drugs include glycosaminoglycan polysulfate ester, pentosan polysulphate, and hyaluronic acid. Nutraceuticals and other dietary supplements have also become important tools in the management of OA in dogs and cats. These supplements appear to have the best effect in patients that have mild or moderate OA (Figs. 2–4). Mild OA can be treated initially with a nutraceutical and supplemented with as NSAID as needed (Fig. 5). Moderate OA is more likely to require concomitant therapy with an NSAID and nutraceutical.

Nutraceuticals

Glucosamine

Glucosamine salt supplements are most commonly found as glucosamine hydrochloride or glucosamine sulfate. Both forms are readily available, but the hydrochloride form provides more glucosamine per unit weight than the sulfate form. Another form, N-acetyl glucosamine, appears to have less activity than the hydrochloride and sulfate forms [10]. Glucosamine is commonly found in combination products containing other products including CS and manganese ascorbate. Glucosamine is an amino sugar that is a precursor to GAGs present in the extracellular matrix of articular cartilage. Normal chondrocytes have the ability to synthesize glucosamine; however, osteoarthritic cartilage appears to have a decreased ability to synthesize it [1,11]. Exogenous glucosamine stimulates the production of proteoglycans and collagen by chondrocytes in cell culture [12,13].

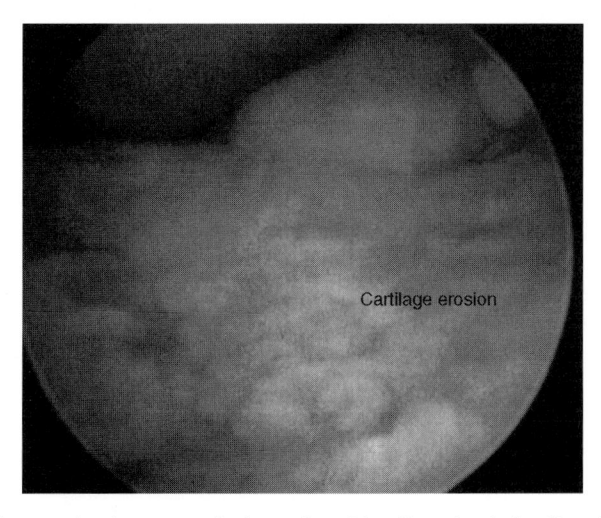

Fig. 2. Cartilage erosion is common in dogs affected by elbow dysplasia. Chondroprotectants and nutraceuticals can be used to help provide substrate for chondrocyte metabolism and potentially suppress inflammation.

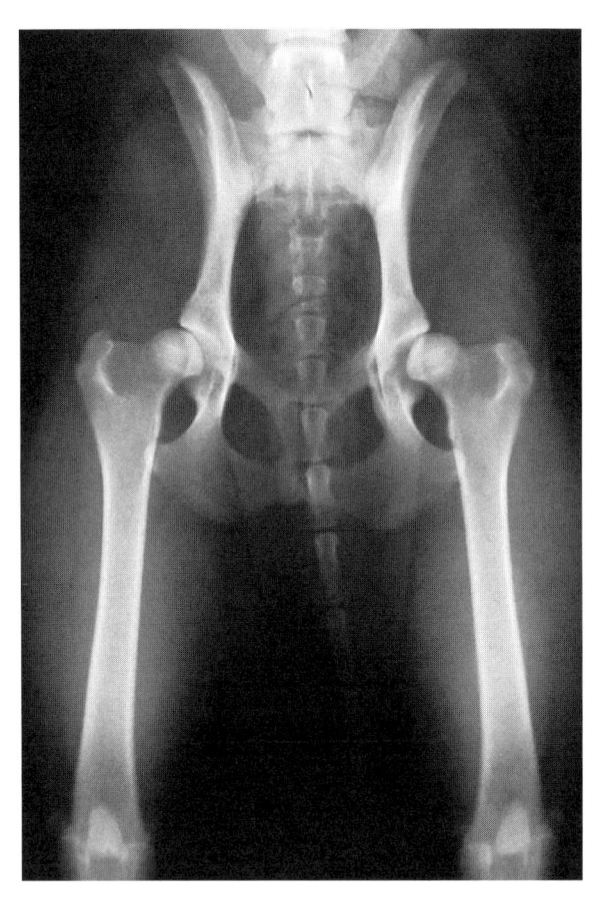

Fig. 3. Dogs and cats that have mild or moderate OA are more likely to benefit from chondroprotectant or nutraceutical therapy. This dog was diagnosed with mild bilateral OA secondary to hip dysplasia.

Glucosamine has good bioavailability when administered orally or parenterally, having good distribution to all body tissues and reaching highest concentrations in the liver, kidney, and articular cartilage [14–16]. Oral glucosamine has been shown to have an intestinal absorption rate of 87% [17]. Orally administered glucosamine sulfate has been associated with relief of clinical signs of DJD and chondroprotection in clinical and experimental studies in humans [18–21]. Although glucosamine has a slower onset of relief of clinical signs associated with DJD compared with ibuprofen, two clinical trials in humans found that it has equal long-term efficacy [18]. Oral glucosamine was found to improve clinical performance in humans who had OA [22]. Use of this product as an individual agent in animals has been proposed, but adequately controlled clinical studies have not been performed to substantiate its efficacy.

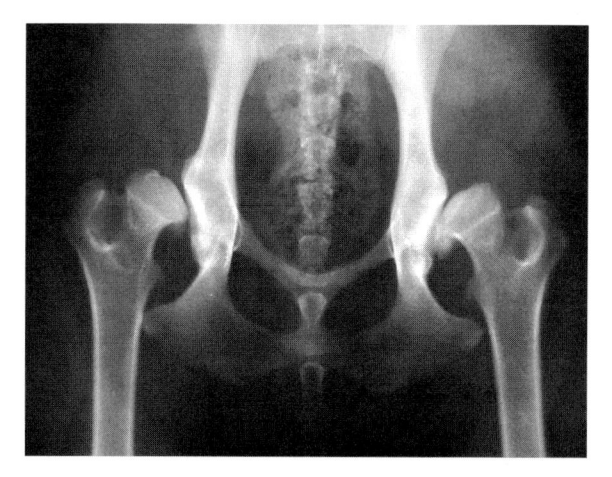

Fig. 4. This dog has severe bilateral OA of the hips secondary to dysplasia. A favorable response to nutraceuticals in this patient is less likely because of the advanced osteoarthritic condition. Nutraceuticals probably have their most beneficial effect in joints having less damage to the articular surface and a higher population of viable chondrocytes.

Chondroitin sulfate

CS is a predominant glycosaminoglycan found within the extracellular matrix of articular cartilage. Oral supplementation of exogenous CS has been advocated anecdotally for many years as a treatment for OA in humans and animals. This compound is often found in combination with other

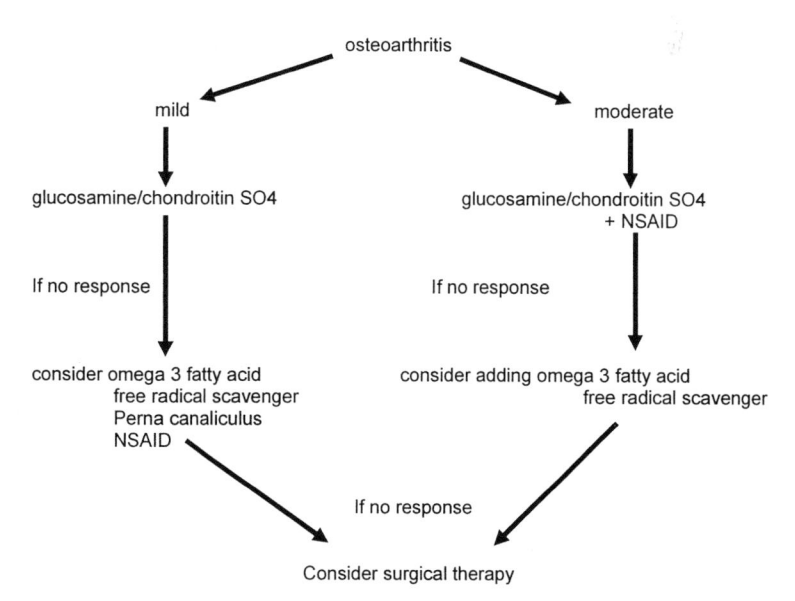

Fig. 5. Flowchart for nutraceutical usage in osteoarthritic dogs and cats.

nutraceuticals such as glucosamine and free radical scavengers. CS has been found to decrease interleukin-1 production, block complement activation, inhibit metalloproteinases, inhibit histamine-mediated inflammation, and stimulate glycosaminoglycan and collagen synthesis [4,23]. Oral absorption of CS has been reported using a variety of techniques. Some controversy exists regarding the fate of CS following oral administration. Various methods have been used to show that CS can be absorbed intestinally, but uncertainty remains regarding whether the majority of CS is absorbed intact or as a subunit of CS [4,24,25]. A highly pure, low molecular weight (LMW) form of CS has been found to have good absorption and bioavailability [14]. Clinical studies have shown improvement in clinical signs associated with OA in human patients receiving CS supplementation [5,24,25].

Combination products

The combination of high-purity glucosamine hydrochloride, LMW CS, and manganese ascorbate (GCM) might be the most commonly used nutraceutical combination in osteoarthritic companion animals (Cosequin, Nutramax Labs) [26]. The effects of the individual components are described below. The combined action of glucosamine and CS is synergistic [27]. This combination has been described as a preferential substrate and stimulant of proteoglycan biosynthesis, including hyaluronic acid and CS [4]. CS appears to inhibit degradative enzymes associated with OA, including metalloproteases and collagenases. These degradative enzymes break down the cartilage and hyaluronan in synovial fluid. Manganese is a cofactor in the synthesis of GAGs and its supplementation might aid in cartilage matrix synthesis. Manganese is also necessary for the synthesis of synovial fluid. It is possible that manganese might also have antioxidant properties. Overdose safety studies have been conducted in the dog, cat, and horse and no persistent abnormality in hematology, serum chemistry, or hemostatic parameters were observed [23,28,29]. No known side effects of clinical significance have been seen in the cat or dog.

Clinical and experimental studies support the use of GCM in combination or as individual components. Leeb et al performed a meta-analysis of the clinical efficacy of CS in humans [30]. Sixteen published studies were examined, with seven trials of 372 patients selected for the meta-analysis. All selected studies were randomized, double-blinded designs in parallel groups; however, rescue medication (analgesics or NSAIDs) were permitted, which is typical of human clinical studies of OA. CS was shown to be significantly superior to placebo with respect to the Lequesne index (a validated, subjective assessment of pain associated with OA). Patients showed at least a 50% improvement in study variables in the CS group compared with placebo. A double-blind clinical study in horses showed GCMs efficacy for treatment of DJD associated with navicular disease [31]. Administration of GCM to dogs that had experimentally induced OA by way of transection of the cranial cruciate ligament showed increased concentration of OA markers, indicative of cartilage matrix synthesis [32]. Glucosamine, CS, and manganese ascorbate might act as signaling molecules for upregulation of the genes for aggrecan and collagen II, not just as substrates for cartilage production [33]. This combination has also been found to suppress the inflammatory affects of chemically induced acute synovitis and experimental immune-mediated arthritis [34,35].

The fate of orally administered CS appears to be affected by the molecular weight of the molecule. LMW CS is absorbed in approximately 2 hours and accumulates in the serum over time, having an estimated bioavailability of 200% [14,36]. Glucosamine hydrochloride is also absorbed in less than 2 hours, but it does not accumulate over time [14]. Orally administered glucosamine has been found to be absorbed readily, and it reaches highest concentrations in articular cartilage [14]. A recent study showed good bioavailability of glucosamine and CS after oral dosing [36].

Mixed glycosaminoglycan products

Most oral GAGs or glucosamine products are available as single- or multiple-ingredient products. Most of the glycosaminoglycan products contain CS or mixed GAGs. Different glucosamine salts are available. Much controversy exists regarding the necessary purity, concentration, and type of glycosaminoglycan or glucosamine product necessary to provide beneficial effects to cartilage. The New Zealand green-lipped mussel (GLM; *Perna canaliculus*) is known to contain GAGs, omega-3 fatty acids, amino acids, vitamins, and minerals [37]. This product is available as a sole dietary supplement or as an additive in canine diets. *Perna canaliculus* is purported to have mild anti-inflammatory and chondroprotective actions, but these effects have not been substantiated unequivocally in humans and animals. Beneficial effects have been purported in one study in humans suffering from rheumatoid arthritis and OA. A recent study in dogs found improvement in joint pain and swelling in arthritic dogs fed a complete diet containing 0.3% GLM [37]. No effect was seen on joint crepitus, range of motion, or mobility scores. Although the study concluded that a GLM supplemented diet could alleviate symptoms of arthritis in dogs, several points about the study can be questioned. The dogs used in the study were not definitively diagnosed as having OA. Joint swelling, which is not a consistent finding in osteoarthritic joints, was significantly improved; however, joint mobility, range of motion, and crepitus, commonly associated with OA, showed no improvement. Additionally, control dogs showed a marked worsening in joint pain and swelling over the 6-week period of the study, which is inconsistent with dogs selected for a chronic, slowly progressive condition such as OA. This study also included a subjective scoring system with parameters added across joints for a total score within the animal. It is difficult to envision that certain scores, such as the measurement of joint swelling of the hip and shoulder, could be obtained accurately or consistently. The validity of the scoring system can be questioned. Further study is warranted before unequivocal acceptance of this substance as a chondroprotective agent or nutraceutical useful in osteoarthritic dogs.

Free radical scavengers

Another class of nutraceutical that has been promoted to reduce inflammation is the free radical scavengers such as superoxide dismutase (SOD), bioflavonoids, glutathione, and dimethylsulfoxide (DMSO). Oxygen-derived free radicals (superoxide, hydrogen peroxide, hydroxyl radical) are thought to play a role in the progression of DJD through their ability to damage cells by oxidative injury. Oxidative injury leads to depolymerization of hyaluronic acid, destruction of collagen, and decreased production of proteoglycans [38–40]. Superoxide dismutase and glutathione are endogenous antioxidants present in mammalian cells that inhibit production of oxygen free radicals. This enzyme acts to stabilize phagocyte cell membranes and lysosomes and reduce superoxide radical levels in tissues, with a resultant decrease in free radical generation. The efficacy, bioavailability, and safety of many oral antioxidants are unknown. This product might also have potential manufacturing or storage problems, which might lead to less active ingredient being available to the pet than is labeled on the product. A recent study found discrepancies in certificate of analysis and labeled contents in six SOD products [8]. Since this study several new products have become available that might have resolved this problem.

DMSO, which is used as a topical agent when treating musculoskeletal problems, has the ability to penetrate most tissues, including skin [41]. Topical application of 20 mL/day of medical-grade DMSO (70–90% solution) every 6 to 8 hours for up to 14 days has been recommended to treat local inflammation [41]. Side effects with topical use are minimal but include a garlic odor to the breath.

Superoxide dismutase is an endogenous antioxidant present in mammalian cells that inhibits production of oxygen free radicals. This enzyme acts to stabilize phagocyte cell membranes and lysosomes and reduce superoxide radical levels in tissues, with a resultant decrease in free radical generation [39–41]. The efficacy of exogenous superoxide dismutase is unknown. One author recommends giving 5 mg subcutaneously for 6 days in the dog followed by alternate day therapy for 8 days [2,41]. The manufacturer recommends giving 2.5 mg/kg subcutaneously five times per week for 2 weeks for treatment of spondylitis or disc disease.

Bioflavanols are also purported to have strong antioxidant properties. Grape seed meal has a rich source of bioflavanols. Bioflavanols are purported to scavenge free radicals, alleviate inflammation induced by oxidative damage, and inhibit degradative enzymes released by oxidative cells [42–45]. One double-blind, randomized study in dogs found improvement in clinical signs attributable to hip OA in dogs supplemented with a product containing bioflavanoids, SOD, and glutathione [42]. Other clinical studies have reported improvement in function and decreased pain in osteoarthritic dogs and horses [43–45]. These studies also reported improvement after 2 to 3 weeks of product administration. Bioflavanols are available commercially, usually in combination with glucosamine and hydrolyzed collagen or with an assortment of other antioxidants including selenium, vitamin E, and superoxide dismutase.

Methyl-sulfonyl-methane

Methyl-sulfonyl-methane (MSM) has been suggested as an agent for management of pain, inflammation, and as an antioxidant [46]. The rationale behind its use, according to the manufacturer and others, is the possibility of a dietary sulfur deficiency. MSM is a white, crystalline, water soluble, odorless, tasteless compound that is sold as a supplement. It is actually a metabolite of industrial-grade DMSO. MSM is found naturally in certain foods, but it is destroyed during processing. DMSO is a byproduct of the wood pulp processing industry and is also available in a medical grade, which is approved only for the treatment of interstitial cystitis in the United States. Radiolabeled sulfur from MSM has been found in amino acids (methionine and cysteine) of proteins in guinea pigs following experimental oral administration. There are no controlled experimental or clinical studies available to support the use of MSM for management of OA in dogs. Companies supplying MSM base their claims of relief of pain and inflammation on results of studies conducted with DMSO. Little is known about safety of the product. Sold in capsules for human use, MSM is available in powder form, tablets, and capsules for use in horses and small animals. Manufacturer recommendations for dosage should be followed. Its use cannot be recommended at this time, however, because of the previously mentioned lack of studies and knowledge about safety.

Omega-3 fatty acids

Omega-3 fatty acids have gained popularity recently for their potential use in pets that have DJD. These products are available naturally in fish and plant sources and commercially as nutraceutical supplements. Omega-3 fatty acids are desaturated in the body to produce eicosapentaenoic acid, which is an analog of arachidonic acid. Prostaglandins, thromboxanes, and leukotrienes are produced from these compounds through the action of cyclo-oxygenase and lipoxygenase. The products resulting from arachidonic acid metabolism are proinflammatory, proaggregatory, and immunosuppressive compared with the metabolic byproducts of eicosapentaenoic acid, which are less inflammatory, vasodilatory, antiaggregatory, and not immunosuppressive. The use of omega-3 fatty acids could theoretically benefit dogs and cats suffering from DJD by decreasing inflammation and reducing the occurrence of microthrombi; however, objective data are lacking to attest to this product's efficacy. The ideal ratio of N6:N3 fatty acids for canine diets is controversial; the current recommendation is between 10:1 and 5:1. A recent study reported lower PGE_2 and reduced clinical and radiographic signs of OA in experimental dogs undergoing cranial cruciate ligament transection while being fed a diet low in N6 fatty acids [47]. Future studies would be useful to evaluate the role of fatty acid therapy in osteoarthritic patients more critically.

Chondroprotectants

Polysulfated glycosaminoglycan

Chondroprotection is achieved by the inhibition of various destructive enzymes and prostaglandins associated with synovitis and DJD. Polysulfated GAGs (GAGPS) have been found to inhibit neutral metalloproteinases (stromelysin, collagenase, elastase), serine proteases, hyaluronidase, and a variety of lysosomal enzymes [40,48–51]. GAGPS have also been discovered to inhibit PGE_2 synthesis, generation of oxygen-derived free radicals, and the complement cascade [48,49]. Protection of articular cartilage has also been seen on gross and histologic examination in numerous experimental studies [50–52]. GAGPS have also been found to stimulate anabolic activity in synoviocytes and chondrocytes. Chondrostimulatory effects are characterized by increased synoviocyte secretion of hyaluronate and enhanced proteoglycan, hyaluronate, and collagen production by articular chondrocytes [53–57]. GAGPS also have anticoagulant and fibrinolytic properties that facilitate clearing of thrombotic emboli deposited in the subchondral and synovial blood vessels [40,57,58]. While the majority of experimental and clinical studies support the premise that GAGPS possesses properties of chondroprotection and chondrostimulation, some studies have found that GAGPS have no beneficial effect or a detrimental effect on cartilage metabolism [40,57].

A clinical study in hip dysplastic dogs found the greatest improvement in orthopedic scores at a dose of 4.4 mg/kg (2 mg/lb Adequan) given intramuscularly every 3 to 5 days for eight injections [59]. Use in cats has also been reported at the same dose. Another study found that twice-weekly intramuscular administration of 5.0 mg/kg GAGPS from 6 weeks to 8 months of age in growing pups that were susceptible to hip dysplasia resulted in less coxofemoral subluxation [60]. The longevity of relief provided by GAGPS is unknown. Most studies have evaluated its effect in the short-term only. Anecdotal reports of duration of amelioration of clinical signs range from days to months. It is also not known whether the complete series of injections are needed when clinical signs return or whether a shorter regimen would suffice.

Side effects of GAGPS in dogs include short-term inhibition of the intrinsic coagulation cascade and inhibition of platelet aggregation when given at doses of 5 mg/kg or 25 mg/kg intramuscularly [1,61]. GAGPS has also been found to inhibit neutrophils and complement, which might predispose to infections, especially when injected intra-articularly under contaminated conditions [62,63]. GAGPS has been reported to cause sensitization reactions in humans, but this effect has not been reported in dogs.

Pentosan polysulphate (Cartrophen-Vet, Biopharm Australia, Sydney, Australia) is a polysaccharide sulfate ester (mean molecular weight 6000 Daltons) prepared semisynthetically from beech hemicellulose [64]. The drug is approved for use in dogs and horses in Australia and is used in a similar manner as Adequan for relieving clinical symptoms of DJD. Pentosan polysulphate can be administered intra-articularly, intramuscularly, subcutaneously, or orally. The recommended dose for intra-articular use is 5 to 10 mg per joint weekly as necessary. The intramuscular or subcutaneous dose in dogs is 3 mg/kg once weekly for 4 weeks. This regimen can be repeated as necessary. A double-blind study evaluating the efficacy of this product for treatment of DJD in dogs found this dose to be ideal [64]. This dose has also been used anecdotally in cats. Oral calcium pentosan polysulphate given at a dose of 10 mg/kg weekly for 4 weeks then repeated every 3 months was found to reduce the presence of cartilage breakdown products in osteoarthritic cartilage [65].

Sodium hyaluronate has been touted to promote joint lubrication, increase endogenous production of hyaluronate, decrease prostaglandin production, scavenge free radicals, inhibit migration of inflammatory cells, decrease synovial membrane permeability, protect and promote healing of articular cartilage, and reduce joint stiffness and adhesion formation between tendon and tendon sheaths [66,67]. The molecule lines the synovial membrane and acts like a sieve, preventing bacteria and inflammatory cells from reaching the synovial compartment by steric hindrance [66,67]. The actions of exogenous and endogenous hyaluronan appear to be similar. Presently, sodium hyaluronate is generally recommended for mild to moderate synovitis and capsulitis rather than DJD. The drug appears to have a chondroprotective effect, but it is unclear whether this is a direct effect or a result of its effect on the articular soft tissues. Sodium hyaluronate is administered intra-articularly or intravenously. Hyaluronate was used in experimental dogs at a dose of 7 mg per joint intra-articularly once weekly with success in slowing DJD [66,67].

Chondroprotectant use during the postoperative period and physical rehabilitation

Rehabilitation programs are developed to improve function and decrease pain in dogs and cats that have musculoskeletal compromise (or following orthopedic surgery). Rehabilitation can involve many physical modalities designed to improve strength, flexibility, and coordination. Chondroprotectants can be used concurrently to accelerate and enhance recovery possibly by several mechanisms:

1. Pain relief to increase willingness of patient to perform rehabilitation exercises
2. Reduction of degradative and inflammatory enzymes might help protect cartilage
3. Stimulation of synovial fluid, proteoglycan, and collagen production to promote cartilage matrix repair

Agents that reduce the expression of inflammatory mediators or upregulate normal chondrocyte expression might provide a microenvironment favorable for optimal cartilage and connective tissue homeostasis. A recent study evaluated the effect of a nutraceutical on intra-articular graft ligamentization dogs undergoing unilateral cranial cruciate ligament transection. Cosequin appeared to have two primary effects in this study: (1) return of the joint capsule/reconstructed CCL complex to a more physiological state, and (2) reduction in the severity of OA in operated joints [68]. Translation following transection of reconstructed CCLs from the Cosequin group was similar to the control, which suggested preservation of a more normal physiologic joint capsule. Dogs not receiving Cosequin had less translation after resection of the reconstructed CCL, suggesting joint capsule thickening and fibrosis. OA was less in dogs receiving Cosequin subjectively as judged by morphologic observation and with mean modified Mankin scores.

Limb immobilization can be performed postoperatively as adjunctive support to restrict use, reduce pain, treat open wounds, or control swelling. Whatever the indication, immobilization of joints can have adverse effects on joint health. Joint immobilization reduces synovial fluid production and leads to proteoglycan depletion because of decreased loading. The changes seen are similar to those observed in OA cartilage. Chondroprotectant treatment might help reduce deleterious effects on the joint during periods of immobilization. Immobilization should be limited to the shortest possible time to improve the chances of joint recovery.

References

[1] Anderson MA. Oral chondroprotectant agents. Part 1. Compend Contin Educ Pract Vet 1999;21(7):601–9.
[2] Boothe DM. Drug management of osteoarthritis (parts 1 and 2). Proc TNAVC 1998;586–91.
[3] Boothe DM. Nutraceuticals in veterinary medicine. Part 1. Compend Contin Educ Pract Vet 1997;19(11):1248–55.
[4] McNamara PS, Johnston SA, Todhunter RJ. Slow-acting, disease-modifying osteoarthritic agents. Vet Clin Small Anim 1997;27(4):863–7 951–2.
[5] Verbruggen G, Goemaere S, Veys EM. Chondroitin sulfate: S/DMOAD (structure/disease modifying anti-osteoarthrosis drug) in the treatment of finger joint, O.A. Osteoarth Cartil 1998;Suppl A:39–46.
[6] Bucsi L, Poor G. Efficacy and tolerability of oral chondroitin sulfate as a symptomatic slow-acting drug for osteoarthritis (SYSADOA) in the treatment of knee osteoarthritis. Osteoarth Cartil 1998;6(Suppl A):31–6.

[7] Adebowale A, Cox D, Liang Z, et al. Analysis of glucosamine and chondroitin sulfate content in marketed products and the Caco-2 permeability of chondroitin sulfate raw materials. JANA 2000;3:37–44.
[8] Beale BS. Evaluation of active enzyme in six oral superoxide dismutase products. Proc Vet Ortho Society. 1998;65.
[9] Smith G. Influence of diet and age on subjective hip score and hip OA: a life long study in Labrador retrievers. Proceedings Veterinary Orthopedic Society, 2002.
[10] Karzel K, Domenjoz R. Effect of hexosamine derivatives and uronic acid derivatives on glycosaminoglycan metabolism on fibroblast cultures. Pharmacology 1971;5:337–45.
[11] Jimenez SA, Dodge GR. The effects of glucosamine on human chondrocyte gene expression. Proc 9th Eular Symposium, 1996. p. 8–10.
[12] Hellio MP, Vigron E, Annefeld M. The effects of glucosamine on the human osteoarthritic chondrocyte. In vitro investigations. Proc 9th Eular Symposium, 1996. p. 11–2.
[13] Basleer C. Stimulation of proteoglycan production by glucosamine sulfate in chondrocytes isolated from human osteoarthritic articular cartilage in vitro. Osteoarth Cartil 1998;6(6): 427–34.
[14] Du J, Adebowale A, Liang A, Eddington ND. Bioavailability and disposition of the dietary supplements, FCHG49 glucosamine and TRH122 chondroitin sulfate in dogs after single and multiple dosing. AAPS PharmSci 2001;Suppl 3(3):W417.
[15] Davidson G. Glucosamine and chondroitin sulfate. Compend Contin Educ Pract Vet 2000; 22(5):454–8.
[16] Setnikar I, Giacchetti C, Zanolo G. Pharmakitetics of glucosamine in dog and in man. Arzneim-Forsch/Drug Res 1986;36(4):703–5.
[17] Setniker I, Giaccheti C, Zanolo G. Pharmacokinetics of glucosamine in the dog and in man. Arzneimittelforschung 1991;36:729.
[18] Vaz AL. Double-blind clinical evaluation of the relative efficacy of ibuprofen and glucosamine sulphate in the management of osteoarthrosis of the knee in outpatients. Curr Med Res Opin 1982;8:145–9.
[19] Hungerford D, Navarro R, Hammad T. Use of nutraceuticals in the management of osteoarthritis. JANA 2000;3(1):23–7.
[20] Leffler CT, Philippi AF, Leffler SG, et al. Glucosamine, chondroitin and manganese ascorbate for degenerative joint disease of the knee or low back: a randomized, double-blind, placebo-controlled pilot study. Mil Med 1999;164(2):85–91.
[21] Das AK, Hammad TA. Efficacy of a combination of FCHG49^{TM} glucosamine hydrochloride, TRH122^{TM} low molecular weight sodium chondroitin sulfate and manganese ascorbate in the management of knee osteoarthritis. Osteoarthr and Cartil 2000;8(5):343–50.
[22] D'Ambrosio E, Casa B, Bompani R, et al. Glucosamine sulfate: a controlled clinical investigation in arthrosis. Pharmacotherapeutica 1981;2(8):504–8.
[23] McNamara PS, Barr SC, Erb HN. Hematologic, hemostatic and biochemical effects in dogs receiving an oral chondroprotective agent for thirty days. AJVR 1996;57(9):1390–4.
[24] Li Hirondel JL. Double-blind clinical study with oral administration of chondroitin sulfate versus placebo in tibiofemoral gonarthrosis. Litera Rheumatol 1992;14:77–82.
[25] Bourgeois P, Chales G, Dehais J, et al. Efficacy and tolerability of chondroitin sulfate 1200 mg/day vs 3×400 mg/day vs placebo. Osteoarth Cartil 1998;6(Suppl A):25–30.
[26] Hulse DS. Treatment methods for pain in the osteoarthritic patient. Vet Clin Small Anim 1998;28(2):361.
[27] Lippiello L, Woodward J, Karpman R, et al. Chondroprotection and metabolic synergy of glucosamine and chondroitin sulfate. Clin Orth Rel Res 2000;381:229–40.
[28] McNamara PS, Barr SC, Erb HN, et al. Hematologic, hemostatic and biochemical effects in cats receiving an oral chondroprotective agent for thirty days. Vet Ther 2000;1(2): 108–17.
[29] Kirker-Head RP. Safety of an oral chondroprotective agent in horses. Vet Therap 2001; 2(4):345–53.

[30] Leeb BF, Schweitzer H, Montag K, Smolen J. A metaanalysis of chondroitin sulfate in the treatment of osteoarthritis. J Rheumatol 2000;27:205–11.
[31] Hansen RR, Smalley LR, Huff GK, et al. Oral treatment with a glucosamine-chondroitin sulfate compound for degenerative joint disease in horses: 25 cases. Equine Pract 1997;19(9):16–22.
[32] Johnson KA, Hulse DA, Hart RC, et al. Effects of an orally administered mixture of chondroitin sulfate, glucosamine hydrochloride and manganese ascorbate on synovial fluid chondroitin sulfate 3B3 and 7D4 epitope in a canine cranial cruciate transection model of osteoarthritis. Osteoarth Cartil 2001;9(1):14–21.
[33] O'Grady CP, Marwin SE, Grande DA. Effects of glucosamine hydrochloride, chondroitin sulfate, and manganese-ascorbate on cartilage metabolism. Proceedings of the AAOS 68th Annual Meeting, 2001. p. 157.
[34] Beren J, Hill SL, Diener-West M, et al. The effect of pre-loading oral glucosamine/chondroitin sulfate/manganese ascorbate combination on experimental arthritis in rats. Experim Biol Medic 2001;226(2):144–52.
[35] Canapp SO, McLaughlin RM, Hoskinson JJ, et al. Scintographic evaluation of glucosamine HCL and chondroitin sulfate as treatment for acute synovitis in dogs. AJVR 1999;60(12):1552–7.
[36] Adebowale A, Du J, Liang Z, et al. The bioavailability and pharmacokinetics of glucosamine hydrochloride and low molecular weight chondroitin sulfate after single and multiple doses to beagle dogs. Biopharm Drug Dispos 2002;23:217–25.
[37] Bui LM, Bierer TL. Influence of green lipped mussels (*Perna canaliculus*) in alleviating signs of arthritis in dogs.
[38] Simon SR. Oxidants, metalloproteases and serine proteases in inflammation. Proteases, protease inhibitors and protease-derived peptides. Basel: Birkhauser Verlag; 1993. 27–37.
[39] Auer DE, Ng JC, Seawright AA. Effect of palosein (superoxide dismutase) and catalase upon oxygen derived free radical induced degradation of equine synovial fluid. Equine Vet J 1990;22:13–7.
[40] Ghosh P, Smith M, Wells C. Second-line agents in osteoarthritis. In: Dixon JS, Furst DE, editors. Second-line agents in the treatment of rheumatic diseases. New York: Marcel Dekker; 1993. p. 363–427.
[41] Beale BS, Goring RL. Degenerative joint disease. In: Bojrab MJ, editor. Disease mechanisms in small animal surgery. Philadelphia: Lea & Febiger; 1993. p. 727–36.
[42] Impellizeri JA, Lau RE, Azzara FA. A 14 week clinical evaluation of an oral antioxidant as a treatment for osteoarthritis secondary to canine hip dysplasia. Vet Q 1998;20(Suppl 1):S107–S108.
[43] Kuck JC, Mulnix JA. Clinical evaluation of an antioxidant joint nutrient and relief of the signs of pain associated with osteoarthritis in the dog. Proprietary data. Golden (CO): Animal Health Options; 2001.
[44] Mulnix JA. Promotion study, canine formula. Proprietary data. Golden (CO): Animal Health Options; 2001.
[45] Kuck JC, Mulnix JA. Clinical evaluation of an antioxidant joint nutrient and relief of the signs of pain associated with osteoarthritis and gait irregularities in the horse. Proprietary data. Golden (CO): Animal Health Options; 2001.
[46] Jones WE. MSM reviewed. J Equine Vet Sci 1987;7(2).
[47] Budsberg S, Barteges J, Schoenherr W et al. Effects of different N6:N3 fatty acid diets on canine stifle osteoarthritis. Proc Vet Ortho Society2001;40.
[48] Egg D. Effects of glycosaminoglycan polysulfate and two nonsteroidal anti-inflammatory drugs on prostaglandin E_2 synthesis in Chinese hamster ovary cell cultures. Pharmacol Res Commun 1983;15:709–17.
[49] Altman RD, Dean DD, Muniz OE, et al. Therapeutic treatment of canine osteoarthritis with glycosaminoglycan polysulfuric acid ester. Arthr Rheum 1989;32(10):1300–7.

[50] Carreno MR, Muniz OE, Howell DS. The effect of glycosaminoglycan polysulfuric acid ester on articular cartilage in experimental osteoarthritis: effects on morphological variables of disease severity. J Rheum 1986;13(3):490–7.
[51] Hannen N, Ghosh P, Bellenger C, et al. Systemic administration of glycosaminoglycan polysulphate provides partial protection of articular cartilage from damage produced by menisectomy in the canine. Ortho Research 1987;5(1):47–59.
[52] Altman RD, Dean DD, Muniz OE, et al. Prophylactic treatment of canine osteoarthritis with glycosaminoglycan polysulfuric acid ester. Arthr Rheum 1989;32(6):759–66.
[53] Verbruggen G, Veys EM. The effect of sulfated glycosaminoglycan on the proteoglycan metabolism of synovial lining cells. Acta Rheumatol Belgica 1971;1:75–92.
[54] von der Mark K. Collagen synthesis in cultures of chondrocytes as effected by arteparon. In: IX Europ cong rheumatol. Basel: Euler; 1980. p. 39–50.
[55] Nishikawa H, Mori I, Umemoto J. Influences of sulfaed glycosaminoglycans on hyaluronic acid in rabbit knee synovia. Arch Biochem Biophys 1985;240:146–8.
[56] Smith MM, Ghosh P. The effect of polysulfated polysaccharides on hyaluronate (HA) synthesis by human synovial fibroblasts. Agents Actions 1986;18:55–62.
[57] Verbruggen G, Veys EM. Treatment of chronic degenerative joint disorders with a glycosaminoglycan polysulfate. In: IX Europ cong rheumatol. Basel: Euler; 1980. p. 51–69.
[58] Dettmer N, Nowack H, Raake W. Platelet aggregation by heparin and arteparon. Munch Med Wschr 1983;125:540–2.
[59] de Haan JJ, Goring RL, Beale BS. Evaluation of polysulfated gllycosaminoglycan for the treatment of hip dysplasia in dogs. Vet Surg 1994;23:177–81.
[60] Lust G, Williams AJ, Burton-Wurster N, et al. Effects of intramuscular administration of glycosaminoglycan polysulfates on signs of incipient hip dysplasia in growing pups. Am J Vet Res 1992;53(10):1836–43.
[61] Beale BS, Clemmons RM, Goring RL. The effect of a semi-synthetic polysulfated glycosaminoglycan on coagulation and primary hemostasis in the dog. Vet Surg 1990.
[62] Rashmir-Raven AM, Coyne CP, Fenwick BW, et al. Inhibition of equine complement activity by polysulfated glycosaminoglycans. Am J Vet Res 1992;53(1):87–90.
[63] Tsuboi I, Matsuura T, Shichijo, et al. Effects of glycosaminoglycan polysulfate on human neutrophil function. Japanese J Inflamm 1988;8:131–5.
[64] Read R, Cullis-Hill D. The systemic use of the chondroprotective agent pentosan polysulfate in the treatment of osteoarthritis- results of a double-blind clinical trial in dogs. J Small Anim Pract 1996;37(3):108–14.
[65] Innes JF, Barr AR, Sharif M. Efficacy of oral calcium pentosan polysulphate for the treatment of osteoarthritis of the canine stifle joint secondary to cranial cruciate ligament deficiency. Vet Rec 2000;146(15):433–7.
[66] Howard RD, McIlwraith CW. Sodium hyaluronate in the treatment of equine joint disease. Compend Cont Educ 1993;15(3):473–81.
[67] Schiavinato A, Lini E, Guidolin D, et al. Intraarticular sodium hyaluronate injections in the pond-nuki experimental model of osteoarthritis in dogs. II. Morphological findings. Clin Orthop 1989;241:286–99.
[68] Hulse DA, Hart RC, Beale BS, Slater M, Weeks B, Kochevar D. The effect of Cosequin in cranial cruciate deficient and reconstructed stifle joints in dogs.

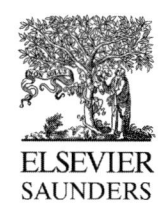

Pharmacognosy: phytomedicines and their mechanisms

Nicholas Larkins, DSc, MRCVS[a],*, Susan Wynn, DVM[b]

[a]*Nutritional Laboratories, High House, Penrhos, Raglan, Monmouthshire NP15 2DJ, UK*
[b]*334 Knollwood Lane, Woodstock, GA 30188, USA*

Since the earliest of times, man and animals have had to distinguish between those plants that are poisonous and those that are not. This starting point shaped the evolution of naturally occurring drugs, which was initially communicated orally; later, in written form, such as papyri, baked clay tablets, parchments, manuscript herbals, printed herbals, pharmacopoeias, and other works; and, most recently, by computerized information-retrieval systems.

The plant kingdom continues to hold many species of plants containing substances of value yet to be discovered. Much of the most recent investigative work owes its existence to pure scientists who would not normally regard themselves as researchers in the field of pharmacognosy.

Plants and the phytochemicals within them are still the major source of medicine for most of the world's population [1]. Artemisinin (Fig. 1), for example, the active antimalarial phytochemical isolated from *Artemesia annua*, is the most powerful and rapidly acting schizonticidal agent of all antimalarial drugs in the treatment of falciparum malaria. The World Health Organization (WHO) reports that there are more than 1.5 million malaria patients in Southeast Asia and Latin America being treated with this compound [2].

The undertaking of this article is to bring together this ancient traditional herbal lore and modern scientific analytic methods to pave the way for a common pathway of understanding. We review some phytochemical groups in terms of their chemical composition and pharmacologic action, relating them to their therapeutic uses.

---

* Corresponding author.
E-mail address: nlarkins@nutri.org (N. Larkins).

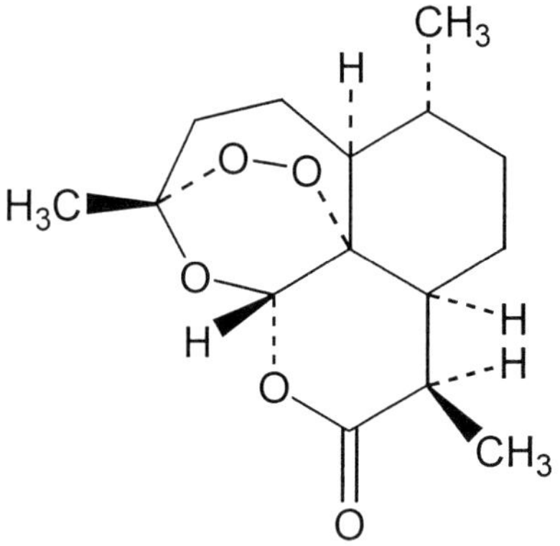

Fig. 1. Artemisinin.

How do plant medicines work? The primary site of phytochemicals consumed orally is the digestive tract. A central functioning mechanism is that they provoke their effect through reflex responses, in many if not all cases, from their activity within the gastrointestinal tract (GIT), for instance, bitter tasting phytochemicals that are capable of strongly stimulating the bitter taste bud receptor switch on the upper digestive system, causing the release of the gastrin interrelated peptide hormones from the G cells of the pyloric antral mucosa and the proximal small intestine. Gastrin is known to increase digestive secretions (pancreatic enzymes and acid secretion by the gastric mucosa), trigger the appetite center in the hypothalamus, and promote bile flow [3].

Phytochemicals: biologically active food components

Are plant materials, such as pineapples, mushrooms, soybeans, and garlic, dietary ingredients or medicines? A dividing line is not always clear. The simple answer is that they are both. Mammals have evolved with plants over tens of thousands of years. As such, mammals have digestive systems and a physiology geared to digesting and using plant-based diets, which often provide a medicinal value as well as sustenance.

Compelling evidence now supports a link between nutrition and numerous acute and chronic diseases. Nutritional science, frequently incorporating the phytochemical constituents of plants and plant materials (leaves, fruits, pollens, seeds, oils, and bark), has advanced from a model targeting the prevention of clinical deficiencies of nutrients to the assessment of nutrient intakes, phytochemical intakes that promote the prophylaxis of cancers, cardiovascular diseases, autoimmune diseases, cataracts, and specific diseases, such as gastrointestinal disturbances, atopy, osteoarthritis, osteochondrosis desiccans, and respiratory diseases [4,5].

Prime principles of nutritional veterinary medicine incorporating nutrients like the conditionally essential amino acid L-glutamine (found in *Aloe vera, Citrus sinensis, Ribes nigrum, Ananas comosus,* and *Camellia sinensis*) and the chondroprotective amino-sugar glucosamine (found in *Rehmannia glutinosa, A vera, Capsicum annum,* and *Glycine max*) conceives that:

- Diets may often have only a borderline or low content of certain essential ingredients. As such, a "normal" diet does not necessarily mean a healthy or optimal one.
- Requirements for essential nutrients vary from individual to individual depending on genetic, physiologic, activity, and other influences. What is adequate for one animal may not be for another.
- Illness is invariably linked with an abnormal biochemistry and an alteration in the metabolism of nutrients and their byproducts.
- Specific nutrients, such as vitamins, provitamins, minerals, trace elements, essential fatty acids, amino acids, and their precursors found in a wide variety of plant species, provide a potent means of influencing body chemistry and thus the disease process via dietary manipulation.
- By correcting fundamental biochemical abnormalities using nutritional means, one can prevent certain diseases or alter the course of a disease for the better.

Some basic metabolic pathways seem to be similar in plants and animals. It is to the secondary plant metabolites, those not necessarily involved in the essential metabolism of the cell, that most phytochemicals owe their therapeutic activity. Primary metabolites, archetypal plant constituents necessary to sustain life, include carbohydrates, proteins, fats, fibers, vitamins, amino acids, minerals, and trace elements.

Why should these secondary metabolites have biologic activity in animals? One suggestion put forward is that enzymes in animals can share a common ancestry with enzymes and proteins in plants [6]. This evolutionary kinship, when combined with the multiple structural similarities between plant and animal substrates, explains, for example, the hormone-like or hormone-modulating effects of several phytochemicals in animals.

Phytochemicals, as secondary plant metabolites, are chemically diverse components. Several groups of these secondary metabolites, for example, antioxidant chemicals like the flavonoids, can function as protective repair mechanisms induced by infection and traumas, such as wounding or insect invasion. Purpurogallin (showing greater activity as a xanthine oxidase inhibitor than the pharmaceutical allopurinol), found in various nutgalls, is produced as part of the defensive/repair mechanisms against invading insect attack. Glucosinolates play a role in protecting against insect attack. Tannins act to preserve against microbial decomposition and insect invasion [7].

Is there any advantage in these chemically complex medicines? Life is indeed chemically complex, involving some trillions of biochemical reactions each second to survive. It seems logical that just as food is chemically complex, so should be the therapeutic approach. Synergy is an important concept in the pharmacology of phytochemicals of botanical medicines. In the context of chemical complexity, it applies when the action of the chemical mixture provides a significantly more pronounced therapeutic benefit than the actions of any individual components. In pharmacology, this can be clearly demonstrated in the antibiotic mixtures of amoxicillin with clavulanic acid, where the sum of the two provides antibacterial therapeutic benefits that are not possible when either component is used individually. Other components within plants may not be demonstrably active but can act to improve stability, solubility, bioavailability, or the half-life of the active components. Again and again, when the composition of an herbal remedy is examined experimentally, it is found to have activity that is apparently more than the sum of the active ingredients [8].

Phytochemicals have been shown to [9–29]:

- Facilitate cell-to-cell communication
- Modify cellular receptor uptake of hormones
- Biotransform carotenoids to vitamin A (all-transretinol)
- Repair DNA damage from toxic exposure
- Detoxify carcinogens through the activation of the cytochrome P450 and phase II liver enzyme systems
- Function as antioxidants
- Induce apoptosis in cancer cells
- Enhance immune response
- Help to prevent cardiovascular disease
- Help to prevent osteoporosis
- Help to prevent macular degeneration and cataracts
- Help to prevent various forms of cancer and metastasis
- Occlude tumor-feeding vessels

Phenols and phenolic glycosides

Plants contain a huge range of phenol groups, such as the flavonoids, of which more than 4000 naturally occurring compounds have been identified. Five major flavonoid groups dominate plants: flavones/flavonols, flavonols and the related procyanidins, anthocyanins, hydroxycinnamates, and flavanones. Fruit, leaves, and roots contain a wide variety of individual phenolics in differing amounts; berries are rich in anthocyanins, and all fruits are rich in hydroxycinnates [30].

From a pharmacologic perspective, the best-known simple phenol is salicylic acid. It has been shown to be antipyretic, anti-inflammatory, and a platelet-activating factor (PAF) inhibitor. Its ester precursors are found in the bark of the willow (*Salix* spp) and poplar (*Populus* spp). Salicylic acid is subsequently formed on ingestion. The O-acetyl derivative is aspirin (Fig. 2).

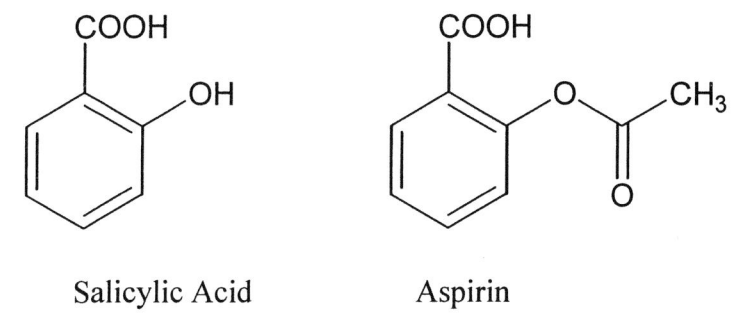

Fig. 2. Salicylic acid and aspirin.

Flavonoids have been shown to display a bewildering array of pharmacologic and biochemical actions:

- Anti-inflammatory
- Antiallergic
- Antimicrobial
- Antihelmintic
- Hepatoprotective
- Antithrombic
- Antiviral
- Ascorbate sparing [31]

Silybin (Fig. 3), formerly called silymarin (a flavonoid isolated from the seeds of the milk thistle [*Silybum marianum*]), is frequently recommended in the treatment of liver disease, giving hepatic protective action against toxin, CCl_4, or ethionine-induced fatty hepatic degeneration. Such toxic insults result in the excessive production of reactive oxygen species (ROS), other toxic nitrogen compounds, and eicosanoids [32].

In sheep, silybin has been shown to exhibit favorable effects in preventing larvae-induced ruminant hepatotoxicosis [33]. This hepatoprotective effect was a result of selective inhibition of leukotriene formation by the liver

Fig. 3. Silybin.

Kupffer cells [34]. Silybin clinically not only displays hepatoprotective properties but might be cytoprotective in other organs and tissues, increasing the secretion of bile into the duodenum and exerting a gastroprotective effect preventing ischemic mucosal injury [35]. In a double-blind, placebo-controlled, clinical trial in patients with acute viral hepatitis, silybin-treated patients showed significant ($P < 0.05$) improvements in bilirubin, glutamate-oxaloacetate transaminase (GOT), and glutamate-pyruvate transaminase (GPT) [36].

Silybin has been studied in dogs poisoned with toxic *Amanita phalloides* mushroom extracts. Florsheim et al [37] administered 85 mg/kg of *Amanita* lyophilizate orally to five groups of 6 to 10 dogs each. Dogs received either no treatment, prednisone, cytochrome C, penicillin, or silymarin (30–50 mg/kg at 5 and 24 hours). Blood was sampled at 5, 24, 48, 96, and 192 hours, and liver enzymes (alkaline phosphatase, gamma glutamyl transferase (GGT), GOT, and GPT) were measured. At 24 hours after intoxication, control dog GPT levels increased by an average of 4479%, whereas those dogs receiving silymarin had GPT increases of only 16%. GGT increased 265% in control dogs, whereas those dogs receiving silymarin had increases of 131%. GOT increased in control dogs by 4335% at 24 hours, whereas those dogs receiving silymarin had increases of only 56% [37]. Dogs given the same dose of *Amanita* toxin and treated with silibinin (50 mg/kg intravenously at 5 and 24 hours) had improved histopathology scores, liver enzyme changes, prothrombin times, and survival compared with control dogs. In this study, 4 of the 12 control dogs died, whereas none of the silibinin-treated dogs died. The silibinin-treated dogs had nearly normal liver histology, whereas control dogs exhibited extensive hepatic necrosis [38].

Silybin inhibits hepatic damage by:

- Acting as a direct antioxidant and free radical scavenger
- Increasing the intracellular content of glutathione (GSH) and superoxide dismutase (SOD)
- Inhibiting the formation of leukotrienes
- Activity at the nuclear level, enhancing synthesis of RNA and proteins, cellular regeneration

Human pharmacokinetic data suggest that the sugar moiety of these flavonoid groups is an important determinant of their bioavailability. Bioavailability may be defined as the fraction of the ingested component that enters the blood circulation intact and can be used for physiologic functions or storage. In one study, the bioavailability of quercetin-β-rutinoside was found to be only 20% that of pure quercetin-β-glucoside [39,40]. Biotransformation enzymes in body tissues, located mainly in the liver, act on absorbed flavonoids and their absorbed colonic metabolites. The kidney and the small intestine may also contain enzymes capable of biotransforming flavonoids [41]. In the colon, microorganisms degrade unabsorbed flavonoids and the flavonoids that have been absorbed and secreted with bile [42].

The subsequent degradation products include a variety of phenylcarboxylic acids, which, depending on their hydroxylation pattern, are antioxidants themselves and thus may contribute to the biologic effects of dietary flavonoids [43].

Flavonoids have additionally been shown to have effects on the various stages of signal transduction, influencing the mechanisms triggered by cytokines, growth factors, or hormones, which leads to changes in gene expression in cells. The phytochemical quercetin has been shown to have effects on all aspects of signal transduction, such as cell surface and intracellular receptors. Myricetin, a phytochemical, affects intracellular mediators, kinases, the cell cycle, DNA replication–related enzymes, and gene expression. Nuclear factor κB (NF-κB) is a ubiquitous transcription factor playing a pivotal role in the induction pathways of inflammatory stimuli, such as tumor necrosis factor(TNF)-α, interferon (IFN)-γ, interleukin (IL)-1, and other agents. NF-κB marshals the "stress" response by activating a mixture of offensive (inflammatory) and defensive (antioxidant) genes. As such, NF-κB can be a central component of a number of mechanisms that lead to pathologic changes. NF-κB activation is an essential factor in inducible nitric oxide synthetase (iNOS) expression in macrophages. iNOS plays an important role in inflammatory reactions via the production of nitric oxide (NO). Antioxidants have been shown to inhibit monocyte adhesion by suppressing NF-κB mobilization and induction of vascular cell adhesion molecule-1 in endothelial cells stimulated to generate radicals [44]. Silymarin, extracted from the seeds of *S marianum*, has metabolic and cell-regulating effects at concentrations found in clinical conditions, namely, carrier-mediated regulation of cell membrane permeability, inhibition of the 5-lipoxygenase pathway, scavenging of ROS, and action on DNA expression (eg, via suppression of NF-κB) [45].

NO is the smallest molecule known to act as a biologic messenger in mammals. Its particular features and its free radical nature make its metabolism extremely complex, and highly regulated control of NO production seems to be more and more important for mammalian health. Plant polyphenols seem to be promising tools for the nonpharmacologic control of NO overflow during chronic inflammation and could act as a preventative treatment against different pathologic conditions that have been proposed to be associated with dysregulated NO production, which has been shown to be involved in arteriosclerosis, cardiovascular disease, and arthritis [46].

Tannins and oligomeric procyanidins

Tannins, secondary metabolites and like flavonoids, are a large group of polyphenols found widely throughout the plant world. Their role in the plant is a matter for conjecture. There is evidence to suggest that they act to deter insect and fungal attack. In the oak, there is increased tannin production in the leaves in late summer that can be closely related to diminished insect attack; oak galls, the richest source of tannins, are themselves manufactured in response to insect attack. Their high concentration found in those tissues lost from the plant (ie, old and dying leaves, outer cork, heartwood, galls) also suggests that they might represent metabolic waste products.

Tannins may be divided into two groups: (1) hydrolyzable tannins, which are esters of a sugar, usually glucose and (2) condensed tannins that are derivatives of flavonols. Tannins which consist of catechin and epicatechin molecules are referred to as monomers. Tannins containing two to four monomers are referred to as oligomeric procyanidins (OPC) with a protein-binding capacity that increases markedly with the degree of polymerization. It is difficult to define the point at which OPC end and true tannins start, however. OPC and their monomers behave like flavonoids (and resemble them chemically); as such, they are sometimes classified alongside them).

Pharmacodynamically when tannins come into contact with mucous membranes, they react with and cross-link collagen proteins in the mucous and epithelial cells of the mucosa, creating an antisecretory effect on the mucous membrane. Topical application of polyphenol-containing plant extracts (eg, tannic acid) to wounds has traditionally been used not only as an antibacterial agent but to help seal the surface skin with an impervious layer (collagen/tannin) (Fig. 4). This cross-linking also renders the mucosa less permeable, providing an astringency that affords increased protection to the mucosal layers against microorganisms, toxins, and irritant chemicals. Because tannins are large polar molecules, they are poorly absorbed through the GIT. One of the most noticeable effects in the gut is their use in controlling diarrhea. Tannins can also affect bowel flora composition. Tea tannins (*Camilla* spp) fed to chicks significantly changed the levels of

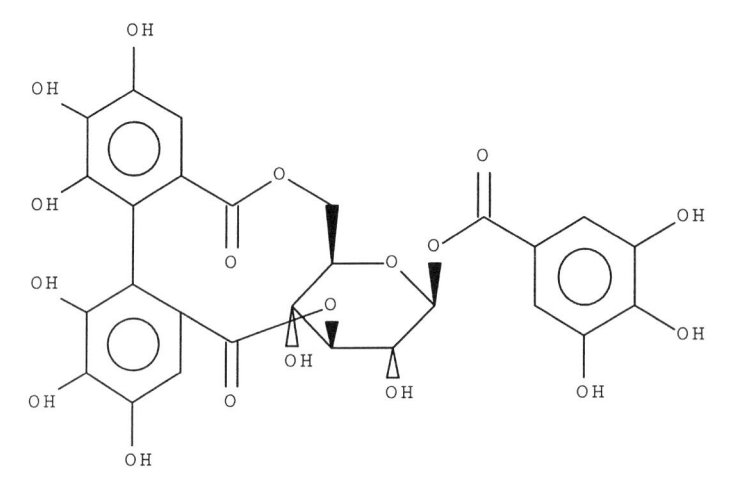

Fig. 4. Tannic acid.

microflora. It is not surprising, given that they are polyphenols, that tannins show a wide range of antioxidant activity. Hamamelitanin (Fig. 5) from *Hamamelis virginiana* and gallic acid, a tannin from nutgalls used as an intestinal astringent in veterinary medicine [47], were more active than ascorbic acid, vitamin C, in scavenging ROS [48].

Vaccinium myrtillus (bilberry) contains 0.5% anthocyanins, catechins (Fig. 6), epicatechins, condensed tannins, OPCs (procyanidin B1–B4), flavonoids, phenolic acids, and pectins. Therapeutic benefits for the following have been supported by clinical trials: gastrointestinal disorders, peripheral vascular disorders, capillary fragility, ischemic injury protection via antioxidant activity, inhibition of lipid peroxidation [49]. Bilberry anthocyanosides reduce microvascular impairments caused by reperfusion injury, with preservation of endothelium, attenuation of leukocyte adhesion, scavenging of the superoxide anion, and improvement of capillary perfusion [50]. Treatment of rats with *V myrtillus* kept the blood-brain barrier permeability normal and limited the increase in vascular permeability in the skin and the aorta wall [51]. Antiulcer activity by anthocyanidins from *V myrtillus* has also been demonstrated to show antioxidant activity, including scavenging of the superoxide anion [52].

Phytochemicals: their function in free radical homeostasis

What is a free radical? A free radical may be defined as any species capable of independent existence that contains one or more unpaired electrons. Hence, we have the term *free*, which relates to the free/unpaired electron. The free radical nature of an atom or molecule is usually denoted by a superscript dot (eg, H$^\bullet$ [hydrogen radical], O$_2^{\bullet-}$ [superoxide anion], and OH$^\bullet$ [hydroxyl radical]). Other examples of free radicals are oxides of nitrogen ($^\bullet$NO), ozone ($^\bullet$O$_3$), and singlet oxygen (with a rearrangement of

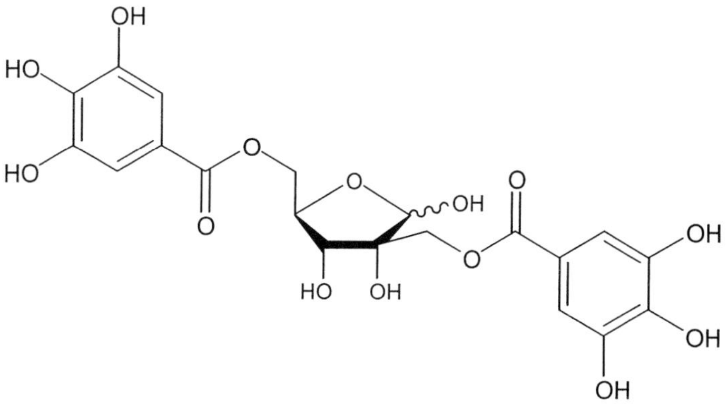

Fig. 5. Hamamelitanin.

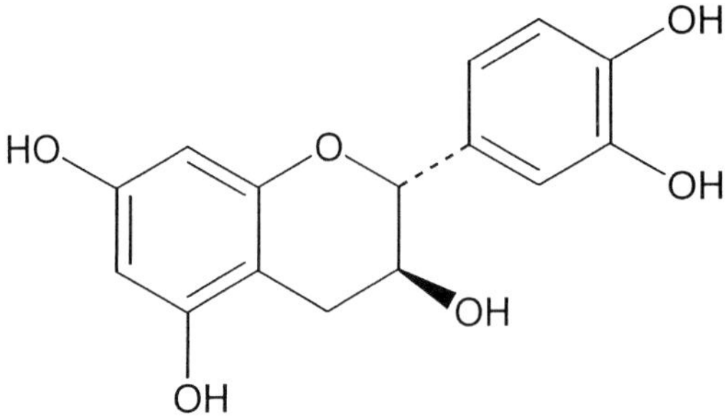

Fig. 6. Catechin.

electrons that produces rapid oxidation). Hydrogen peroxide (H_2O_2), although not a free radical because there are no unpaired electrons, is a ROS. ROS refers not only to oxygen radicals but to some nonradical derivatives of O_2.

Under normal conditions, the mammalian body needs oxygen but also finds oxygen toxic. As a normal byproduct of respiration, highly ROS and toxic ROS are produced. As a result, we are stuck with the conundrum of having essential life-giving chemicals in themselves causing toxicity by way of oxidation [53,54].

ROS are formed in the mammalian body by "accidents of chemistry" as well as for specific metabolic purposes. The reactivity of different free radicals varies, but excessive production has been found to cause severe damage to biologic molecules, especially to DNA, lipids, and proteins. Excessive production of ROS has been linked to cancer, cardiovascular diseases, atherosclerosis, diabetes, cataracts, arthritis, toxic liver injury, adverse drug reactions, immune hypersensitivity, inflammation, ischemia/reperfusion (anoxia/reoxygenation) injuries (eg, those involved in the laminitic syndrome), neurologic disease, and aging. This is only to mention the most heavily investigated entities [55].

It is well known that the immune response in the killing mechanism of phagocytes, which is triggered by a 10- to 20-fold increase in oxygen uptake by resting neutrophils (often called the respiratory burst), releases cytokines (IL-1, IL-6, and TNF), free radicals like the oxide radical and hydroxy radical, and the reactive oxygen molecule H_2O_2 [56].

Activated phagocytic cells, such as monocytes, neutrophils, eosinophils, and macrophages, generate the superoxide anion. This radical production by phagocytes is extremely important for their bactericidal and tumoricidal functions. The superoxide anions generated by phagocytes dismutase to H_2O_2 (an essential but toxic metabolite), which is a fairly unreactive molecule but gives rise to the highly toxic hydroxyl radical (OH^-) by reaction with transition metal ions

Mammalian cells produce antioxidant defenses, which, among others, include transferrin, lactoferrin, ceruloplasmin, albumin, haptoglobin-haemoplexin, and urate. SOD, which is present in the cytosol, is responsible for decreasing superoxide levels to less than 10^{11} M. Catalase, which is found in peroxisomes, breaks down H_2O_2 to give O_2 and H_2O. The GSH antioxidant family groups, such as GST peroxidase, a selenium-containing enzyme, are found in the mitochondria and cytosol, reducing organic hydroperoxidase and H_2O_2.

In the extracellular fluids, such as plasma and synovial fluid, SOD activities are low and catalase and GST peroxidase are essentially absent. The antioxidants in the aqueous phase of plasma include ceruloplasmin, albumin (the protein itself and possibly the albumin-bound bilirubin), ascorbic acid, elastoferrin, transferrin, haptoglobin, and hemopexin. The antioxidants in the lipid phase include tocopherols, retinols, and SOD [53].

Endogenous antioxidant defense systems scavenge and minimize the formation of oxygen-derived species; however, they are inadequate to prevent damage completely. Exogenous antioxidants can be particularly important in diminishing this cumulative oxidative damage [57–59]. Phytochemical antioxidants, with polyphenol nuclei and extended hydroxyl side chain groups, can react to form a resonance-stabilized phenoxy radical "quenching" the oxygen radicals (Fig. 7) [60].

Reactive oxygen species: immune system

ROS (oxidants) are produced by the immune system. These substances include cytokines and oxidant molecules, such as hydrogen peroxide (H_2O_2) and hypochlorous acid (HOCl). The purpose of these immune cell products is to destroy invading organisms and damaged tissue, bringing about recovery. Oxidants and cytokines can also damage healthy tissue, however. Excessive or inappropriate production of these substances can result, with mortality and morbidity after infection and trauma and in inflammatory diseases. ROS enhance IL-1, IL-8, and TNFα production in response to inflammatory stimuli by activating the nuclear transcription factor NF-κB. Sophisticated antioxidant defenses directly and indirectly protect the host against the influence of cytokines and oxidants. Indirect protection is afforded by specific antioxidants that reduce activation of NF-κB, thereby preventing upregulation of cytokine production by oxidants [61].

Cytokines increase oxidant production and antioxidant defenses, thus minimizing damage to the host. Although antioxidant defenses interact when a component is compromised, the nature and extent of the defenses are influenced by dietary intake of certain specific sulfur amino acids (for GST synthesis) and vitamins E and C. In animal studies, in vivo and in vitro responses to inflammatory stimuli are influenced by dietary intake of copper, zinc, selenium, *N*-acetylcysteine, cysteine, methionine, taurine, and vitamins E and C, which comprise some of the primary metabolites found in plants and their phytochemical secondary metabolites. Plants are both food and medicine [53].

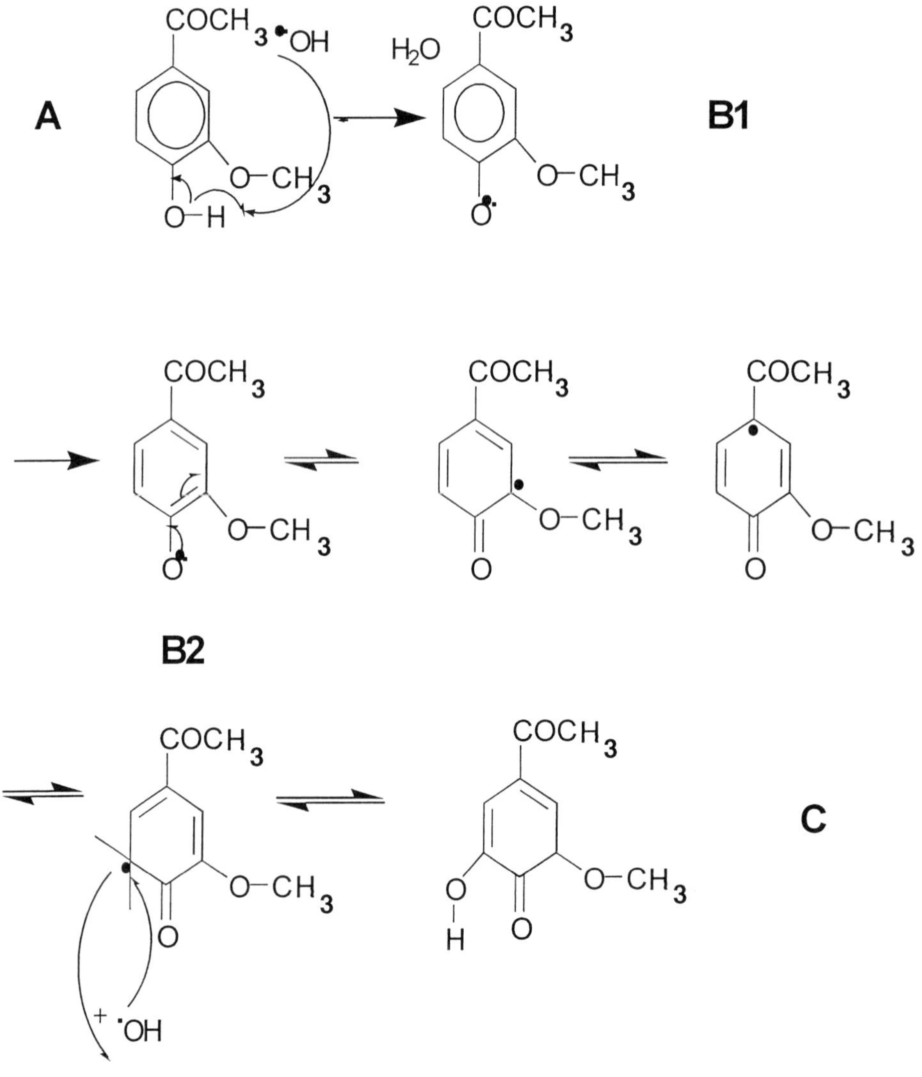

Fig. 7. Radical scavenging (antioxidant activity) by a plant phenol, acetovanillone, showing the essential roles that the hydroxyl (−OH) groups play as proton (H+) donors. Molecule A traps a free radical electron from a hydroxyl radical, OH·. The antioxidant molecule in this free radical form (molecules B1 and B2) can delocalize the free electron by moving it around the ring. This delocalization has the effect of making the species less reactive than the other OH· species, which structurally have no means to delocalize. Eventually, the free radical form of the antioxidant molecule may react with another free radical species (eg, another OH·), and a stable molecule is formed (molecule C). It should be noted that molecule C has fewer C=C bonds than molecule A, is less able to delocalize an electron, and is thus less effective as an antioxidant.

The most effective of these phytochemicals are the low-molecular-weight simple phenolic compounds, flavonoids, anthocyanidins, catechins, tannins, and coumarins. Phenols with two adjacent −OH groups or other chelating structures can also bind transition metal ions, especially iron and copper, in forms poorly active in promoting free radical reactions [62]. Phenols/ polyphenols can also directly scavenge ROS, such as OH•, ONOOH, and HOCl [63].

Anti-inflammatory activity

The phytochemicals genistein, kaempferol, quercetin, resorcinol, and resveratrol, which show cyclooxygenase (COX)-2 inhibition activity, have demonstrated significant dose-dependent decreases in TNFα, which is an inflammatory-mediating cytokine [64]. Plant-based COX-2 inhibitors, unlike pharmacologic nonsteroidal anti-inflammatory drugs (NSAIDs), have a slow onset of pain relief [65]. For many years, inflammation represented the only process in which ROS produced during the oxidative burst of activated neutrophils could be considered beneficial [66]. Today, much progress has been achieved in understanding the complex role of ROS in inflammatory reactions. Rather than simply beneficial or detrimental, the eventual effects of these ROS depend on a number of factors, such as the integrated involvement of different cells, the chronology and the type of microvascular changes, and the interaction with other reactive species [67–69].

The phytochemical apocynin (Fig. 8) can be found in *Picrorrhiza kurroa*, *Apocynum androsaemifolium*, *Apocynum cannabinum*, and the rhizomes of *Iris* spp. Apocynin is a potent intracellular inhibitor of superoxide anion (O_2^-) production in neutrophils [70]. The effects of apocynin on the regulation of the antioxidant GSH and activation of the transcription factor AP-1 in human alveolar epithelial cells (A549) indicate that apocynin displays antioxidant properties, in part, by increasing GSH synthesis through activation of AP-1 [71,72].

Apocynin concentration dependently inhibited the formation of thromboxane A2, whereas the release of prostaglandins E2-α and F2-α was

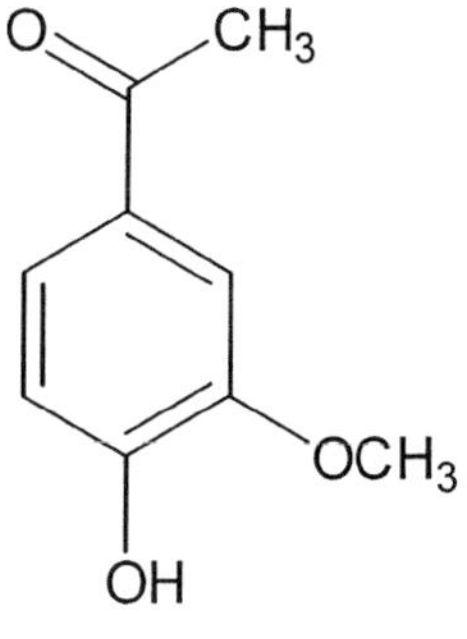

Fig. 8. Apocynin.

stimulated. Apocynin also potently inhibited arachidonic acid–induced aggregation of bovine platelets, possibly through inhibition of thromboxane formation [73]. Apocynin in vitro inhibits inflammation-mediated cartilage destruction without having adverse effects on cartilage. The latter may be an advantage of apocynin over many other nonsteroidal drugs [74]. Apocynin has been shown to be a potent and selective inhibitor of neutrophil oxyradical production. The mechanism of action involves metabolic activation in a myeloperoxidase-dependent reaction. The reaction product(s) prevent(s) the assembly of the superoxide anion–generating NADPH: oxidoreductase by conjugation to essential thiol groups [75]. Different neutrophil functions that are essential to their bactericidal activity, however, remain intact. When administered orally, a potent anti-inflammatory activity was found in rats with experimentally induced local or systemic inflammation [75].

Using its phytochemical marker substance harpagoside, *Harpagophytum procumbens* has been shown to exert anti-inflammatory effects by interacting with the eicosanoid biosynthesis, strongly indicating a close relation between serum harpagoside levels and the inhibition of leukotriene biosynthesis [76]. The active constituents are widely held to be the iridoid glucosides, although, of these, it has not been definitively established whether harpagoside is the most important pharmacologically active constituent of the whole extract. Other compounds present in the root may contribute to the pharmacologic activities of devil's claw. It has also been suggested that harpagogenin, formed by in vivo acid hydrolysis of harpagoside, may have biologic activity. Harpagophytum has been shown to be as effective as the NSAID diacerein in the treatment of knee or hip osteoarthritis. A reduced need for analgesic and NSAID therapy was observed [77]. Harpagophytum extract has been show to have a significant influence on sensory and vascular muscular response, resulting in a reduction in muscle stiffness [78].

In *Vitis vinifera* and *Polygonum* spp, the phytochemical resveratrol has been shown to inhibit COX-2 activity directly. The synthesis of resveratrol in various plant species is induced by stress conditions, such as infection or trauma, ultraviolet radiation, or exposure to ozone [79]. The addition of pure resveratrol to human mammary and oral epithelial cells exposed to phorbol esters, which induce COX-2 expression and the production of prostaglandin E2, inhibited both these effects, reversing the increases in COX-2 mRNA and protein [80].

The phytochemical curcumin (Fig. 9), from *Curcuma longa*, inhibits the 5-lipoxygenase activity in rat peritoneal neutrophils as well as the 12-lipoxygenase and COX activities in human platelets, providing a dual inhibition of arachidonic acid metabolism. In a cell-free peroxidation system, curcumin exerted strong antioxidative activity. The clinical efficacy of rhizomes of *C longa* produced a significant drop in severity of osteoarthritic pain ($P < 0.001$) and in disability score ($P < 0.05$) [81]. Curcumin causes an increase in glutathione S-transferase (GST) activity in rodent liver that may contribute to its anticancer and anti-inflammatory activities. Turmeric

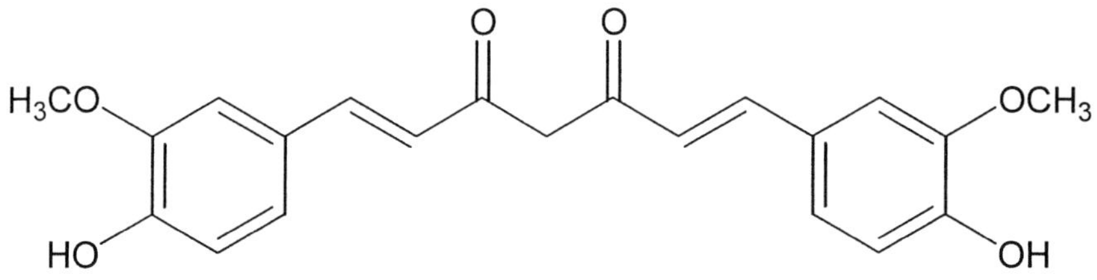

Fig. 9. Curcumin.

(4 g/kg) and curcumin (0.4 g/kg) have been shown to induce significant increases in hepatic levels of GST [82]. An additional study presented at the 1999 American Association for Cancer Research (AACR) conference showed that curcumin could suppress COX-2 expression in human colon cancer cells. The researchers found that the compound not only inhibited cell growth but reduced the expression of COX-2 mRNA [83].

Lipids

Plant lipids include saturated and unsaturated fatty acids, oils, fat-soluble vitamins, and fatty acid esters. These groups of phytochemicals can act on cellular membranes, thus affecting signaling, transport, and receptor function. Some lipids also act as enzyme cofactors (a prominent vitamin activity) and are antioxidants. The group includes isoprenoids, which consist of multiple 5-carbon isoprene units and a long unsaturated side chain, such as the ω-3 and ω-6 fatty acids, and the fatty acid ester linoleic acid. The polyunsaturated fatty acids (PUFAs) of the ω-3 (α-linolenic) and ω-6 (linoleic) series acids are found in dark green leafy vegetables, grains, legumes, nuts, and seeds.

γ-Linolenic acid and eicosapentaenoic acid (found in *Portulaca oleracea* [purslane]) disrupt the proinflammatory prostaglandin E2 cascade, reducing inflammation and platelet aggregation and modulating immune response. A human patient with osteoclastoma was injected with a γ-linoleic acid lithium salt mixture, which was observed to give abrupt and complete occlusion of tumor-feeding vessels. A follow-up angiogram performed after 8 years showed the original tumor-feeding vessel still occluded. The property of this injection technique to occlude tumor-feeding vessels selectively has been confirmed in another four patients: two with hepatomas, one with osteoclastoma, and one with renal cell carcinoma [84].

Alkaloids

With more than 10,000 alkaloids already documented in scientific literature, it is clear that scientific and medical research groups are aware of this large, diverse, pharmacologically active class of phytochemicals. With

> **Plants containing γ-linolenic acid**
>
> *Borago officinalis* (borage): seed
> *Daucus carota* (carrot): seed
> *Humulus lupulus* (hops): seed
> *Oenothera biennis* (evening primrose): seed
> *R nigrum* (black currant): seed
> *Ribes uva-crispa* (gooseberry): seed
> *Stellaria media* (chickweed): plant
> *Valeriana officinalis* (valerian, common valerian): plant

the alkaloids, pharmacognosy comes closest to conventional pharmacology. At least 40% of all plant families produce at least 1 alkaloid, with the greatest number found among the flowering plants. In rare cases, alkaloids have been found in bacteria and fungi. Alkaloid concentrations can also vary significantly from minute traces up to as high as 15% by dry weight. Most alkaloids, often structurally dissimilar groups containing one or more nitrogen atoms, are synthesized in the plant from amino acids.

The ability to cross the blood-brain barrier and the ability to interact with various neurotransmitter receptors are two key alkaloid properties that determine much of their pharmacology. Examples of familiar alkaloids include morphine (from opium), cocaine (from coca), mescaline (from mescal), nicotine (from tobacco), coniine (from hemlock), and caffeine (from tea and coffee) [85].

Berberine (Fig. 10) and berbamine (Fig. 11), among the numerous phytochemical alkaloids detected in *Berberis aquifolium*, *Berberis vulgaris*, *Hydrastis canadensis*, and numerous other species of the *Berberis* genus, exhibit numerous pharmacologic effects, including antibacterial, antifungal, and anti-inflammatory activity [86]. Interestingly, in 1886, Parke Davis and Company made *B aquifolium* commercially available for the treatment of skin diseases.

Berberine can inhibit the carbohydrate metabolism and protein synthesis of bacteria, thus stabilizing immune function and the phagocytic process [87–89]. Berberine is reported to be effective against diarrheas caused by enterotoxins, such as *Vibrio cholerae* and *Escherichia coli* [90].

Saponins/phytosterols

Saponin phytochemicals produce foam when dissolved in water. Like detergents, they are large molecules that contain hydrophilic and lipophilic parts. Saponins are glycosides with the sugar moiety attached to the hydrophilic end. Two classes are recognized. They are the steroidal saponins, which contain the characteristic four-ringed steroid nucleus, and the triterpenoid saponins, which have a five-ringed structure.

Plants containing α-linolenic acid

Allium schoenoprasum (chives): leaf
Beta vulgaris (beet): leaf, root
Capsicum frutescens (cayenne): fruit
Carica papaya (papaya): fruit
Cichorium intybus (chicory): leaf, root
Citrus aurantiifolia (lime): fruit
Citrus paradisi (grapefruit): fruit
Citrus reticulata (mandarin, tangerine): fruit
C sinensis (orange): fruit
Cucurbita pepo L (pumpkin): flower, fruit, seed
D carota (carrot): seed
Fragaria spp (strawberry): fruit
Ginkgo biloba (ginkgo, maidenhair tree): seed
G max (soybean): seed
Juglans cinerea (butternut): seed
Linum usitatissimum (flax, linseed): seed
Malus domestica (apple): fruit
Origanum vulgare (marjoram, wild oregano): plant
Piper nigrum L (black pepper, pepper): fruit
P oleracea (purslane): herb
R nigrum (black currant): fruit
Thymus vulgaris (common thyme, garden thyme, thyme): plant
V vinifera (European grape, grape, wine grape): fruit
Zea mays (corn): seed
Zingiber officinale (ginger): rhizome

Saponins and phytosterols differ only in the groups attached to the five-membered ring. The best-known mammal sterol is cholesterol, which is essential for life and a critical component of cell membranes, organs, the brain, and the nervous system. Just as cholesterol is the mammal precursor to all steroid hormones, such as cortisol, estrogen, progesterone, and testosterone, β-sitosterol (BSS; Fig. 12) is the plant's precursor to growth and reproductive hormones. *Dioscorea* spp contain variable amounts of the sapogenin diosgenin (Fig. 13), which can be converted into the corticosteroids dehydroepiandrosterone (DHEA), estrogen, and progesterone in vitro. Diosgenin in vivo does not convert into steroid hormones, however. Diosgenin has a weak estrogenic or progesteronic effect, which may account for its traditional use. Studies show that its effects do not replicate those of sex hormones or any synthetic drugs used for hormone replacement [91].

BSS and its glycoside (BSSG) are sterol molecules that are synthesized by plants. In animals, BSS and BSSG have been shown to exhibit

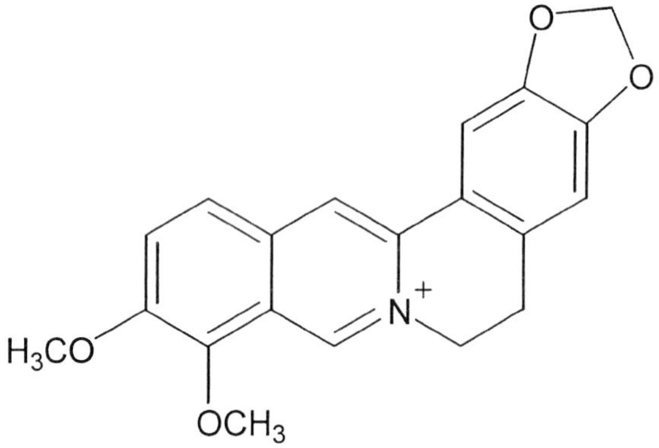

Fig. 10. Berberine.

anti-inflammatory, antineoplastic, antipyretic, and immune-modulating activity [92]. BSS has been isolated from wheat germ oil, corn oil, rye germ oil, cottonseed oil, soy and calabar beans, rice embryos, and cinchona bark. Animal studies have demonstrated that BSS possesses anti-inflammatory, antipyretic, antineoplastic, and immune-modulating properties. Algae and fungi also manufacture phytosterols. For example, ergosterol and other sterols from red yeast grown on rice have been shown to lower cholesterol. Clinical efficacy has been demonstrated in treatment of type II hyperlipoproteinemia [93], inhibition of cholesterol absorption [94], and inhibition of induced carcinogenesis [95].

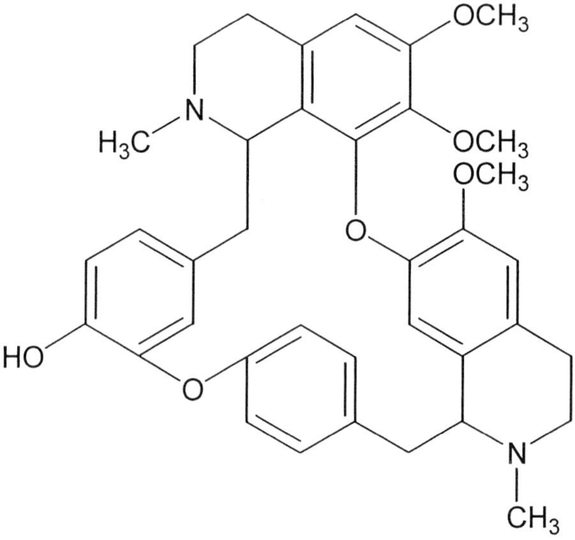

Fig. 11. Berbamine.

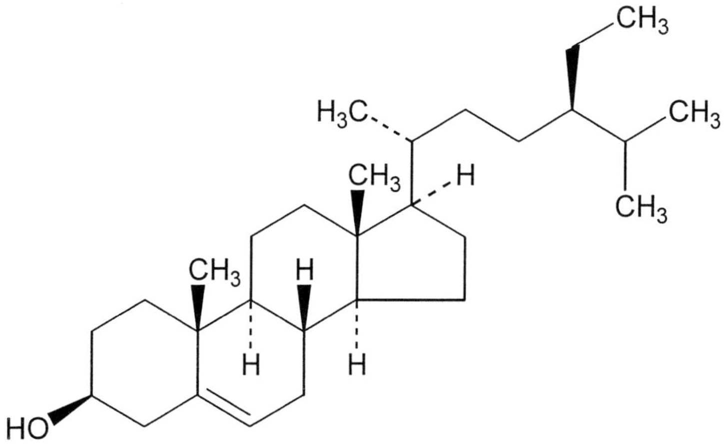

Fig. 12. β-Sitosterol.

Plant sterols may improve the T helper (Th) 1/Th2 ratio and natural killer (NK) cell function. A clinical trial with feline immunodeficiency virus (FIV)–infected cats resulted in enhanced survival times and stable CD4 levels compared with cats given placebo [96]. Plant stanols and plant sterols suppress intestinal cholesterol absorption by inhibiting cholesterol incorporation into micelles [97]. Fatty acid esters of plant sterols and plant stanols easily dissolve in the fats of foods, effectively reducing plasma cholesterol and low-density lipoprotein (LDL) cholesterol levels as a result of the suppression of intestinal cholesterol absorption showing significantly reduced plasma levels of total cholesterol and LDL cholesterol [98].

Quite novel and original, however, is the molecular evidence of a proinflammatory role played by hypercholesterolemia through the

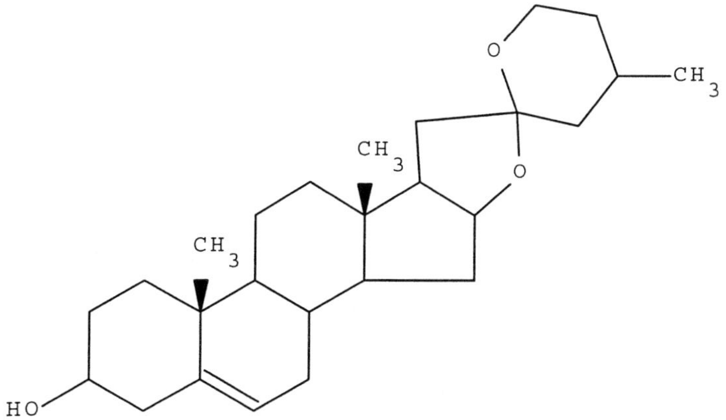

Fig. 13. Diosgenin.

excessive generation of ROS [99]. Unlike cholesterol, BSS is rapidly secreted into the bile and is esterified outside the intestinal wall at a much slower rate. In vitro, animal, and human studies have shown that BSS is capable of influencing several aspects of the immune response by selectively enhancing activity of Th1 cells and leaving unchanged or dampening the effect of Th2 cells. BSS administration results in a significant rise in IL-2 and IFNγ, which enhances direct NK cell activity. Dampening the effects of Th2 cells leads to decreased levels of the interleukins (IL-4, IL-6, and IL-10) involved in B-lymphocyte differentiation and inflammation [100,101].

Hypoglycemic properties of phytosterols were elucidated in an animal study using normo- and hyperglycemic rats. It is thought that phytosterol administration increases circulating insulin levels via stimulation of insulin secretion from pancreatic β-cells [102]. Randomized, placebo-controlled, clinical studies have been conducted on benign prostate hypertrophy (BPH). Although the exact mechanism is still unclear, BSS administration resulted in an improved peak urinary flow rate as well as an improvement in subjective symptoms of BPH [103]. Phytomedicines for BPH include saw palmetto (*Sabal serrlulata*), *Pygeum africanus*, and pumpkin (*Curcubita maxima*) seeds. BSS and other phytosterols for use in the treatment of BPH have been available in Germany for the past 20 years [104,105]. A study to investigate the effects of plant sterols and sterolins (BSS/BSSG mixture) on selected immune parameters in marathon runners showed less neutrophilia, lymphopenia, and leukocytosis compared with marathon runners on placebo capsules The placebo-treated individuals showed significant increases in their total white blood cell numbers as well as in their neutrophils ($P > 0.03$ and $P > 0.03$, respectively). Statistically significant increases within lymphocyte subsets were observed in the runners who received the active capsules: CD3+ cells increased ($P > 0.02$), as did CD4+ cells ($P > 0.03$) [106].

Phytoestrogens

Phytoestrogens, isoflavones, and lignans are phytochemicals that have estrogenic activity. They possess key structural features in common with estradiol, the major endogenous estrogen, which enable them to bind to and activate the estrogen receptor in target tissues. The relative molar-binding affinities of the isoflavones are considerably lower than those of estradiol, however [107]. These phytochemicals include genistein, quercetin, and daidzein as well as their glucosides. Tamoxifen (a nonsteroidal estrogen antineoplastic antagonist) and quercetin have been shown to interact with type II estrogen binding sites and inhibit the growth of human melanoma cells [108]. Synergism between tamoxifen and genistein shows downregulation of signal transduction in breast cancer cells [109]. It was observed in Australia in the 1940s that grazing sheep developed infertility when grazing on various species of clover (*Trifolium* spp). Isoflavone glycosides were identified as being responsible. Other animal studies have shown that isoflavones influence mammalian reproductive processes and sex hormone metabolism [110].

Although many isoflavones are weak estrogens, they can function as both estrogen agonists and antagonists depending on the hormonal milieu, target tissue, and species being examined. Evidence now points to the ability of these compounds to influence not only sex hormone metabolism and associated biologically activity but intracellular enzymes, protein synthesis, growth factors, malignant cell proliferation, differentiation, and angiogenesis (Fig. 14) [110–112].

Genistein (Fig. 14) has shown a marked capacity to inhibit endothelial cell proliferation and in vitro angiogenesis at concentrations of 50 and 150 µM, respectively. The conclusion reached was that genistein might represent a member of a new class of dietary-derived antiangiogenic compounds [113]. Isoflavone intake may prevent the development of cancer. Genistein has been shown to inhibit the growth of human prostrate cells in vitro [114]. Isoflavones, particularly genistein, exhibit anticancer potential that is independent of their hormonal effects and seem to inhibit tumor cell growth regulation. Genistein can inhibit several enzymes, including protein kinases and those involved in signal transduction [115].

The anticarcinogenic action of isoflavonoids is correlated with binding to estrogen receptors, antiproliferative action with regard to cancer cells, or inhibition of tyrosine kinases [116]. Flavonoids (genistein, naringenin, hesperetin, quercetin, apigenin, nobiletin, and tangeretin) have been found to act synergistically with tocotrienols (vitamin E groups found in palm oil, similar to tocopherols but their side chain contains three double bonds, whereas the side chain of tocopherols is saturated) and with the anticancer drug tamoxifen in the inhibition of estrogen receptor–negative and estrogen receptor–positive cancer cells, possibly inhibiting proliferation by different mechanisms [117].

The wide distribution of isoflavonoids and flavonoids in the plant kingdom, together with their antiangiogenic and antimitotic properties, suggests that phytoestrogens may contribute to the preventive effect on chronic diseases, including solid tumors. Certain flavonoids structurally

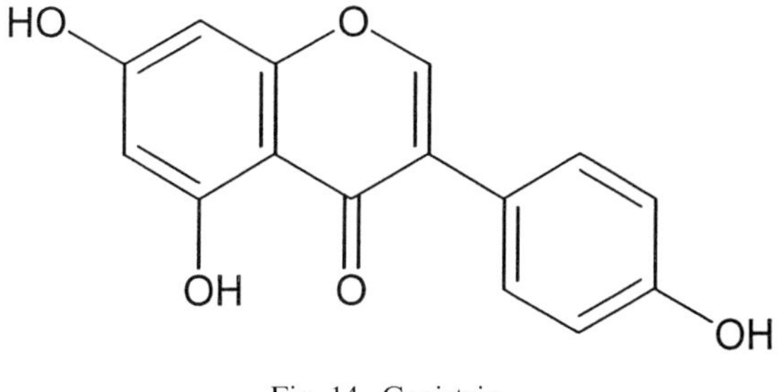

Fig. 14. Genistein.

related to genistein have been shown to be more potent inhibitors. Fisetin, apigenin, and luteolin inhibit the proliferation of normal and tumor cells as well as in vitro angiogenesis at half-maximal concentrations in the lower micromolar range [114,118,119].

The synthetic isoflavone ipriflavone (Fig. 15) has been shown to reverse osteoporosis [120–123].

Clinical effects of herbs: adaptogenic activity

Schisandra chinensis and *Eleutherococcus senticosus*, both of which are herbal adaptogens, are discussed. The term *adaptogen* was first coined by Lazarev and elaborated by Brekhman. According to Brekhman and Dardymov [124], an adaptogen is a substance that can produce a nonspecific increase in the resistance of an organism to noxious influences.

Ideally, an adaptogen has the following properties:

- It is nontoxic and relatively free from side effects.
- It is nonspecific; it can increase the resistance to a wide range of physical, chemical, and biologic stressors.
- It may have a normalizing action irrespective of whether the pathologic state is hypo- or hyperfunctional.

Schisandra chinensis

Scientific studies have shown hepatoprotective, adaptogenic, nervine, antitussive, and antioxidant activity of *S chinensis*. [125,126]. The fruit contains dibenzocyclooctene lignans (about 2% weight), with the main constituents being schisandrin (Fig. 16), schisandrin A, schisandrin B, schisandrin C, γ-schisandrin (racemic form of schisandrin B), gomesin A, and gomesin N.

Treatment of rats with a lignan-enriched extract of the fruit of *S chinensis* enhanced the hepatic antioxidant/detoxification system, as indicated by increases in the hepatic-reduced GSH level as well as in hepatic glutathione reductase (GRD) and GST activities [127]. *S chinensis* seems to be more

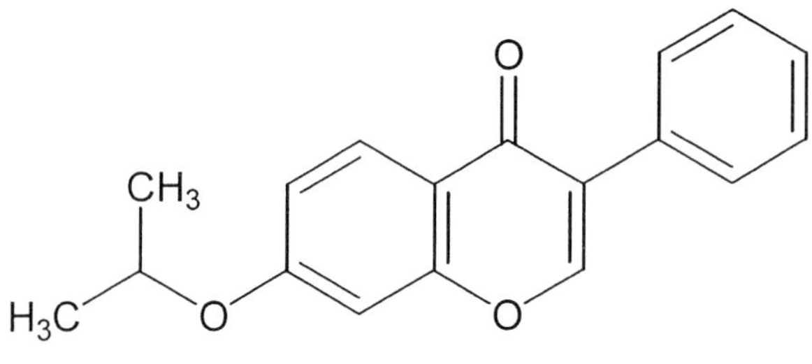

Fig. 15. Ipriflavone.

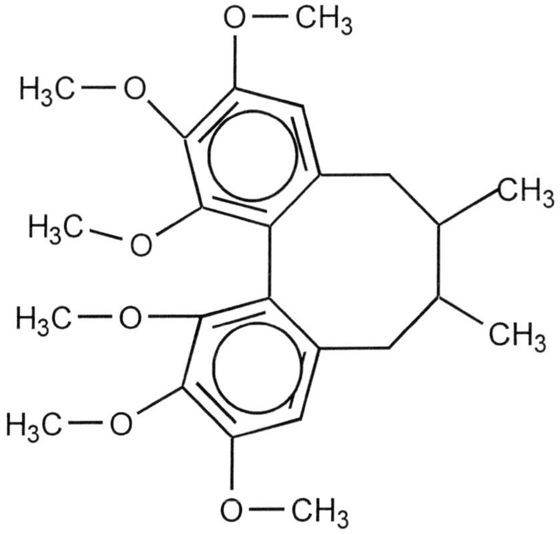

Fig. 16. Schisandrin.

effective than vitamin E in protecting against aflatoxin B1 and cadmium toxicity. The mechanism of hepatoprotection afforded by *S chinensis* pretreatment may involve facilitation of antioxidant and detoxification processes in the liver. The antioxidant activity within the liver sustains hepatic GSH, ascorbic acid, and α-tocopherol levels [128].

S chinensis has been shown to cause a dose-dependent enhancement in hepatic GSH status. This was evidenced by significant increases in the hepatic GSH level and activities of hepatic glucose-6-phosphate and GRD as well as a decreased susceptibility of hepatic tissue homogenates to in vitro peroxide-induced GSH depletion. The scavenging effects of schizandrins on hydroxyl radicals (OH•) in Fenton's reaction and the scavenging effects on superoxide anions ($O_2^{-•}$) in the riboflavin/EDTA and xanthine/xanthine oxidase systems were also observed [129].

GSH is a tripeptide (γ-glutamylcysteinylglycine) that contains an important thiol (sulfhydryl) group within the central cysteine amino acid. GSH is involved in numerous vital processes in which the reducing potential of thiol is used. These metabolic processes include detoxification of xenobiotics, reduction of hydroperoxides, synthesis of leukotrienes, synthesis of prostaglandins, maintenance of protein structure, maintenance of membrane structure, and regulation of numerous enzyme activities. Functioning as an essential endogenous antioxidant, GSH is widely distributed in most if not all cells where it is abundant in the cytoplasm, nuclei, and mitochondria. GSH liver levels have been shown to be increased by *S chinensis*, and *C longa* [130–132]. *S chinensis* enhanced the hepatic antioxidant/detoxification system, as indicated by increases in the hepatic reduced GSH level as well as hepatic GRD and GST activities [125,133].

In a randomized, double-blind, crossover study, 18 healthy horses received a single dose of *Schizandra* concentrate (equivalent to about 50 g of dried berries, containing 1.2% schizandrins) or placebo 30 minutes before a test race. For the Thoroughbred horse group, the exercise consisted of an 8-minute race over 5.6 km. The show jumpers were taken over a 700-m obstacle course with 12 jumps. Treatment with *Schizandra* reduced heart rate and respiratory frequency, increased plasma glucose, and decreased lactate levels in both groups. The effects were more marked in the racehorse group. The *Schisandra*-treated show jumpers completed the circuit in a shorter time than the controls [134]. In an earlier study involving Thoroughbred horses, a single dose of extract equivalent to 192 g of *Schisandra* fruit produced similar results to those of the previous study. The horses were, on average, 1.8 seconds faster over 800 m. It was postulated that the *Schizandra* might cause a lower synthesis of lactate in muscles under anaerobic conditions and stimulate lactate clearance by the liver [135]. Significant reductions in serum GPT, GOT and creatine kinase (CK) were observed in poorly performing horses at 7 and 14 days after oral administration of standardized *Schisandra* extract ($P < 0.01$–0.05) compared with baseline values. The horses selected had persistently high enzyme levels. Those treated with placebo did not experience any significant reductions in enzyme levels [136].

Eleutherococcus senticosus

The key constituents of *E senticosus* include eleutherosides (0.6%–0.9%) A, B, B1, C, D, and E; triterpenoid saponins (BSS glucoside); and glycans (eleutherans A, B, C, D, E, F, and G). The eleutherosides are unique to *Eleutherococcus*.

Indications supported by clinical trials have shown *E senticosus* to improve physical performance, minimize the effects of stress in athletes, enhance immune function (NK cells and Th cells), and reduce convalescence time after antibiotic therapy [137,138]. *Eleutherococcus* has displayed a marked antidiabetic effect in diabetic rats, increasing insulin and lowering glucagons [139]. The eleutherosides had an insulin-like activity in diabetic rats [140], and the eleutherans have been shown to be hypoglycemic [141].

In an equine study a standardized *E senticosus* extract was shown to favor an optimal response to vaccination [142–144].

A placebo-controlled study on the effect of an eleutherococcus extract on the immune system involving 36 volunteers showed a highly significant increase in the absolute number of immunocompetent cells, especially T lymphocytes ($P < 0.00001$), predominantly on the Th subtype but also on cytotoxic and NK cells. Pharmacokinetic studies indicate that eleutheroside B (Fig. 17) is enriched in the adrenal cortex. This suggested a complicated network involving effects on steroidogenesis, which, in turn, causes

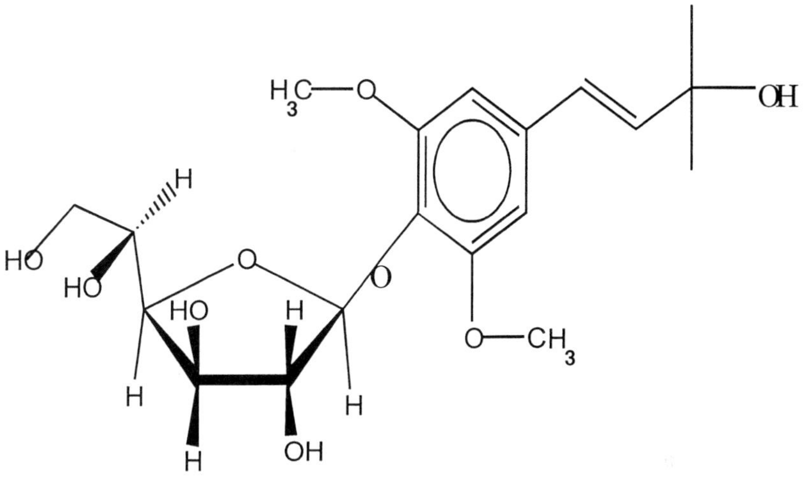

Fig. 17. Eleutheroside B.

interactions with the immune system, leading to the conclusion that *E senticosus* was capable of nonspecific immunostimulation [145].

Immune support

Most plants or their extracts with claims to stimulating the immune system enhance nonspecific immunity and not antigen-specific adaptive immune functions. They increase resistance by mobilizing effector cells that act against all foreign particles rather than just one specific type by:

- Stimulation of the nonspecific immune system with activation of macrophages and granulocytes to eliminate nonphysiologic substances
- Enhancement of the sensitivity and reactivity of the immune system to seize and eliminate weak antigens
- Inhibition of inflammation by incorporation of lipids into the lipid matrix of damaged cell membranes
- Selective inhibition of growth of malignant cells by simultaneous improvement of erythrocyte and macrophage function
- Enhancement of the growth inhibitory effect of (pharmaceutical) cytostatics by an intact immune system
- Selective growth inhibition of virus-transformed cells
- Enhanced movement of white blood cells into areas of infection; solubilization of immune complexes; and destruction of bacteria, viruses, and other microorganisms
- Stimulation of phagocytosis
- Inhibition of the enzyme (hyaluronidase), which is secreted by bacteria, helping them to gain access to healthy cells

An estimated 100,000 varieties of mushrooms exist; some 700 are used for food, and about 50 seem to have medicinal value. Medicinal properties have been attributed to mushrooms for thousands of years. Polysaccharides or polysaccharide-protein complexes derived from fungi have received much attention in biomedical research. These bioactive biopolymers are mainly present as glucans with different types of glycosidic linkages, such as (1→3), (1→6)-β-glucans and (1→3)-α-glucans, whereas others mostly bind to protein residues as polysaccharide-protein complexes. The most promising activities of these polysaccharides are their immunomodulation and anticancer effects. Three antitumor polysaccharides (lentinan, schizophyllan, and protein-bound polysaccharide or polysaccharopeptide) were isolated from *Lentinus edodes*, *Schizophyllum commune*, and *Coriolus versicolor*, respectively. These polysaccharides have been shown to have various potent pharmacologic properties, such as antioxidant, free radical scavenging, antiviral, hepatoprotective, antifibrotic, anti-inflammatory, antidiabetic, and hypocholesterolemic activities (Fig. 18) [146].

It is believed that the antitumor mechanisms of several species of whole mushrooms as well as those of polysaccharides isolated from *L edodes*, *S commune*, *Grifola frondosa*, and *Sclerotinia sclerotiorum* are mediated largely by T cells and macrophages. Despite the structural and functional similarities of these glucans, they differ in their effectiveness against specific tumors and in their ability to elicit various cellular responses, particularly cytokine expression and production [147]. TNFα (a cytokine regulating inflammatory and immune responses) release by macrophages is likely to be induced only by β-glucans with high molecular weights and lower branching ratios [148]. *L edodes* and *G frondosa* have been shown to have increased TNFα production from approximately 300 to 700 pg/mL and NO production from 4 to 7 μM [148]. Lentinan stimulates the antioxidant activity of SOD and macrophages in vitro. Other active phytochemicals also occur in *Shiitake*, namely, KS-2, a glycoprotein that is isolated in what is called a D-fraction from *Shiitake mycelia* and in RNA isolated from spores. The former stimulates IFN production in animal models when administered orally. IFN, produced by white blood cells, prevents viral protein synthesis [149–151].

The D-fraction has been found to activate NK cells, macrophages, and memory T cells. A second study by the same researchers showed that T cells are responsible for maitake's ability to help the body resist cancer

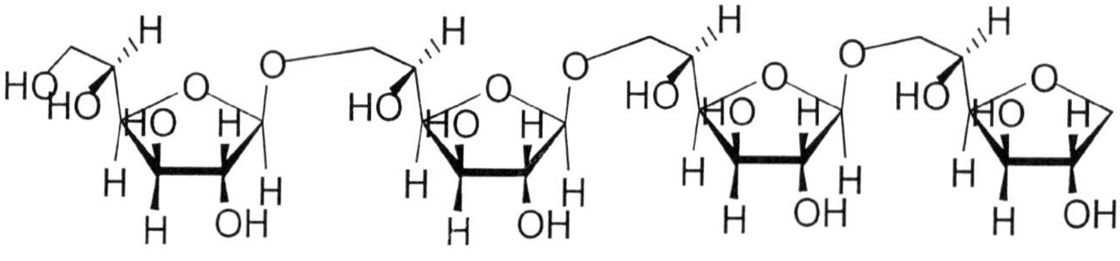

Fig. 18. β-Glucans: unbranched polysaccharides of linked β-(1→6)-D-glucopyranose units.

metastases. Maitake also activates several cytokines (ie, IL-1, IL-2) that attach to T-cell lymphocytes, essentially helping them to clone themselves into an army of cells that attack promoting-promoting cells [152]. Increases in the number of peritoneal macrophages and the third component of complement (C3)–positive fluorescent cells in mice treated with IV-1 suggested that the inhibitory effect on tumor growth is caused by immunologic host-mediated mechanisms [153,154].

In a study on collagen-induced arthritis in mice, a *G frondosa* extract demonstrated immunoregulating activities, IL-1β, granulocyte-macrophage colony-stimulating factor, and TNFα production from splenic macrophages, which were significantly increased to 2.0, 4.7, and 1.9 times the control group level, respectively [155]. Another study on the effect of administration of oat β-glucan on immune parameters of healthy and immunosuppressed beef steers indicated that β-glucans did not influence immune responses of naive cells in vitro or of healthy steers in vivo; however, β-glucans significantly restored some of the specific and nonspecific immune parameters studied [156]. A study on the effect of intramammary infusions of β-1,3-glucan, or IL-2 on leukocyte subpopulations in mammary glands of sheep demonstrated that intramammary infusion of β-1,3-glucan modulated nonspecific immunity in the udder of sheep [157]. Another study using a single intramammary infusion of β-1,3-glucan into the bovine udder during the dry period demonstrated the numbers of lymphocytes and polymorphonuclear leukocytes, the proportions of IL-2 receptor–positive lymphocytes, the proportions of CD14+ or major histocompatibility complex (MHC) class II–positive leukocytes, and the concentrations of IgG1 and IgG2 increased in comparison with untreated controls [158].

The broad spectrum of immunopharmacologic activities of β-D-glucans have been shown to:

- Enhance macrophage activity
- Enhance T-cell activity
- Enhance NK cell activity
- Increase IL-1 production
- Activate complement pathway
- Inhibit tumor growth
- Enhance immune response in sheep and cattle

Astragalus membranaceus

Phytochemicals isolated include the triterpenoid saponins astragalosides I through VIII, acetylastragalosides, astragenol, and others [159]. Approximately 2% of the root consists of coumarin and flavonoid derivatives. The polysaccharides show considerable immune-enhancing activity [160]. *Astragalus membranaceus* increases the number of stem cells in the marrow and lymph tissue and stimulates their development into active immune cells.

A membranaceus has been found to stimulate the production of IFN. The combined effect of IFN and astragalus root resulted not only in decreased common cold incidence but in shortening the course of illness. The polysaccharides have antirhinoviral activity by promoting and potentiating IFN function on antiviral activity [161]. The saponins can activate the peritoneal macrophages and enhance lipopolysaccharide (LPS)-induced TNF activity two- to threefold [162].

A membranaceus reduces the autoimmune response and stimulates B cells and antibody production. Animal in vitro research studies confirm enhanced T-cell activity and stimulated macrophages, which produce cytokine TNF and IL-6, which mediate the acute-phase response. *A membranaceus* suppressed tumor growth and restored immune function compromised by tumor growth. *Astragalus* polysaccharides have been shown to potentiate the antitumor activity of IL-2, enhance NK cell activity, and potentiate the activity of lymphocytes and monocytes [163]. Mononuclear cells obtained from myasthenia gravis patients show that *Astragalus* saponins are immunomodulating, reducing the titer of nicotinic acetylcholine receptor antibodies significantly. This can explain why the plant has been shown to be effective in the treatment of autoimmune disorders [164].

A membranaceus whole-root extracts have been shown to increase antibodies, IgE, and IgM; to increase proliferation of splenocytes; and to enhance IFN production [165]. The anti-herpes simplex virus activity of *A membranaceus* alone or in combination with recombinant human IFNα-2b (produced by *E coli*) exhibited more potent anti-herpes simplex virus activity than IFN alone [166]. The root of *A membranaceus* has been used for the treatment of hypertension, chronic hepatitis, duodenal ulcers, and chronic nephritis as well as in the promotion of immunity in folk remedies. COX-2 is responsible for the production of large amounts of proinflammatory prostaglandins at these inflammatory sites. Two isoflavone glycosides isolated from *A membranaceus*, 7,2′-dihydroxy-3′,4′-dimethoxyisoflavan-7-O-β-D-glucoside and calycosin-7-O-β-D-glucoside, inhibited COX-2 activity [167].

In an analysis of the practical problems existing in current swine production in China, it was argued that widespread use of large-dose and high-concentration nutrient additives and antibiotics in the feed results in excessive fat deposit and water accumulation in the pork and disturbs the growth of the animals. *A membranaceus* root and rhubarb (*Rheum officinale*) were used in feeding experiments that resulted in an increased daily weight gain and raised the lean meat percentage (4.8% and 6.5%, respectively) compared with the control groups [168]. In a study on the effect of adding Chinese herb polysaccharide preparations to a Newcastle disease–inactivated vaccine on the development of the immune organs in chickens, 7-day-old chicks were immunized with the inactivated vaccine alone, the vaccine plus *Astragalus* polysaccharide, the vaccine plus lentinan (a β-1,3-D-glucan polysaccharide isolated from the edible mushroom *L edodes*), or the vaccine plus compound Chinese herb polysaccharides. The results showed that the vaccines with herb polysaccharides increased the weights of the immune organs [169].

Summary

The more a critical look at the medicinal properties of plants is undertaken, the more it will be realized that nature does not make it easy to find all there is to know about them and the complexities of their interactions. An illustration of this can be found in one of the earlier scientific studies on phytomedicines, the Nobel laureate Albert Szent-Györgyi and his colleagues [170] found that flavanone extracts from the *Capsicum* spp contain an ascorbate-protective factor. It has now been repeatedly shown that the electron-donating properties of the phytochemical flavonoids, providing both nutritive and chemotherapeutic benefits, are the basis of their antioxidant action [171–175].

Studies by zoologists have demonstrated that animals, by selectively choosing specific plants, soils, and clays, maintain their health and treat themselves in times of ill health. The term *zoopharmacognosy*, now well researched, has been coined to describe the study of this recognized phenomenon. Long ago, Isaac Newton stated that for every action, there is an equal and opposite reaction. The same may be seen in plants and plant material. The same may be said of life in general. At the most basic concept, we are talking of electrons and their activities.

References

[1] Newman DJ, Cragg GM, Snader KM. The influence of natural products on drug discovery. Nat Prod Rep 2000;17:219–20.
[2] Huang KC. The pharmacology of Chinese herbs. Boca Raton: CRC Press; 1999. p. 450–2.
[3] Schmid W. Pflanzliche Bitterstoffe. Planta Med 1996;(Suppl):34–40.
[4] Halliwell B. Establishing the significance and optimal intake of dietary antioxidants. The biomarker concept. Nutr Rev 1999;57:104–13.
[5] Van Acker SA, Tromo MN, Haenen GR, van der Vijgh WJ, Bast A. Flavonoids as scavengers of nitric oxide radical. Biochem Biophys Res Commun 1995;214:755–79.
[6] Baker ME. Endocrine activity of plant-derived compounds: an evolutionary perspective. Proc Soc Exp Biol Med 1995;208:131–8.
[7] Evans CW. Trease and Evans' pharmacognosy. 13th edition. Philadelphia: Bailliere Tindall; 1989.
[8] Knight J, Larkins NJ, Ganderton M, Armstrong K. The use of Pholasin-based assays to evalute anti- and pro-oxidant capacity of extracts of certain functional foods: the effect of these foods on leucocytes in blood [abstract]. Free Radic Biol Med 2003;35(Suppl 1):s38.
[9] Das UN. Abrupt and complete occlusion of tumor-feeding vessels by gamma-linoleic acid. Nutrition 2002;18(7/8):662–3.
[10] Naidu MR, Das UN, Kishan A. Intratumoral gamma-linolenic acid therapy of human gliomas, prostaglandins. Prostaglandins Leukot Essent Fatty Acids 1992;45:181–4.
[11] Begin ME, Das UN, Ells G. Cytotoxic effects of essential fatty acids (EFA) in mixed cultures of normal and malignant human cells. Prog Lipid Res 1986;25:573–8.

[12] Kelly GS. Larch arabinogalactan: clinical relevance of a novel immune-enhancing polysaccharide. Altern Med Rev 1999;4(2):96–103.
[13] Potter SM. Overview of proposed mechanisms for the hypo-cholesterolemic effect of soy. J Nutr 1995;125(3 Suppl):606S–11S.
[14] Shils ME, Olson JA, Shike M. Modern nutrition in health and disease. 8th edition. Philadelphia: Lea & Febiger; 1994. p. 290.
[15] Jenkinson AM, et al. The effect of increased intakes of polyunsaturated fatty acids and vitamin E on DNA damage in human lymphocytes. FASEB J 1999;13(15):2138–42.
[16] Mo H, Elson CE. Apoptosis and cell-cycle arrest in human and murine tumor cells are initiated by isoprenoids. J Nutr 1999;129(4):804–13.
[17] Zhang R, et al. Enhancement of immune function in mice fed with high doses of soy daidzein. Nutr Cancer 1997;29:24–8.
[18] Gaziano JM, et al. A prospective study of consumption of carotenoids in fruits and vegetables and decreased cardiovascular mortality in the elderly. Ann Epidemiol 1995; 5(4):255–60.
[19] Head KA. Ipriflavone: an important bone-building isoflavone. Altern Med Rev 1999;4(1):10–22.
[20] Seddon JM, et al. Dietary carotenoids, vitamin A, C, and E, and advanced age-related macular degeneration: eye disease case-control study group. JAMA 1994;272(18):1413–20.
[21] Saija A, Scalese M, Lanza M, et al. Flavonoids as antioxidant agents: importance of their interaction with biomembranes. Free Radic Biol Med 1995;19:481–6.
[22] Skaper SD, Fabris M, Ferrari V, et al. Quercetin protects cutaneous tissue-associated cell types including sensory neurons from oxidative stress induced by glutathione depletion: cooperative effects of ascorbic acid. Free Radic Biol Med 1997;22:669–78.
[23] Kim HP, Mani I, Ziboh VA. Effects of naturally-occurring flavonoids and biflavonoids on epidermal cyclooxygenase from guinea pigs. Prostaglandins Leukot Essent Fatty Acids 1998;58:17–24.
[24] Bronner C, Landry Y. Kinetics of the inhibitory effect of flavonoids on histamine secretion from mast cells. Agents Actions 1985;16:147–51.
[25] Kaul TN, Middleton E Jr, Ogra PL. Antiviral effect of flavonoids on human viruses. J Med Virol 1985;15:71–9.
[26] Stavric B. Quercetin in our diet: from potent mutagen to probable anticarcinogen. Clin Biochem 1994;27:245–8.
[27] Scambia G, Raneletti FO, Panici PB, et al. Quercetin induces type-II estrogen-binding sites in estrogen-receptor-negative (MDA-MB231) and estrogen-receptor-positive (MCF-7) human breast-cancer cell lines. Int J Cancer 1993;54:462–6.
[28] Castillo MH, Perkins E, Campbell JH. The effects of the bioflavonoid quercetin on squamous cell carcinoma of head and neck origin. Am J Surg 1989;158:351–5.
[29] Beil W, Birkholz C, Sewing KF. Effects of flavonoids on parietal cell acid secretion, gastric mucosal prostaglandin production and Helicobacter pylori growth. Arzneimittelforschung 1995;45:697–700.
[30] Rice-Evans C. Wake up to flavonoids. International Congress and Symposium series 226. Oxford, UK: Royal Society of Medicine Press; 2000.
[31] Bors W, Michel C, Schikora S. Interaction of flavonoids with ascorbate and determination of their univalent redox potentials; a pulse radiolysis study. Free Radic Biol Med 1995;19:45–52.
[32] Bosisio E, et al. Effect of the flavanolignans of Silybum marianum L. on lipid peroxidation in rat liver microsomes and freshly isolated hepatocytes. Biotechnol Ther 1993;4:263–70.
[33] Thamsborg SM, et al. Putative effect of silymarin on sawfly (Arge pullata)-induced hepatotoxicosis in sheep. Vet Hum Toxicol 1996;35:89–96.
[34] Dehmlov C, Erhard J, De Groot H. Inhibition of Kupffer cell functions as an explanation for the hepatoprotective properties of silybin. Hepatology 1996;23(4):749–54.

[35] Alarcon de la Lastra AC, Martin MJ, Motilva V. Gastroprotection induced by silymarin, the hepatoprotective principle of *Silybum marianum* in ischemia-reperfusion mucosal injury: role of neutrophils. Planta Med 1995;61:116–25.
[36] Magliulo E, Gaglardi B, Fiori GP. Results of a double blind study on the effects of silymarin in the treatment of acute viral hepatitis, carried out at two medical centers. Med Klin 1978;73(28–29):1060–5.
[37] Florgheim GL, Eberhard M, Tschumi P, Duckert F. Effects of penicillin and silymarin on liver enzymes and blood clotting factors in dogs given a boiled preparation of Amanita phalloides. Toxicol Appl Pharmacol 1978;46(2):455–62.
[38] Vogel G, Tuchweber B, Trost W, Mengs U. Protection by silibinin against Amanita phalloides intoxication in beagles. Toxicol Appl Pharmacol 1984;73(3):355–62.
[39] Hollman PCH. Wake up to flavanoids. In: International Congress and Symposium, series 226. Oxford, UK: Royal Society of Medicine Press; 2000.
[40] Hollman PCH. Absorption, metabolism and bioavailability of flavonoids. In: Rice-Evans C, Packer L, editors. Flavonoids in health and disease. New York: Marcel Dekker; 1997. p. 483–522.
[41] Hollman PCH, Katan MB. Absorption, metabolism, and bioavailability of flavonoids. In: Rice-Evans C, Packer L, editors. Flavonoids in health and disease. New York: Marcel Dekker; 1999. p. 483–516.
[42] Rice-Evans CA, Miller NJ, Paganga G. Structure-antioxidant activity relationships of flavonoids and phenolic acids. Free Radic Biol Med 1996;20:933–56.
[43] Weber C, Erl W, Pietsch A, Strobel M, Ziegler-Heitbrock HW, Weber PC. Antioxidants inhibit monocyte adhesion by suppressing NF-κB mobilization and induction of vascular cell adhesion molecule-1 in endothelial cells stimulated to generate radicals. Arterioscler Thromb 1994;14(10):1665–73.
[44] Saller R, Meier R, Brignoli R. The use of silymarin in the treatment of liver diseases. Drugs 2001;61(14):2035–63.
[45] Van Acker SA, Tromo MN, Haenen GR, van der Vijgh WJ, Bast A. Flavonoids as scavengers of nitric oxide radical. Biochem Biophys Res Commun 1995;214:755–9.
[46] Virgili F, Kobuchi H, Packer L. Nitogen monoxide (NO) metabolism. In: Rice-Evans C, Packer L, editors. Flavonoids in health and disease. New York: Marcel Dekker; 1997. p. 421–36.
[47] Budavari S, O'Neil M, Smith A, Heckelman P, Obenchain J, editors. Merck Index. 12th edition. NJ: Merck and CO; 2000.
[48] Haslam E. Natural polyphenols (vegetable tannins) as drugs: possible modes of actions. J Nat Prod 1996;59:205–15.
[49] Colantuoni A, Bertuglia S, Magistretti MJ. Effects of *Vaccinium myrtillus* anthocyanosides on arterial vasomotion. Arzneimittelforschung 1991;41:905–9.
[50] Bertuglia S, Malandrino S, Colantuoni A. Effect of *Vaccinium myrtillus* anthrocyanosides on ischemic-reperfusion injury in hamster cheek pouch microcirculation. Pharmacol Res 1995;31:183–7.
[51] Detre Z, Jellinek H, Miskulin M, et al. Studies on vascular permeability in hypertention: action of anthrocynanosides. Clin Physiol Biochem 1986;4:143–9.
[52] Magistretti MJ, et al. Antiulcer activity of an anthocyanidin from *Vaccinium myrtillus*. Arzneimittelforschung 1988;38:686–90.
[53] Larkins NJ. Free radical biology and pathology. J Equine Vet Sci 1999;9(2):84–9, 134–5.
[54] Halliwell B, Gutteridge JM. Antioxidant defences. In: Free radicals in biology and medicine. 3rd edition. Oxford, UK: Oxford Science Publications; 1999. p. 105–245.
[55] Madhave DL, et al, editors. Food antioxidants. Technological, toxicological and health perspectives. New York: Marcel Dekker; 1996.
[56] Babior BM. Superoxide: a two-edged sword. Braz J Med Biol Res 1997;30:141–50.
[57] Halliwell B. Free radicals and antioxidants: a personal view. Nutr Rev 1994;52(8 Part 1): 253–65.

[58] Gutteridge JM. Antioxidants, nutritional supplements and life-threatening diseases. Br J Biomed Sci 1994;51(3):288–95.
[59] Halliwell B. Oxidative stress, nutrition and health: experimental strategies for optimisation of nutritional antioxidant intake in humans. Free Radic Res 1996;25(1): 57–74.
[60] Halliwell B, Gutteridge JM. Antioxidant defences. Free radicals in biology and medicine. 3rd edition. Oxford, UK: Oxford Science Publications; 1999. p. 229–30.
[61] Halliwell B, Gutteridge JM. Reactive species as useful biomolecules. Free radicals in biology and medicine. 3rd edition. Oxford, UK: Oxford Science Publications; 1999. p. 430–536.
[62] Morel I, Cillard P, Cillard J. Role of flavonoids and iron chelation in antioxidant action. Methods Enzymol 1994;234:437–43.
[63] Torel J, et al. Antioxidant activity of flavonoids and reactivity with peroxyl radical. Phytochemistry 1986;25:383–7.
[64] Mutoh M, et al. Suppression of cyclooxygenase-2 promoter-dependent transcriptional activity in colon cancer cells by chemopreventive agents with a resorcin-type structure. Carcinogenesis 2000;21(5):959–63.
[65] Maekawa K, et al. The molecular mechanism of inhibition of interleukin-1beta-induced cyclooxygenase 2 expression in human synovial cells by Tripterygium wilfordii Hook F extract. Inflamm Res 1999;48(11):575–81.
[66] Foreman HJ, Thomas MJ. Oxidant production and bactericidal activity of phagocytes. Annu Rev Physiol 1986;48:669–80.
[67] Babior BM. Phagocytes and oxidative stress. Am J Med 2000;109:33–4.
[68] Lentsh AB, Ward PA. Regulation of inflammatory vascular damage. J Pathol 2000;190: 434–48.
[69] Poli G. Serial review: reactive oxygen and nitrogen in inflammation. Free Radic Biol Med 2002;33:301–2.
[70] Müller AA, et al. Plant-derived acetophenones with antiasthmatic and anti-inflammatory properties: inhibitory effects on chemotaxis, right angle light scatter and actin polymerization of polymorphonuclear granulocytes. Planta Med 1999;65(7):590–4.
[71] Lapperre TS, Jimenez LA, Antonicelli F, Drost EM, Hiemstra PS, Stolk J, et al. Apocynin increases glutathione synthesis and activates AP-1 in alveolar epithelial cells. FEBS Lett 1999;443(2):235–9.
[72] Pearse DB, Dodd JM. Ischemia-reperfusion lung injury is prevented by apocynin, a novel inhibitor of leukocyte NADPH oxidase. Chest 1999;116(1 Suppl):55S–6S.
[73] Engels F, Renirie BF, Hart BA, Labadie RP, Nijkamp FP. Effects of apocynin, a drug isolated from the roots of Picrorrhiza kurroa, on arachidonic acid metabolism. FEBS Lett 1992;305(3):254–6.
[74] Lafeber FP, Beukelman CJ, van den Worm E, van Roy JL, Vianen ME, van Roon JA, et al. Apocynin, a plant-derived, cartilage-saving drug, might be useful in the treatment of rheumatoid arthritis. Rheumatology (Oxf) 1999;38(11):1088–93.
[75] Hart BA, Simons JM. Metabolic activation of phenols by stimulated neutrophils: a concept for a selective type of anti-inflammatory drug. Biotechnol Ther 1992;3(3–4): 119–35.
[76] Loew D, Mollerfeld J, Schrodter A, Puttkammer S, Kaszkin M. Investigations on the pharmacokinetic properties of Harpagophytum extracts and their effects on eicosanoid biosynthesis in vitro and ex vivo. Clin Pharmacol Ther 2001;69(5):356–64.
[77] Leblan D, Chantre P, Fournie B. Harpagophytum procumbens in the treatment of knee and hip osteoarthritis. Four-month results of a prospective, multicenter, double-blind trial versus diacerhein. Joint Bone Spine 2000;67(5):462–7.
[78] Gobel H, Heinze A, Ingwersen M, Niederberger U, Gerber D. Effects of Harpagophytum procumbens LI 174 (devil's claw) on sensory, motor and vascular muscle agility in the treatment of unspecific back pain. Schmerz 2001;15(1):10–8.

[79] Langcake P, et al. The production of resveratrol by Vitis vinifera and other members of the Vitaceae as a response to infection or injury. Physiol Plant Pathol 1976;9:77–8.
[80] Subbaramaiah K, et al. Resveratrol inhibits cyclooxygenase-2 transcription and activity in phorbol ester-treated human mammary epithelial cells. J Biol Chem 1998;273(34): 21875–82.
[81] Flynn DL, Rafferty MF, Boctor AM. Inhibition of 5-hydroxy-eicosatetraenoic acid (5-HETE) formation in intact human neutrophils by naturally occurring diaryheptanoids: inhibiting activities of curcuminoids and yakuchinones. Prostaglandins Leukot Med 1986; 22(3):357–60.
[82] Piper JT, Singhal SS, Salameh MS, Torman RT, Awasthi YC, Awasthi S. Mechanisms of anticarcinogenic properties of curcumin: the effect of curcumin on glutathione linked detoxification enzymes in rat liver. Int J Biochem Cell Biol 1998;30(4):445–56.
[83] Kawamori T, Lubet R, Steele VE, Kelloff GJ, Kaskey RB, Rao CV, et al. Chemopreventive effect of curcumin, a naturally occurring anti-inflammatory agent. Cancer Res 1999;59(3):597–601.
[84] Das UN. Abrupt and complete occlusion of tumor-feeding vessels by gamma-linoleic acid. Nutrition 2002;18(7/8):662–3.
[85] Duke JA. Handbook of phytochemical constituents of GRAS herbs and other economic plants. Ann Arbor: CRC Press; 1992.
[86] Duke JA. Handbook of biologically active phytochemicals and their activities. Ann Arbor: CRC Press; 1992.
[87] Huang KC. The pharmacology of Chinese herbs. 2nd edition. Ann Arbor: CRC Press; 1999. 381–3.
[88] Takasuna K, et al. Protective effects of kampo medicines and baicalin against intestinal toxicity of a new anticancer comptothecin derivative, irinotecam hydrochloride (CPT-II), in rats. Jpn J Cancer Res 1995;86:978–84.
[89] Sheng WD, et al. Clinical evaluation in Malaria. East Afr Med J 1997;74:283–4.
[90] Preininger V. The pharmacology and toxicology of the papaveraceae alkaloids. In: Mankse RH, Holmes HL, editors. The alkaloids, vol. 15. New York: Academic Press; 1975. p. 239–50.
[91] Evans WC. Trease and Evans' pharmacognosy. 13th edition. Philadelphia: Bailliere Tindall; 1989. p. 480–517.
[92] Lees RS, et al. Lipoprotein metabolism. New York: Springer-Verlag; 1976.
[93] Ikeda I, et al. Some aspects of mechanism of inhibition of cholesterol absorption by beta-sitosterol. Biochim Biophys Acta 1983;732:651.
[94] Nigro ND. Combined inhibitors of carcinogenesis: effect of azoxymethane-induced intestinal cancer in rats. J Natl Cancer Inst 1982;69:103.
[95] Bouic PJ, Lamprecht JH. Plant sterols and sterolins: a review of their immune-modulating properties. Altern Med Rev 1999;4(3):170–7.
[96] Bouic PJ. Immunomodulation in HIV/AIDS: the Tygerberg/Stellenbosch University experience. AIDS Bull 1997;6:18–20.
[97] Wilson MD, et al. Review of cholesterol absorption with emphasis on dietary and bilary cholesterol. J Lipid Res 1994;35:943–55.
[98] Ishiwata K, et al. Influence of apolipoprotein E phenotype on metabolism of lipids and lipoproteins after plant stanol ingestion in Japanese subjects. Nutrition 2002;18:561–5.
[99] Poli G. Serial review: reactive oxygen and nitrogen in Inflammation. Free Radic Biol Med 2002;33:301–2.
[100] Gupta MB, et al. Anti-inflammatory and antipyretic activities of beta-sitosterol. Planta Med 1980;39:157–63.
[101] Bouic PJ, Etsebeth S, Liebenberg RW, et al. Beta-sitosterol and beta-sitosterol glycoside stimulate human peripheral blood lymphocyte proliferation: implications for their use as an immunomodulatory vitamin combination. Int J Immunopharmacol 1996;18: 693–700.

[102] Ivorra MD, D'Ocon MP, Paya M, Villar A. Antihyperglycemic and insulin-releasing effects of β-sitosterol 3-β-D-glucoside and its aglycone, β-sitosterol. Arch Int Pharmacodyn Ther 1988;296:224–31.
[103] Szutrely HP. Clinical trials in treatment of prostate adenoma. Med Klin 1982;77:520–8.
[104] Klippel KF, et al. A multi-centric, placebo controlled, double-blind clinical trial of beta-sitosterol for the treatment of benign prostatic hyperplasia. Br J Urol 1997;80:427–32.
[105] Berges RR, et al. Randomised, placebo controlled, double blind clinical trial of beta-sitosterol in patients with benign prostatic hyperplasia. Lancet 1995;345:1529–32.
[106] Bouic PJ, Clark A, Lamprecht J, Freestone M, Pool EJ, Liebenberg RW, et al. The effects of B-sitosterol (BSS) and B-sitosterol glucoside (BSSG) mixture on selected immune parameters of marathon runners: inhibition of post marathon immune suppression and inflammation. Int J Sports Med 1999;20(4):258–62.
[107] Shutt DA, et al. Steroid and phytoestrogen binding to sheet uterine receptors in vitro. J Endocrinol 1972;52:299–310.
[108] Piantelli M, Maggiano N, Ricci R, Iarocca LM, Capelli A, Scambia G, et al. Tamoxifen and quercetin interact with type II estrogen binding sites and inhibit the growth of human melanoma cells. J Invest Dermatol 1995;105:248–53.
[109] Shen F, Xue X, Weber G. Tamoxifen and genistein synergistically down-regulate signal transduction and proliferation in estrogen receptor negative human breast carcinoma MDA-MD-435 cells. Anticancer Res 1999;19(3A):1657–62.
[110] Kuiper GG, Lemmen JG, Carlsson B. Interaction of estrogenic chemicals and phytoestrogens with estrogen receptor beta. Endocrinology 1998;139(10):4252–63.
[111] Molteni A, Brizio-Molteni L, Persky V. In vitro hormonal effects of soybean isoflavones. J Nutr 1995;125(Suppl):751s–6s.
[112] Herman C, Adlercreutz T, Goldin BR. Soybean phytoestrogens intake and cancer risk. J Nutr 1995;125(Suppl):757s–70s.
[113] Barnes S. Effect of genistein on in vitro and in vivo models of cancer. J Nutr 1995;125(Suppl):177s–783s.
[114] Fotsis T, Pepper M, Adlercreutz H, Hase T, Montesano R, Schweigerer L. Genistein, a dietary ingested isoflavonoid, inhibits cell proliferation and in vitro angiogenesis. J Nutr 1995;125(Suppl):790s–7s.
[115] Onozawa M, Fukuda K, Ohtani M. Effects of soybean isoflavones on cell growth and apoptosis of the human prostatic cancer cell line LNCaP. Jpn J Clin Oncol 1998;58(17):3833–8.
[116] Peterson G. Evaluation of the biochemical targets of genistein in tumor cells. J Nutr 1995;125(Suppl):784s–9s.
[117] Herman C, Adlercreutz T, Goldin BR. Soybean phytoestrogen intake and cancer risk. J Nutr 1995;126(Suppl):757s–70s.
[118] Carroll K, Guthrie N, So FV, Chambers AF. Anticancer properties of flavonoids. In: Rice-Evans C, Packer L, editors. Flavonoids in health and disease. Philadelphia: Marcel Dekker; 1990. p. 437–46.
[119] Fotsis T, Montesano R, Pepper M, Adlercreutz H. Phytoestrogens and inhibition of angiogenesis. Baillieres Clin Endocrinol Metab 1998;12(4):649–66.
[120] Bassleer CT, Franchimont PP, Henrotin YE, Franchimont NM, Geenen VG, Reginster JY. Effects of ipriflavone and its metabolites on human articular chondrocytes cultivated in clusters. Osteoarthritis Cartilage 1996;4(1):1–8.
[121] Reginster JY. Ipriflavone: pharmacological properties and usefulness in postmenopausal osteoporosis. Bone Miner 1993;23(3):223–32.
[122] Scheiber MD, et al. Isoflavones and postmenopausal bone health: a viable alternative to estrogen therapy? Menopause Fall 1999;6(3):233–41.
[123] Head KA. Ipriflavone: an important bone-building isoflavone. Altern Med Rev 1999;4(1):10–22.

[124] Brekhman I, Dardymov IV. New substances of plant origin which increase nonspecific resistance. Annu Rev Pharmacol 1969;9:419–30.
[125] Panossian AG, Oganessian AS, Ambartsumian M, et al. Effects of heavy physical exercise and adaptogens on nitric oxide content in human saliva. Phytomedicine 1999; 6(1):17–26.
[126] Chang HM, But PP. Pharmacology and applications of Chinese materia medica, vol. 1. Singapore: World Scientific Publishing; 1987. p. 199–209.
[127] Ip SP, Ko KM. The crucial antioxidant action of schisandrin B in protecting against carbon tetrachloride hepatotoxicity in mice: a comparative study with butylated hydroxytoluene. Biochem Pharmacol 1996;52(11):1687–93.
[128] Mak DH, Ip SP, Li PC, et al. Effects of Schisandrin B and alpha-tocopherol on lipid peroxidation, in vitro and in vivo. Mol Cell Biochem 1996;165(2):161–5.
[129] Zhu M, Lin KF, Yeung RY, et al. Evaluation of the protective effects of Schisandra chinensis on phase I drug metabolism using a CCl_4 intoxication model. J Ethnopharmacol 1999;67:61–8.
[130] Ko KM, Ip SP, Poon MK. Effect of a lignan-enriched fructus schisandrae extract on hepatic glutathione status in rats: protection against carbon tetrachloride toxicity. Planta Med 1995;61(2):134–7.
[131] Kawamori T, Lubet R, Steele VE, Kelloff GJ, Kaskey RB, Rao CV, et al. Chemopreventive effect of curcumin, a naturally occurring anti-inflammatory agent. Cancer Res 1999;59(3):597–601.
[132] Piper JT, Singhal SS, Salameh MS, Torman RT, Awasthi YC, Awasthi S. Mechanisms of anticarcinogenic properties of curcumin: the effect of curcumin on glutathione linked detoxification enzymes in rat liver. Int J Biochem Cell Biol 1998;30(4):445–56.
[133] Ip SP, Mak DH, Li PC. Effect of a lignan-enriched extract of Schisandra chinensis on aflatoxin B1 and cadmium chloride-induced hepatotoxicity in rats. Pharmacol Toxicol 1996;78(6):413–6.
[134] Hancke J, Burgos R, Wikman G, et al. Schizandra chinensis, a potential phytodrug for recovery of sport horses. Fitoterapia 1994;65(2):113–8.
[135] Ahumada F, Hermosilla J, Hola R, et al. Studies on the effect of Schizandra chinensis extract on horses submitted to exercise and maximum effort. Phytother Res 1989;3(5): 175–9.
[136] Hancke J, Burgos R, Caceres D, et al. Reduction of serum hepatic transaminases and CPK in sport horses with poor performance treated with a standardized Schizandra chinensis fruit extract. Phytomedicine 1996;3(3):237–40.
[137] Zykov MP. Prospects of immunostimulating vaccination against influenza including the use of *Eleutherococcus senticosus* and other preparations of plant origin. In: Proceedings of the Far East Science Center Symposium. Vladivostok: Far East Science Center, USSR Ac. Sci. 1986. p. 164–9.
[138] Wagner H. In: Chang HM, et al, editors. Advances in Chinese medicinal materials. Singapore: World Scientific Publishing; 1985. p. 159–70.
[139] Kupin VI, et al. *Eleutherococcus senticosus* demonstrates nonspecific immunity in patients undergoing anti-tumor treatment. Vopr Onkol 1986;32:21–6.
[140] Molokovskii DS, et al. The action of adaptogenic plant preparations in experimental alloxan diabets. Probl Endokrinol (Mosk) 1989;35:82–7.
[141] Dardymov IV, et al. New substances of plant origin which increase non-specific resistance Annu Rev Pharmacol 1969;9:419–30.
[142] Hikino H, et al. Isolation and hypoglycaemic activity of eleutherans A, B, C, D, E, F and G: from *Eleutherococcus senticosus* roots. J Nat Prod 1986;49:293–7.
[143] Debarcy B, Sironval C. Fortifying immunological defences by adaptogens and their practical use in horses. HPH Scientific News1991;17–25.
[144] Wong OW, et al. Effect of strenuous exercise stress on chemiluminescence response of equine alveolar macrophages. Equine Vet J 1990;22(1):33–5.

[145] Bohn B, Nebe CT, Birr C. Flow-cytometric studies with Eleuterococcus senticosus extract as an immunomodulatory agent. Arzneimittelforschung 1987;10:1193–6.
[146] Ooi VEC, Liu F. A review of pharmacological activities of mushroom polysaccharides. International Journal of Medicinal Mushrooms 1999;1(3):195–206.
[147] Borchers AT, Stern JS, Hackman RM, Keen CL, Gershwin ME. Mushrooms, tumors, and immunity. Proc Soc Exp Biol Med 1999;221(4):281–93.
[148] Okazaki M, Adachi Y, Ohno N, Yadomae T. Structure-activity relationship of (1→3)-beta-D-glucans in the induction of cytokine production from macrophages, in vitro. Biol Pharm Bull 1995;18(10):1320–7.
[149] Adachi Y, et al. The effect enhancement of cytokine production by macrophages stimulated with 1, 3 beta D glucan, grifolan, isolated from Grifola frondosa. Biol Pharm Bull 1994;17:1554–60.
[150] Ohno N, et al. Effect of beta-glucan on the nitric oxide synthesis of peritoneal macrophage (sic) in mice. Biol Pharm Bull 1996;19:608–12.
[151] Nakano H, et al. A multi-institutional prospective study of lentinan in advanced gastric cancer patients with unresectable and recurrent disease: effects on prolongation of survival and improvement of quality of life. Kanagawa Research Group. Hepatogastroenterology 1999;46:2662–8.
[152] Matsuoka H, et al. Lentinan potentiates immunity and prolongs the survival time of some patients. Anticancer Res 1997;17:2251–5.
[153] Williams DL, et al. Therapeutic efficacy of glucan in a murine model of hepatic metastatic disease. Hepatology 1985;5:198–206.
[154] Ukawa Y, Ito H, Hisamatsu M. Antitumor effects of (1→3)-beta-D-glucan and (1→6)-beta-D-glucan purified from newly cultivated mushroom, Hatakeshimeji (Lyophyllum decastes Sing.). J Biosci Bioeng 2000;90(1):98–104.
[155] Shigesue K, Kodama N, Nanba H. Effects of maitake (Grifola frondosa) polysaccharide on collagen-induced arthritis in mice. Jpn J Pharmacol 2000;84(3):293–300.
[156] Estrada A, van Kessel A, Laarveld B. Effect of administration of oat beta-glucan on immune parameters of healthy and immunosuppressed beef steers. Can J Vet Res 1999;63(4):261–8.
[157] Waller KP, Cloditz IG. The effect of intramammary infusion of beta-1,3-glucan or interleukin-2 on leukocyte subpopulations in mammary glands of sheep. Am J Vet Res 1999;60(6):703–7.
[158] Inchaisri C, Waller KP, Johannisson A. Studies on the modulation of leucocyte subpopulations and immunoglobulins following intramammary infusion of beta 1, 3-glucan into the bovine udder during the dry period. J Vet Med B Infect Dis Vet Public Health 2000;47(5):373–86.
[159] Chang HM, But PP. Pharmacology and applications of Chinese materia medica, vol. 1. Singapore: World Scientific Publishing; 1987.
[160] Chu D, et al. Fractionated extract of Astragalus membranaceus, a Chinese medicinal herb, potentiates LAK cell cytotoxicity generated by a low dose of recombinant interleukin-2. J Clin Lab Immunol 1988;26(4):183–7.
[161] Zang LL, et al. Pharmacology and applications of Chinese materia medica. Chin J Exp Clin Virol 1996;10:77.
[162] Zhang WH, et al. Cellular proteins that bind to the hepatitis B virus post-transcriptional regulatory element. Shanghai J Immunol 1996;16:224–8.
[163] Zee-Cheng RK. Shi-quan-da-bu-tang, SQT. A potent Chinese biological response modified in cancer immunotherapy, potentiating and detoxification of anti-cancer drugs. Methods Find Exp Clin Pharmacol 1992;14:725–36.
[164] Tu LH, et al. CD83 expression influences CD4+ T-cell development in the thymus. Chin Med J 1994;107:300–12.
[165] Chang H, et al. Pharmacology and applications of Chinese materia medica, vol. 2. Singapore: World Scientific Publishing; 1987.

[166] Zhang LL, et al. Study on the anti-herpes simplex virus activity of a suppository or ointment form of Astragalus membranaceus combined with interferon alpha 2b in human diploid cell culture. Chinese J Exp Clin Virol 1998;12(3):269–71.
[167] Kim EJ, et al. Inhibitory effect of Astragali Radix on COX-2 activity. Korean Journal of Pharmacognosy 2001;32(4):82–5.
[168] Ge CR, et al. Research of feed additive formulations for swine with Chinese traditional medicinal herbs as their ingredients. Journal of Yunnan Agricultural University 2002; 17(1):45–50.
[169] Zhang LC, et al. Effect of adding Chinese herb polysaccharide preparations to a Newcastle disease inactivated vaccine on the development of the immune organs in chickens. Chin J Vet Sci 1998;18(4):378–81.
[170] Benthsath A, Rusznak S, Szent-Györgyi A. Vitamin nature of flavone. Nature 1936;138: 27–35.
[171] Huguet AI, Manez S, Alcaraz MJ. Superoxide scavenging properties of flavonoids in non-enzymatic systems. Z Naturforsch 1990;45:19–24.
[172] Gyorgy I, Antus S, Foldiak G. Pulse radiolysis of silybin: one electron oxidation of the flavonoid at neutral pH. Radiat Phys Chem 1992;5:39–81.
[173] Rice-Evans C, Miller NJ, Bolwell PG, Bramley PM, Pridham JB. The relative antioxidant activities of plant-derived polyphenolic flavonoids. Free Radic Res 1995;22:375–83.
[174] Salah N, Miller NJ, Paganga G, Tijburg L, Bolwell PG, Rice-Evans C. Polyphenolic flavonoids as scavengers of aqueous phase radicals and chain-breaking antioxidants. Arch Biochem Biophys 1995;322:339–46.
[175] Simic MG, Jovanovic SV. Interaction of oxygen radicals by dietary phenolic compounds in anticarcinogenesis.. Cancer Res 1994;54(Suppl):2044s–51s.

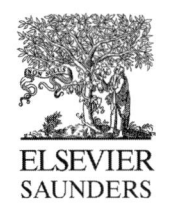

Regulatory issues of functional foods, feeds, and nutraceuticals

Maureen L. Storey, PhD

Center for Food and Nutrition Policy, Virginia Polytechnic Institute and State University, 1101 King Street, Suite 611, Alexandria, VA 22314, USA

The purpose of this article is to: (1) familiarize readers with the United States public policy process that affects the functional food and nutraceutical industry; (2) illustrate the complex United States regulatory infrastructure and rulemaking process; and (3) provide a few pertinent examples of functional foods that have used claims.

Public policy process

The public policy process directly affects the regulation of functional foods, feeds, and nutraceuticals. The legislative process establishes the laws that form the framework for regulation, the executive branch implements the laws with detailed regulations and enforces the regulations, and the judiciary adjudicates disputes arising from regulations. The judiciary is a critical component of the public policy process, especially when the law, or implementation of the law by the executive branch, is challenged in some way. Although the judicial branch of the government is not discussed in detail here, it has and will continue to have profound effects on implementation of the regulations governing health messages made by food and dietary supplement manufacturers.

The legislative branch is represented by the Senate and the House of Representatives, which comprise Congress. Lawmakers elected by the democratic process identify public policy problems that theoretically can be rectified by enacting a new law or amending an old one. The public policy process begins by identifying a significant societal problem and taking the necessary steps to correct it. Setting an agenda, identifying options, and implementing a policy that solves the problem are part of this process, which

E-mail address: mstorey@vt.edu

seldom proceeds without controversy and debate. Evaluation is a critical part of the public policy process to assess whether the problem was resolved in an efficient, effective, and targeted manner, or if the policy should be terminated [1].

Implementation of the policy is the responsibility of the executive branch of the government, which is led by the president and vice president. The secretaries of the president's cabinet—including the vice president—are responsible for "executing" or interpreting and enforcing the law through detailed regulations [2].

Within this branch of the government, there are two cabinet-level departments that regulate food: the Departments of Health and Human Services (DHHS) and Agriculture (USDA). Other agencies and commissions play a role, however. For example, the Federal Trade Commission (FTC), an independent commission of the federal government, participates in developing regulations on advertising to protect the public from unsafe products and false or misleading claims. The Environmental Protection Agency (EPA) protects the public health by safeguarding the water, air, and land. The Food and Drug Administration (FDA) of the DHHS, the Food Safety and Inspection Service (FSIS) of the USDA, and the FTC hold complementary jurisdiction over claims made by food and dietary supplement makers. A memorandum of understanding established in 1954 made the FTC the primary authority for regulating food advertising, while the FDA retained responsibility for food labeling. The USDA regulates meat, poultry products, and egg products by the authority of the Federal Meat Inspection Act [3], the Poultry Products Inspection Act [4], and the Egg Products Inspection Act [5]; the FDA regulates all other foods, including animal feeds and pet foods, shell eggs, seafood, dietary supplements, cosmetics, drugs, and medical devices.

The FDA's regulatory authority was established early in the twentieth century when Congress enacted two key pieces of legislation to protect the public health: the Pure Food Act of 1906 and the Federal Food, Drug, and Cosmetic Act (FFDCA) of 1938 [6]. The 1906 statute signed into law by President Theodore Roosevelt for the first time addressed adulteration, misbranding, and mislabeling of foods [1]. The original law was seriously flawed, because Congress provided no funds to enforce it and did not set up standards against which to measure whether or not a food was adulterated.

In 1938, President Franklin D. Roosevelt signed the FFDCA, which amended the 1906 statute, and authorized the US Department of Health and Human Services to protect the public health by developing and enforcing regulations for manufacturers of pharmaceuticals and most foods. The 1938 statute set forth very broad definitions for drugs and food: "articles used for food or drink for man or other animals, chewing gum, and articles used for components of any other such article." "The term 'drug' means (A) articles recognized in the official United States Pharmacopeia, official Homeopathic Pharmacopeia of the United States, or official National Formulary, or any supplement to any of them; and (B) articles intended for use in the diagnosis, cure, mitigation, treatment, or prevention of disease in man or other animals; and (C) articles (other than food) intended to affect the structure or any function of the body of man or other animals; and (D) articles intended for use as a component of any articles specified in clause (A), (B), or (C); but does not include devices or other components, parts, or accessories" [6]. The definition of a drug, however, did not acknowledge that nutrients found in foods can also affect health.

Nutritive cures for disease

The disease-preventing, health-promoting benefits of foods have been recognized, if not completely understood, since the 1700s. At that time, Dr. James Lind, a British naval surgeon, conducted the first clinical trial during which he fed lemon juice to scorbutic sailors to cure them of the deadly disease scurvy. Years later, lime juice became a staple aboard ships undergoing long sea voyages. These citrus fruits—excellent sources of ascorbic acid or vitamin C—prevented, cured, and treated scurvy, a noncommunicable nutrient deficiency disease. Other micronutrients found in foods were subsequently discovered and recognized as preventative and curative agents of nutrient deficiency diseases.

In 1938, Congress did not foresee the advances in nutrition science and epidemiology that now blur the distinction between the prevention of disease and the promotion of health by foods and drugs. For decades following the enactment of the FFDCA, there was little question that food and nutrients found in food could prevent deadly, classical deficiency diseases such as scurvy, pellagra, and beri-beri. Today, true deficiency diseases are a rarity in the United States and most developed countries, where a wide variety of food is plentiful and fortification helps ensure adequate intake of certain nutrients shown to be consumed at low levels.

Although classical nutrient deficiency diseases are rare, chronic diseases of aging have increased as the population has aged. In the early 1940s, scientists began to discover important links between diet and health. For example, Tannenbaum [7] found that laboratory rats that were fed calorie-restricted diets developed fewer tumors than rats that were fed ad libitum. As more studies conducted in laboratory animals confirmed Tannenbaum's early studies, the public health tool of epidemiology evolved and made other important links between diet and complex, chronic diseases of aging in human populations. As the science of nutrition and epidemiology moved forward, the law was mired in 1938. The explicit language in the FFDCA that prohibits speech about foods mitigating, preventing, curing, or treating disease is now a "Gordian knot" for the FDA and food manufacturers alike. Over 60 years ago, the definition of a drug was based on the scientific knowledge of the day; today, however, the definition restricts communication about the health benefits associated with novel nutrients found in foods.

Recognizing the need for consistency in nutrition labeling, the restrictive nature of communicating health messages, and the scientific understanding of the diet–disease relationship, Congress enacted the Nutrition Labeling and Education Act (NLEA) of 1990 [8], which mandated nutrition labeling on almost all food products and permitted the FDA to promulgate regulations that would allow food manufacturers to communicate important health messages on food labels.

The rulemaking process

The rulemaking process, like the public policy process, has multiple steps and ample opportunity to seek and receive public comment in an open and transparent way [9]. Rulemaking can begin with an advanced notice of proposed rulemaking, but this step is not required. A proposed rule is published in the *Federal Register* (www.archives.gov/Federal_register) thus setting in motion internal and external reviews of the proposed rule, requests for public comment, public hearings, and issuance of a final rule. A concluding step in rulemaking can be a legal challenge to the final rule, such as the 1999 *Pearson v Shalala* case (www.ded.uscourts.gov/cv0596.pdf).

Following the enactment of the NLEA, there was confusion about whether or not the new law and subsequent regulations also applied to dietary supplements that are technically regulated as foods. In 1994, Congress enacted the Dietary Supplement Health and Education Act (DSHEA) [10], which provided for statements of nutritional support or so-called "structure/function claims" on dietary supplements. Claims that have not been approved by the FDA must be accompanied by a disclaimer that the FDA has not evaluated the statement and that the product is not intended to diagnose, treat, cure, or prevent disease.

This 1994 statute was followed by the Food and Drug Administration Modernization Act (FDAMA) of 1997 [11] that allowed health claims in labeling based on official authoritative statements from certain federal agencies or the National Academy of Sciences (NAS). This amendment was intended to expedite the dissemination of health information on food packages by circumventing the lengthy petition process for health claims. Manufacturers must notify the FDA about the intent to use an authoritative statement, and the submission must be successful to use it. Congress did not include dietary supplements in this health claim provision, but the legal challenge brought in 1999 decided that "qualified" health claims could be made on dietary supplements only.

Although the NLEA, DSHEA, and FDAMA created some flexibility in conveying important food and health information to the public, these three legislative actions did not untangle the original knot created by the FFDCA. The original language distinguishing foods and drugs still limited the ability to effectively communicate the health benefits of foods and functional foods to consumers:

A food or dietary supplement for which a claim, subject to sections 403(r)(1)(B) and 403(r)(3) of this title or sections 403(r)(1)(B) and 403(r)(5)(D) of this title, is made in accordance with the requirements of section 403(r) of this title is not a drug solely because the label or the labeling contains such a claim. A food, dietary ingredient, or dietary supplement for which a truthful and not misleading statement is made in accordance with section 403(r)(6) of this title is not a drug under clause (C) solely because the label or the labeling contains such a statement [6].

Labeling claims

Three types of claims—nutrient content, health, and structure/function—allow food and supplement manufacturers to communicate the benefit of consuming their product.

Nutrient content claims

Nutrient content claims allow a manufacturer to state the level of a certain nutrient provided by the product or use a descriptor that has been approved by the FDA; however, these claims do not make a connection to a health benefit. Nutrient content claims may either state directly the level of the nutrient (eg, 200 mg of calcium, 100% of vitamin C) or describe the level of the nutrient using an adjective that has been defined by the FDA. Descriptors are adjectives that modify a nutrient or dietary substance and describe in broad terms the level of the nutrient, such as "high," "good," "low," or "free." For example, to claim that a product is a "good" source of vitamin E, the product must provide at least 10% of vitamin E per reference amount customarily consumed. Criteria to make comparative claims have also been defined by the FDA to reduce consumer confusion about marketing tactics. For example, a popular pet food designed for older cats may state "25% less fat" than the average product. Issues arise, however, when the substance has not been recognized by the NAS as a nutrient and therefore does not have an established dietary reference intake (DRI) or a daily value (DV) for it. Examples of nontraditional nutrients may be lycopene, omega-3 fatty acids, anthocyanins, flavonoids, and lutein.

The FDAMA also allowed nutrient content claims based on authoritative statements by a federal agency or the NAS and can be used on both foods and dietary supplements. Dietary supplements can also make percentage claims and comparative percentage claims of ingredients for which there is no established DV. Examples of this type of claim are: "20% omega-3 fatty acids" and "three times more omega-3 fatty acids per tablet than a serving of salmon."

Health claims

Health claims used on food labels must be preapproved by the FDA. These claims relate a dietary pattern or food to reducing the risk of a certain disease. The preapproval of claims is based on the totality of publicly available literature and significant scientific agreement among qualified scientific experts. Food manufacturers can submit a petition to the FDA requesting approval of a new health claim, but the petition process can be lengthy and does not provide exclusive use of the claim by the petitioner. This may discourage food and supplement manufacturers from using health claims unless the product has significant market leadership in the product category.

To date, 12 health claims have been approved by the FDA; abbreviated versions of these are shown in Box 1. In addition to the preapproval petition process authorized by the NLEA, health claims can be made as a result of an authoritative statement issued by an official body of the federal government. Two claims have been approved based on authoritative statements by federal scientific bodies. Whole-grain foods that contain 51% or more of whole-grain ingredients by weight per reference amount (RA) and that provide a certain level of dietary fiber per RA can use the following claim:

> Diets rich in whole grain foods and other plant foods and low in total fat, saturated fat, and cholesterol may reduce the risk of heart disease and some cancers.

Potassium and the risk of hypertension is the second claim that has been authorized based on an authoritative statement [12].

Until recently, only dietary supplements could make "qualified" health claims. "Qualified" health claims were allowed as a result of the 1999 decision of the US Court of Appeals for the District of Columbia in the case of *Pearson v. Shalala* and do not meet the same significant scientific agreement standard required for foods under the NLEA. In July 2003, the FDA published an interim guidance to the food and supplement industries that would allow qualified health claims on labels that do not rise to the standard of significant scientific agreement [13]. The guidance made clear an evidence-based ranking system against which scientific data could be judged. It also laid out a "grading" system (levels B, C, or D) that would designate the relative strength of the scientific evidence and the language of the qualified health claim (Table 1). The agency will evaluate the success of the new system in 2004.

Structure/function claims

Structure/function claims do not require preapproval and can be used by foods and dietary supplements. These claims do not draw a link to disease but to a structure or function in the body. The distinction between health and structure/function claims is subtle, and there are no data to show that the public can distinguish between the two types of claims. For example, a calcium-rich food may note that calcium helps maintain bone health or builds strong bones, rather than reduces the risk of osteoporosis.

Box 1. Abbreviated FDA-approved health claims

21 CFR 101.72: Calcium may help reduce the risk of osteoporosis in petite, white and Asian women.
21 CFR 101.73: Diets low in fat may help reduce the risk of some cancers.
21 CFR 101.74: Diets low in sodium may help reduce the risk of hypertension.
21 CFR 101.75: Diets low in saturated fat and cholesterol may help reduce the risk of heart disease.
21 CFR 101.76: Low-fat diets rich in fiber-containing grain products, fruits, and vegetables may reduce the risk of some forms of cancer.
21 CFR 101.77: Diets low in saturated fat and cholesterol and rich in fruits, vegetables, and grain products, particularly those in soluble fiber may reduce the risk of heart disease.
21 CFR 101.78: Low fat diets rich in fruits and vegetables may reduce the risk of some cancers.
21 CFR 101.79: Folic acid may help reduce the risk of having a baby with certain birth defects of the spinal cord and brain.
21 CFR 101.80: Sugar alcohols do not promote dental caries.
21 CFR 101.81: Soluble fiber from oats or psyllium may help reduce the risk of heart disease.
21 CFR 101.82: Diets low in saturated fat and cholesterol and providing 25 grams of soy protein may help the risk of heart disease.
21 CFR 101.83: Stanol and sterol esters may help reduce the risk of heart disease.

Data from US Food and Drug Administration, Center for Food Safety and Applied Nutrition. A food labeling guide. September 1994 [editorial revisions: June 1999 and November 2000]. Available at: http://www.cfsan.fda.gov/~dms/flg-6c.html. Accessed November 11, 2003.

Whether a product is categorized as a food or a drug depends on its intended use in the marketplace, but the intended use may be determined by the information provided on the package label or other labeling associated with the product. Hence, placing a health message on a label can lead to circular arguments about whether the product is a food, supplement, or drug. Issues remain surrounding the convoluted system of health and structure/function claims that seems inconsistent when applied to foods and dietary supplements. For example, the regulatory scheme has created a "catch-22" for cranberry juice cocktail. A health claim that cranberry juice

Table 1
FDA guidance on levels of qualified health claims

Scientific ranking	FDA category	Appropriate qualifying language
Second level	B	"…although there is scientific evidence supporting the claim, the evidence is not conclusive."
Third level	C	"Some scientific evidence suggests [insert claim language] …however, the FDA has determined that this evidence is limited and not conclusive."
Fourth level	D	"Very limited and preliminary scientific research suggests [insert claim language] … the FDA concludes that there is little scientific evidence supporting this claim."

Adapted from US Food and Drug Administration, Center for Food Safety and Applied Nutrition. Consumer health information for better nutrition initiative, July 10, 2003, task force final report. http://www.cfsan.fda.gov/~dms/nuttftoc.html#oview. Accessed August 7, 2002.

cocktail helps prevent the recurrence of urinary tract infections would place the food in the drug category, regardless of its intended use as a beverage.

On the other hand, a structure/function claim for the beverage ("cranberry juice cocktail helps maintain urinary tract health") requires that the benefit be derived from the "nutritive value" of the product. Research shows that phytonutrients, such as anthocyanins—not "classical" nutrients—appear to be the agents that reduce bacterial adhesion to the walls of the urinary tract. The active effect of these phytonutrients on the bacteria mitigates reoccurrence of infection. Because the effect is not derived from the nutritive value in the classical sense, the product falls within the definition of a drug, regardless of whether or not the claim is truthful and is not misleading.

Food–drug continuum

As noted previously, functional foods are not a separate regulatory category, but can be thought of as lying along a food-drug continuum, as shown in Fig. 1. This continuum draws upon several characteristics that categorize each broad class of substances; however, there is significant overlap across the food and supplement groupings.

Conventional foods naturally provide nutrients, many of which are capable of preventing and treating classical deficiency diseases. For example, citrus fruits are an excellent source of vitamin C, a phytonutrient that prevents and treats scurvy. Other food categories that are not discussed in detail in this article are foods for special dietary use (FSDUs) and medical foods. FSDUs typically provide nutrients for certain physiological

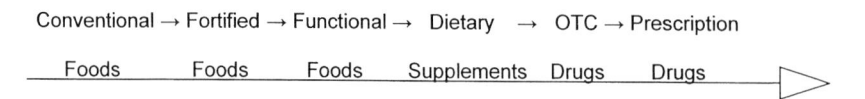

Conventional → Fortified → Functional → Dietary → OTC → Prescription
Foods   Foods   Foods   Supplements   Drugs   Drugs

Fig. 1. Conceptual framework for a food–drug continuum.

conditions, such as pregnancy. Medical foods are designed for people who have specific nutritional requirements and are administered under the supervision of a physician.

Enriched and fortified foods are those that have had nutrients added back to their original levels (enriched foods) or at levels higher than the original (fortified foods). Breakfast cereals are examples of fortified foods that provide several nutrients that have been added through fortification. Some of the fortifying nutrients may not be found naturally in a grain product (eg, vitamin C).

Functional foods have been defined as those providing health benefits beyond basic nutrition [14]. This is not a regulatory definition, however [15]. The NAS Institute of Medicine has defined functional foods as foods "in which concentrations of one or more ingredients have been manipulated to enhance their contributions to a healthful diet" [16]. The "health benefits beyond basic nutrition" implies that the functional foods are not directly intended to mitigate or prevent classical deficiency diseases; rather, the benefits extend to mitigating the risk of chronic diseases of aging, which are multifactorial in nature. The term *nutraceutical* can be thought of as a micronutrient that is associated with reducing the risk of chronic disease and ranges from plant- to animal-derived substances. These substances are sometimes referred to as *phytonutrients* or *zoonutrients*, respectively. For example, lycopene—a carotenoid found naturally in tomatoes and watermelon—is a phytonutrient associated with reduced risk of prostate cancer. Omega-3 fatty acids from fatty fish and conjugated linoleic acid in foods made from ruminants are zoonutrients that have been linked to reduced risk of coronary heart disease and cancer. These substances are not considered to be nutrients in the classical sense and have not been officially recognized by the NAS.

Nutraceuticals raise significant safety issues, especially when isolation and extraction of these novel nutrients are concentrated into products that make overdosing easier (eg, dietary supplements in the form of pills, tablets, or capsules). There is greater potential for abuse of intake because there is no self-regulatory mechanism (eg, feeling full) that allows for an intake check. Dietary supplements range from single nutrients to multivitamins and minerals and are typically delivered in concentrated dosages through pills, capsules, tablets, or some food forms (eg, teas); hence the similarities to the delivery mechanisms of many drugs. The DSHEA defines dietary supplements as vitamins, minerals, herbs or other botanicals, amino acids, and other dietary substances that increase the dietary intake. It would appear that safety considerations of dietary supplements hinge on whether or not the FDA can show the product has been adulterated in some way.

Summary

It is clear that the prospects of functional foods and nutraceuticals already excite the scientific community into discovering new substances that promise to extend healthy life. The greatest challenge will remain in the public policy and regulatory arenas, which will encourage research and development of products providing health benefits and permit marketing of products in truthful, nonmisleading communications while protecting public health and maintaining public confidence.

References

[1] Boyle MA, Morris DH. The art and science of policy making. In: Community nutrition in action: an entrepreneurial approach. 2nd edition. Belmont (CA): Wadsworth Publishing Company; 1999. p. 34–71.
[2] Sparrow MK. The regulatory craft—controlling risks, solving problems, and managing compliance. Washington, DC: Brookings Institution Press; 2000.
[3] Federal Meat Inspection Act, as amended. Public law 59–242. 1907.
[4] Poultry Products Inspection Act. Public law 85–172. 1957.
[5] Egg Products Act, as amended. Public law 91–597. 1970.
[6] Federal Food, Drug, and Cosmetic Act. Public law 75–717. 1938.
[7] Tannenbaum A. The dependence of tumor formation on the degree of caloric restriction. Cancer Res 1945;5:609–15.
[8] Nutrition Labeling and Education Act. Public law 101–535. 1990.
[9] Kerwin CM. 1999. Rulemaking: how government agencies write law and make policy. 2nd edition. Washington, DC: CQ Press (a division of Congressional Quarterly, Inc.); 1999. p. 75–7.
[10] Dietary Supplement Health and Education Act. Public law 103–417. 1994.
[11] Food and Drug Administration Modernization Act. Public law 105–115. 1997.
[12] US Food and Drug Administration, Center for Food Safety and Applied Nutrition. A food labeling guide. September 1994 [editorial revisions: June 1999 and November 2000]. Available at: http://www.cfsan.fda.gov/~dms/flg-6c.html. Accessed November 11, 2003.
[13] US Food and Drug Administration, Center for Food Safety and Applied Nutrition. Consumer health information for better nutrition initiative, July 10, 2003, task force final report. http://www.cfsan.fda.gov/~dms/nuttftoc.html#oview. Accessed August 7, 2002.
[14] International Food Information Council. Food safety and nutrition information. Available at: http://ific.org/glossary/#Fpolicy.net/proactive/newsroom/release.vtml. Accessed August 7, 2002.
[15] Ross S. Functional foods: the Food and Drug Administration perspective. Am J Clin Nutr 2000;71:1735S–8S.
[16] Glinsmann WH. Functional foods in North America. Nutr Rev 1996;54:S33–7.

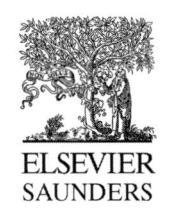

Cellular effects of common nutraceuticals and natural food substances

Lester Mandelker, DVM[a],*, Susan Wynn, DVM[b]

[a]*Community Veterinary Hospital, 1631 W. Bay Drive, Largo, FL 33770, USA*
[b]*334 Knollwood Lane, Woodstock, GA 30188, USA*

Disclaimer

The following information consists of proposed cellular effects regarding the use of certain nutraceuticals (including antioxidants, phytonutrients, and other biological therapies) and herbs. The information was gathered from scientific sources and experimental research. Much of the information is considered controversial and is intended for educational and scientific usage. Some of the volume of references for the proposed cellular mechanisms can be found elsewhere in this issue, while others can be supplied by special request from the authors. It is suggested that practitioners use their best available judgment and sound reasoning when applying these supplements in clinical situations.

---

* Corresponding author.
E-mail address: lestervet2@aol.com (L. Mandelker).

Common name	Represented chemicals	Proposed mechanism of action	Proposed cellular effects	Traditional and potential uses	Adverse effects	Dose
Algae (spirulina)	Phycocyanin, allophycocyanin, amino acids, vitamins, minerals	Antioxidant; may enhance immune function	May inhibit COX-2 enzymes; may reverse DNA damage from peroxynitrite	Food supplement, anticancer and antiviral effects	May be cyagenic at high doses	Proportional to human dose
Alpha lipoic acid	Dihydrolipoic acid (DL-alpha-lipoic acid)	Antioxidant, anti-inflammatory effects, metal chelator; potentiates levels of vitamin C and vitamin E; reduces oxidative stress	Modulates apoptosis; modulates NF-κB activation; increases cellular glutathione levels and improves cellular redox state	Antioxidant, diabetic neuropathy, ischemia-reprofusion injury	Adverse effects may be seen in cats at 30 mg	1–5 mg/kg/d in dogs; unpublished data suggest that supplementing >30 mg/d in cats may not be safe
Arginine	L-arginine	Immune stimulant; reduces cancer growth, assists in urea cycle regulation; may assist protein metabolic waste, vascular regulation, immune system function, and neurotransmission	Helps regulate inflammation through nitric oxide; precursor for urea, creatine, creatinine and nitric oxide; may reduce adhesion molecules	Cancer, diabetes, hepatic encepahalopathy, hepatic lipidosis	None reported	500–3000 mg/d
Androstenedione	4-androstene-3, 17 dione	Adrenal androgen	Modulates IL-6	Increase energy, enhance muscle mass	Liver damage, hormone imbalance	Proportional to human dose

Bioflavonoids	Quercetin, polyphenols, rutin, anthocyanidins, proanthocyanidins, pycnogenol, reservatrol	Antioxidant; anti-inflammatory, antimicrobial, hepatoprotective, antithrombotic, antiviral, and anticancer effects	Modulate apoptosis; may inhibit transcription of NF-κB; may inhibit leukotriene synthesis; may reduce adhesion molecules; promote endothelial nitric oxide synthase; may enhance GJIC; may improve RNA synthesis; some bind estrogen receptors	Capillary integrity, retinopathy, lymph edema; allergies, cancer, anti-aging; improve wound healing	None	Proportional to human dose
Branched chain amino acids	Isoleucine, leucine, valine	Promotes protein synthesis; modifies cytokine production	May modulate Th1 immune response; modulate mRNA protein synthesis	Hepatic encephalopathy, performance enhancers	Unknown	Proportional to human dose; adults normally take 1–5 g/d
Borage oil	Gamma linolenic acid	May reduce inflammation; may regulate eicosanoid production; may modulate tumor cell chemosensitivity	Precursor to PGE1; inhibits conversion of arachondic acid to eukotrienes	Skin disease, immune-mediated arthritis, allergies, asthma, cancer	None reported	Proportional to human dose

(continued on next page)

Table (continued)

Common name	Represented chemicals	Proposed mechanism of action	Proposed cellular effects	Traditional and potential uses	Adverse effects	Dose
Carnitine	L-carnitine	Immune modulator; essential for mitochondrial energy production and vitamin C–dependant synthesis; essential factor in fatty acid metabolism; influences CNS neurotransmitters	May improve lymphocyte proliferative responsiveness to mitogens; may improve mitochondrial oxidation; transports fatty acids into nerve cells; stimulates acetylcholine formation	Heart disease, hepatic lipidosis, wight loss, athletic performance, hepatopathy of American cocker spaniels, senile dementia, neurotoxicity; increases bone density	Unknown	20–150 mg/kg tid
Carnosine	L-carnosine	Antioxidant, free radical and metal ion scavenger	Substrate for nitric oxide synthase; may reduce glycation of proteins	Anti-aging	None reported	Proportional to human dose
Chondroitin	Chondroitin sulfate	May inhibit proteoglycan degradation	Inhibition of aggrecanase activity	Osteoarthritis; may lower cholesterol	Unknown; loss of glycemic control reported in humans for another glycosaminoglycan, glucosamine; animals rarely exhibit diarrhea and nausea	Label dose on veterinary products; proportional to human dose on human products

Coenzyme Q10	Ubiquinone	Antioxidant; supports energy metabolism; catalyst in ATP production	Intracellular oxidation–reduction reactions	Heart disease, cardiomyopathy, hypertension	Rare	2–20 mg/kg/d
Chromium	Chromium	May increase insulin sensitivity; essential component of glucose tolerance factor	Alters mitochondria respiration/oxidation; may lead to cellular NADH depletion	Diabetes mellitus, weight loss; studies in dogs and cats have not been encouraging	Chromium piconilate may be carcinogenic	50–300 µg/d
Creatine	Creatine monohydrate	Supplies phosphocreatine; is the ready energy source for muscle function; may promote protein muscle synthesis	Modulates creatine mitochondrial transport	May enhance athletic performance; may ameliorate progress of neuromuscular diseases; may improve geriatric muscle wasting	Unknown	Label dose on veterinary products
Carotenoids	Alpha-carotene, lutein, lycopene, zeaxanathin, crytpxanthin, beta carotene, and hundreds of others	Antioxidant, immune stimulant	May stimulate NK cells; may reduce DNA damage; may inhibit oxidant-induced cytokine production.; up-regulate connexin genes and may improve GJIC	Cancer prevention, retinal disorders	None	Proportional to human dose
Cetyl myristolate	Cetyl alcohol and myristoleic acid	Anti-arthritic	May modulate immune function	Arthritis, tissue lubricant	Unknown	250–2000 mg/d

(continued on next page)

Table (continued)

Common name	Represented chemicals	Proposed mechanism of action	Proposed cellular effects	Traditional and potential uses	Adverse effects	Dose
Choline	Choline chloride, phosphatidyl choline (lecithin)	Promotes lipid transport; is a structural component of biologic membranes, neurotransmitters, and transmethylation reactions	Precursor to acetylcholine	Heart disease, fatigue, senility, performance enhancer	None	Proportional to human dose
DHA (from fish oil)	Docosahexaenoic acid	Immune modulator, omega-3 fatty acid with anti-inflammatory properties; modulates prostaglandin synthesis	Modulates cell membrane synthesis and mitochondrial membrane phospholipids; may facilitate apoptosis	Cancer, immune-mediated disease	Unknown	~60 mg/kg/d (d/d) or proportional to human dose
DHEA	Dehydroepiandrosterone	Immune modulator, precursor to sex hormones; modulates plasma membrane proteins; cytoprotective of cells	May stimulate Th2 response; may modulate NF-κB activation; modulates GABA activity	Lupus, anti-aging, hypercholesterolemia, mood elevator, obesity	May cause liver abnormalities	5–25 mg/d
DMSO, MSM	Dimethyl sulfoxide (DMSO); mehtylsulfonylmethane (MSM)	Anti-inflammatory hydroxyl radical scavengers, natural solvent	May reduce cell membrane injury; promote GJIC	Arthritis, inflammation, interstitial cystitis, spinal cord injury	Garlic odor (DMSO)	250–1000 mg (MSM)

DMG	N, N, dimethylglycine (pangamic acid)	Antioxidant; may improve oxygen use and promote liver detoxification; may enhance immune function	May modulate homocysteine metabolism (via methionine pump); may enhance both humoral and cell-mediated immune responses; may reduce lactic acid during exercise	Athletic endurance, circulatory stimulant, hyperlipidemias, metabolic enhancer	Unknown	1–3 mg/kg; doses of 50–400 mg/d have been recommended
DMAE	Dimethyl-aminoethanol	Intermediate phospholipid metabolite; may enhance insulin activity	May stimulate DNA synthesis in fibroblasts	Anti-aging, stimulates fibrous tissue	Unknown	Proportional to human dose; rarely used clinically
EPA	Eicoapentaenoic acid	Omega-3 fatty acid with anti-inflammatory activity; modulates immune functions; modulates eicosanoid production; may reduce cancer cachexia	May alter cell membrane phospholipids; down-regulates NF-κB; may reduce CD4/CD8 lymphocyte ratio; may induce apoptosis in cancer cells; may inhibit lipoxygenase; may reduce TNF-α synthesis and IL-2 production	Arthritis, cancer, immune modulator, cardiovascular disease, kidney disease	May reduce blood clotting	60 mg/kg

(continued on next page)

Table (continued)

Common name	Represented chemicals	Proposed mechanism of action	Proposed cellular effects	Traditional and potential uses	Adverse effects	Dose
Enzymes (proteolytic)	Trypsin, chymotrypsin, bromelain, papain	Immune modulator; may exert antiedematous, anti-inflammatory, antithrombotic, and fibrinolytic activities	May modulate T cell response by inhibiting T cell signal transduction; may alter leukocyte migration and activation	Arthritis, digestive aid, musculoskeletal trauma, chronic inflammatory diseases; possibly long-term prevention of pancreatitis	May cause some gastritis, dose-related oral bleeding	Follow label on veterinary products; proportional to human dose
5-HTP	5-hydroxytryptophan	Precursor to serotonin	Serotonergic–endocrine interrelations	Depression, sleep disorders, behavioral disorders	Neurologic signs including seizures and blindness; GI signs, hyperthermia, and death have been reported in dogs receiving doses as low as 2.5 mg/kg (human dose is ~0.7–1.5 mg/kg tid)	Not recommended
Fructooligosaccarides	Fructooligosaccarides	Immunosuppression; helps maintain healthy GI tract	Supports growth of *Bifidobacterium* and *Lactobacillus* sp in GI tract	Weight gain, GI disturbances, intestinal bacterial overgrowth, chronic diarrhea	None	Follow label on veterinary products; proportional to human dose

Glutamine	L-glutamine	Preferred fuel for enterocytes; may enhance cellular immunity, modulate tumor cell metabolism, and improve clinical outcome in stress situations	May stimulate DNA synthesis; essential donor for nucleotide precursor synthesis; may modulate inflammatory activities of IL-8 and TNF-α; precursor to GABA and L-glutamic acid	GI supplement for bowel disease; conditionally essential in chronic debilitating illness	None	500 mg/kg divided daily
GAGs and precursors	Glucosamine Hcl, glucosamine sulfate, chondroitin sulfate	Building block of cartilage (GAGs); modify joint damage; may stimulate synthesis of proteoglycans in vascular endothelium and bladder mucosa	May inhibit degradative enzymes; may inhibit nitric oxide activity; may modulate cytokine activity	Osteoarthritis, rheumatoid arthritis, wound healing, feline lower tract disease	May increase bleeding and partial thromboplastin time; studies done on one brand (Cosequin) show no hematologic adverse events	Veterinary forms labeled for arthritis; proportional to human dose
Glutathione (reduced form)	L-glutathione	Primary intracellular antioxidant; primary agent for detoxifcation of drugs; reduces oxidative stress	Modulates apoptosis; primes DNA synthesis	Anti-aging, immune enhancer, liver disease	Unknown	Dose proportional to human dose; absorption is questionable when dosed orally
Lactoferrin	Siderophillin	Anti-inflammatory, antiviral effects; may enhance immune function	Enhances phagocytic activity; regulates iron activity	Feline stomatitis, immune disorders	Unknown	40 mg/kg topically (mixed in milk, syrup, or food slurry)

(continued on next page)

Table (continued)

Common name	Represented chemicals	Proposed mechanism of action	Proposed cellular effects	Traditional and potential uses	Adverse effects	Dose
Lysine	L-lysine	Assists production of antibodies, hormones and enzymes; reduces blood arginine levels (which is essential for suppressing reactivation of herpesvirus)	May suppress herpes viral replication; precursor to L-carnitine	Herpes infections	Unknown	250–500 mg bid in food
Melatonin	Melatonin	Antioxidant; may enhance T (helper) cell response to antigen; regulates circadian cycles; may up-regulate cell lineage specific stem cell activity	May protect DNA and cellular membranes from oxidative stress; may stimulate IL-2 release by T helper cells and lymphocytes	Insomnia, anticancer effects, alopecia in certain breeds; regulates circadian rhythm; may be used for episodes of thunder-phobia	Mild hypothermia may suppress male infertility; may increase adverse lung effects in asthmatics	0.3–5 mg total, depending on animal size; 6 mg tid for alopecia in boxers
Methionine	DL-methionine	Antioxidant, source of sulfur; essential for energy production and muscle building	Component of glutathione redox system; precursor to S-adenosyl-methionine	Controversial use in liver support	High doses may increase iron levels, cause pancreatic damage, or induce neurological change	Human dose is 800–1000 mg/d
NAC	N-acetyl-L-cysteine	Increases glutathione levels; radical oxygen scavenger	Modulates apoptosis; may inhibit TNF-α and stress-mediated NF-κB activation	Neurodegenerative conditions, bronchitis, liver toxicity, acetaminophen toxicity.	Unknown	25 mg/kg tid

Phenylalanine	L-phenylalanine, DL-phenylalanine combo	Precursor to L-dopa, norepinephrine, epinephrine	Inhibits decarboxylation of endogenous opioids	anti-aging, antioxidant, topically for corneal ulcers Analgesic effects, depression; may enhance acupuncture	Unknown	125–500 mg bid/tid; maintain at lowest effective dose after loading
Phospholipids	Phosphatidylserine, phosphatidyl choline, phosphatidyl inositol phosphatidylethanolamine	Essential components of cell membranes, regulates CNS neurotransmitters	Membrane phospholipid that facilitates signal transduction; may reduce liver damage from toxins; may reduce fibrogenesis, alter lipoproteins, and reduce hyperlipidemias in humans	Cognitive dysfunction, mood enhancer, depression	None reported	25–100 mg/kg bid
Pregnenolone	Pregnenolone	Steroid hormone	Precursor to DHEA and sex hormones (estrogen, testosterone, and progesterone)	Mood enhancer, improved CNS function, chronic fatigue, autoimmune diseases, antistress	Mood swings, insomnia, anxiety, hormonal changes	Unknown (rarely used)

(continued on next page)

Table (continued)

Common name	Represented chemicals	Proposed mechanism of action	Proposed cellular effects	Traditional and potential uses	Adverse effects	Dose
SAM-e	S-adenosyl-methionine	Improves hepatic function; increases bile flow; aids liver detoxification enzyme activity; increases cellular glutathione levels	Involved in three major biochemical pathways (trans-methylation, transsulfuration, and ainopropylation); up-regulates genes for proteoglycan synthesis; may facilitate DNA production and brain neurotransmitters	Anti-aging; liver damage, osteoarthritis, and depression in humans	Very high levels are hepatoxic	18–20 mg/kg/d
Selenium	Sodium selenite, sodium selenate	Antioxidant; modulates thyroid homone; synergy with vitamin E; binds to some toxins	Component of glutathione perioxidase; inhibits oxidation of lipids; scavenges free radicals and protects cellular DNA; hepatic microsomal oxidation and detoxification	Muscular diseases; may help prevent cancer in humans; useful in managing pancreatitis in dogs	High levels are toxic; lethal dose in dogs is 2 mg/kg	5–50 µg/d; 0.3 mg/kg sodium selenite intravenously for acute pancreatitis

SOD	Superoxide dismutase	Endogenous antioxidant enzyme; neutralizes superoxide radicals	Protects mitochondrial membranes from oxidation	Osteoarthritis, heart disease	Unknown	5–20 IU/kg; not well explored yet
Taurine	L-taurine	Regulates heart rhythm; reduces ischemic damage; improves endogenous and exogenous antioxidant defense; modulates CNS activity (osmoregulation, neuroprotection, and neuromodulation)	Modulates intracellular calcium levels; maintains cell membrane stability; vital for the proper use of sodium potassium and calcium; bile acid conjugation	Congestive heart failure, diabetes, liver disease; hypertension, anxiety, CNS disturbances, dilated cardiomyopathy of cats and cocker spaniels	None	250–500 mg bid
Transfer factor	Dialyzable leukocyte extract	Improves cell mediated immune function, modulates immune function	Stimulates activity of NK cells	Cancer, chronic immune-mediated disease	None reported	Should be distinguished from commercial nutraceutical combination products with the same name

(continued on next page)

Table (continued)

Common name	Represented chemicals	Proposed mechanism of action	Proposed cellular effects	Traditional and potential uses	Adverse effects	Dose
Vanadium, vanadyl sulfate	Vanadium	Enhances insulin sensitivity, vital for cellular metabolism, necessary for bone and teeth formation	Modulates glucose-6-phosphatase activity; postinsulin receptor glucose metabolism activator; may activate NF-κB (proinflammatory actions)	Diabetes	High levels can be nephrotoxic and carcinogenic	Vanadium 0.2 mg/kg qd or vanadyl sulfate 1 mg/kg qd
Vitamin C	Ascorbic acid, sodium ascorbate, magnesium ascorbate, esterified ascorbate, and so forth	Antioxidant, pro-oxidant under certain circumstances, aids synthesis of collagen, catecholamines, steroids, carnitine, iron absorption, and improves immune function, antihistamine activity	Reduces TNF-α–induced activation of NF-κB; may modulate apoptosis; may protect DNA via reduction of reactive oxygen species; may reduce oxidation of LDLs; may improve endothelial GJIC	Allergies, chronic inflammation, immune function, macular degeneration, cataracts, cancer prevention; may reduce effectiveness of chemotherapeutic agents	Increases oxalate crystalluria; may interfere with activity of glycosides in urine; depleted by tetracyclines salicylates	50 mg/kg, up to 1000 mg/d in large dogs; doses of 3–5 g/d have been used without adverse effect in large dogs

Vitamin E	D-alpha tocopherol (active form), DL-alpha tocopherol, mixed tocopherrols, tocotrienols	Antioxidant, neuropro-tective and antiatherogenic effects; suppresses lipid peroxidation; modulates synthesis of coenzyme A and ATP; modulates immune response; improves oxygen use	Fat soluble membrane stabilizer; modulates apoptosis; modulates growth factors; may decrease androgen concentrations; may decrease LDL oxidation; may reduce adhesion molecules; may decrease transcription factor NF-κ B	Cancer prevention, cholestatic liver disease, cardiovascular disease, diabetes, inflammatory disorders, immune function enhancement, senility	Rare; potential effects of anticoagulants and digoxin	10–20 IU/kg, up to 800 IU/d for large dogs
Zinc	Zinc gluconate zinc sulfate, zinc methionine	Antioxidant, enzyme system factor; stabilizes cell membranes; aids protein synthesis; component of SOD; enhances immune function and wound repair	Oxygen scavenger through induction of metallothionein, zinc-dependent transcription factor; modulates apoptosis NF-κ B; modulates genetic expression of cytokines (IL-2); modulates T cell function and ratio	Zinc responsive dermatitis, immunity, wound repair, skin disorders, viral infections, mental health, Wilson's disease (binds copper), sexual maturation	High doses can cause gastritis, hemolytic anemia, icterus, hypotension	Zinc methionine, 4 mg/kg/d po; zinc sulfate, 10 mg/kg/d po; zinc gluconate, 5 mg/kg/d po

Abbreviations: DHA, docosahexaenoic acid; DHEA, dehydroepiandrosterone; DMAE, dimethylaminoethanol; DMG, dimethylglycine; DMSO, dimethyl sulfoxide; EPA, eicoapentaenoic acid; GABA, gamma-aminobutyric acid; GAGs, glycoaminoglycans; GJIC, gap junctional intercellular communication; HTP, hydroytryptophan; IL, interleukin; LDL, low-density lipoprotein; MSM, methylsulfonylmethane; NAC, N-acetylcysteine; NF, necrosis factor; SAM, S-adenosylmethionine; SOD, superoxide dismutase; TNF, tumor necrosis factor.

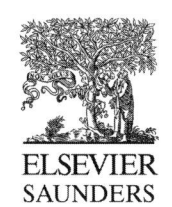

Cellular effects of various herbs and botanicals

Lester Mandelker, DVM[a,]*,
Susan Wynn, DVM[b]

[a]*Community Veterinary Hospital, 1631 W. Bay Drive, Largo, FL 33770, USA*
[b]*334 Knollwood Lane, Woodstock, GA 30188, USA*

Disclaimer

The following information consists of proposed cellular effects regarding the use of certain nutraceuticals (including antioxidants, phytonutrients, and other biologic therapies) and herbs. The information was gathered from scientific sources and experimental research. Much of the information is considered controversial and is intended for educational and scientific usage. Some of the volume of references for the proposed cellular mechanisms can be found elsewhere in this issue, while others can be supplied by special request from the authors. It is suggested that practitioners use their best available judgment and sound reasoning when applying these supplements in clinical situations.

---

* Corresponding author.
E-mail address: lestervet2@aol.com (L. Mandelker).

Common name	Selected ingredients	Proposed mechanism of action	Proposed cellular effects	Traditional and potential uses	Adverse effects	Suggested dose
Aloe vera (Aloe barbadensis)	Polysaccharides, resins, tannins, anthraquinones, L-glutamine, glucosamine	Immune stimulant, anti-inflammatory effects	Stimulates macrophage activity; may inhibit collagenase, cyclo-oxygenase, and metalloproteinase	Wound healing; some practitioners use for inflammatory bowel diseases	Acemannan (aloe vera extract) had no adverse effects topically up to 1500 mg/kg; purgative when some forms are used orally	Follow labeled dose
Ashwagandha (Withania somnifera)	Alkaloids, steroidal lactones, amino acids	Anti-inflammatory, immune-modulating, nootropic-like effects, antistress	May up-regulate hemopoetic cells; may enhance gamma interferon levels and IL-2 and colony-stimulating factors	Adaptogenic ("Indian ginseng"), tonic, sedative, chronic inflammatory conditions, chronic illness	None described	Proportional to human dose
Astragalus (Astragalus membranaceous)	Astragalosides, sterols, flavonoids, minerals	Immunostimulant antiviral effects; may promote TNF-α secretion	May replenish glutathione levels in liver; may modulate T cells; may stimulate B cells and antibody production	Tonic, immune deficiency, cancer support, chronic debility	None known	Proportional to human dose
Bilberry (Vaccinium myrtilis)	Anthocyanins, flavonoids, catechins, rannins, various minerals, B vitamins	Antioxidant, diuretic	Anti-angiogenic, free radical scavenger; may induce apoptosis in cancer cells	Vasculopathy, retinopathy	None	Proportional to human dose

Black walnut (*Juglans nigra*)	Naphthaquinones	Bowel stimulant, antiparasitic effects	May increase GI motility	Laxative; often recommended for deworming and heartworm prevention by lay people	Black walnut toxicosis (horses and dogs)	Proportional to human dose
Boswellia (*Boswellia serrata*)	Boswellic acids	Anti-inflammatory and anti-arthritic effects	May inhibit leukotriene synthesis; may reduce chemotaxis of inflammatory cells; may reduce carcinogenesis	Musculoskeletal pain, arthritis, asthma, colitis, inflammatory bowel disease	GI upset; caution with concurrent nonsteroidal anti-inflammatory drug usage	Proportional to human dose
Calendula (*Calendula officinalis*)	Triterpenes, flavonoids, glycosides, resins	Anti-inflammatory effects	Radical scavenger; may stimulate epithelialization	Astringent, wound care	Focal skin irritation	Use topically
Catnip (*Nepeta cataria*)	Tannins, volatile oils, various phytochemicals	Anti-anxiety, CNS stimulant, antispasmadic antioxidant, immune stimulant	May promote neutrophil chemotaxis; may lower seizure threshold	Aid in behavior modification; traditional for mild gastritis, flatulence	Adverse CNS stimulation with ingestion; can be toxic at high doses	Occasional use topically to obtain desired effects; a distraction (eg, toys, treats) is recommended when administrating

(continued on next page)

Table (continued)

Common name	Selected ingredients	Proposed mechanism of action	Proposed cellular effects	Traditional and potential uses	Adverse effects	Suggested dose
Cat's claw (*Uncaria tomentosa*)	Unique alkaloids, tannins, polyphenols, catechins, beta-sitosterol.	Anti-inflammatory and antimicrobial effects, immune modulator	May enhance T cell and B cell function; may reduce activation of NF-κB; may modulate TNF-α synthesis	Often used for cancer, viral infections, and gastroenteritis	Avoid in pregnancy	Proportional to human dose
Chamomile (*Matricaria recutita, Matricaria chamomilla*)	Flavonoids, including apigenin, various phytochemicals	Antioxidant, anti-inflammatory effects, anxiolytic and spasmolytic effects	May inhibit transcriptional activation of COX-2; may down-regulate adhesion molecules	Skin irritation, stomatitis, gastritis, anxiety, insomnia, appetite stimulant	Allergic reactions; reported to cause coagulopathy, including epistaxis in cats	Proportional to human dose
Cranberry (*Vaccine macrocarpon*)	Proanthocyanidins, carotenes, various phytochemicals	Antioxidant; may reduce oxidation of low-density lipoprotein	Bacterial anti-adhesion activity; may reduce soluble adhesion molecules	Urinary tract infections	None reported	Proportional to human dose
Dandelion (*Taraxacum officinale*)	Sesquiterpene lactones, flavonoid glycosides, triterpenes, various vitamins and minerals	Diuretic, antioxidant, mild cholagogue	May modulate TNF-α production	Liver tonic; aids digestion and promotes diuresis	Contact dermatitis, allergic reactions	Proportional to human dose

Herb	Constituents	Actions	Indications	Adverse effects	Dosage
Devil's claw (*Harpophogytum procumbens*)	Iridoid glycosides, flavonoids, phytosterols	Negative chronotropic and positive inotropic effects, analgesic, anti-inflammatory effects, GI stimulant	May down-regulate TNF-α	Arthritis, GI tonic	Contraindicated where GI ulcers are present	Proportional to human dose
Echinacea (*Echinacea purpurea*, *Echinacea angustifolia*)	Alkamides, caffeic acid, polysaccharides, volatile oils	Nonspecific immune stimulant, antimicrobial effects	May stimulate T cells; may increase phagocytic activity of macrophages	Chronic infections, bacterial infections	Rare leukopenia associated with long-term use; potential for allergic reactions; may be contra-indicated in patients with autoimmune disease	Proportional to human dose
Eleutherococcus (*Eleutherococcus senticosus*), "Siberian ginseng"	Eleutherosides, polysaccharides, triterpenoid saponins, lignans	Antiviral effects, anti-allergy effects; may modulate immune function	May enhance T cell synthesis, cytotoxic and NK cells; may inhibit RNA viruses; may modulate cytokine synthesis	General tonic/adaptogen, chronic illness, physical endurance, mental acuity, chronic allergies	Rare	Proportional to human dose
Ephedra (*Ephedra sinica*), "Ma Huang"	Protoalkaloids (ephedrine, pseudoephedrine), tannins, saponins, flavone	Sympathomimetic agent and bronchodilator	Pressor and hyperglycemic effects	Stimulant, asthma	Cardiac arrythmias, hypertension, seizures; may cause idiosyncratic reactions in cats	Should be used in formulas only under guidance of a trained erbalist

(*continued on next page*)

Table (continued)

Common name	Selected ingredients	Proposed mechanism of action	Proposed cellular effects	Traditional and potential uses	Adverse effects	Suggested dose
Garlic (*Allium sativum*)	Volatile oils (allicin, diallyl sulfide), vitamins/trace minerals	Antioxidant, antimicrobial effects, antithrombotic effects; reduces cholesterol synthesis	May enhance fibrinolytic activity and inhibit platelet aggregation; decreases the activity of HMG-CoA reductase (cholesterol synthesis); may modulate leukocyte cell proliferation and cytokine production	Cancer prevention and treatment, blood lipid reduction, cardio-vascular disease, chronic infections	High doses cause Heinz body formation; anticoagulant effects at higher doses	Proportional to human dose
Ginger (*Zingiber officinale*)	Volatile oils (zingiberene, gingerols), carotenes, caffeic acid, vitamins, minerals	Antioxidant, anti-emetic, antispasmadic, anti-arthritic	May inhibit eicosanoid biosynthesis; may induce apoptosis in certain cancers	Motion sickness, nausea, arthritis.	May increase bleeding times	Proportional to human dose

Ginkgo (*Ginkgo biloba*)	Flavonoids, catechins, glycosides, terpene lactones	Antioxidant, neuroprotective, anticoagulant effects, antistress effects	Anti-apoptotic effects in CNS, free radical scavenger; modulates corticosteroid synthesis and expression; inhibits monoamine oxidase; may antagonize platelet activating factor	Dementia, cardiovascular disease, asthma	May increase bleeding times	Proportional to human dose
Goldenseal (*Hydrastis Canadensis*)	Isoquinoline alkaloids (berberine, hydrastine, canadine) resin, volatile oil	Antibacterial, Antiprotozoan, increases GI motility	May increase antigen-specific immunoglobulin production; may exhibit positive inotropic, negative chronotropic, antiarrhythmic, and vasodilator properties	Intestinal bacterial overgrowth, giardia, chronic diarrhea, stomatitis	Hypotension; dogs have been given 45 mg/kg berberine IV without ill effect	Proportional to human dose
Grape Seed (*Vitis vinifera*)	Proanthocyanidins	Antioxidant, anti-inflammatory effects; inhibits destructive enzymes	Scavenges oxygen radicals, reduces lipid peroxidation; inhibits the formation of inflammatory cytokines; may down-regulate adhesion molecules	Cardiovascular disease, autoimmune disease; reduces inflammation and carcinogenesis	None reported	Proportional to human dose

(continued on next page)

Table (continued)

Common name	Selected ingredients	Proposed mechanism of action	Proposed cellular effects	Traditional and potential uses	Adverse effects	Suggested dose
Green tea (*Camellia sinensis*)	Polyphenols (catechin and epillocatechin gallate)	Antioxidant, anti-inflammatory effects, chemoprotective, hypocholesterolemic effects, anticlotting effects	May inhibit metallo-proteinases; may suppress colony growth factors and NF-κB; may suppress angiogenesis; may inhibit nitric oxide production	Cancer prevention, hyperlipidemia	None reported	Proportional to human dose; high daily doses are needed for desired effects
Hawthorn (*Crataegus oxycantha*)	Flavonoids including quercetin, procyanidins	Antioxidant, cardiovascular tonic	Positive inotrope peripheral vasodilator; may improve coronary blood flow; may act as an angiotensin-converting enzyme inhibitor; may inhibit 3′,5′-cyclic adenosine monophosphate phosphodiesterase	Dilated cardiomyopathy, congestive heart failure, hypertension, hypercholesterolemia	Potential for interaction with cardiovascular drugs; may interact with vasodilating medications	Proportional to human dose

Horsetail (*Equisetum arvense*)	Flavonoids, silicates (silicic acid), sterols, beta carotene, alkaloids (nicotine)	Diuresis	May aid calcium absorption; silica supports regeneration of connective tissue	Cystitis, urinary calculi	GI irritation, dermatitis; uncooked herb has thiaminase, jypoglycemic effect; silica may be carcinogenic (rare)	Proportional to human dose
Kava kava (*Piper methysticum*)	Kavalactones	Central nervous system depressant, anxiolytic, anticonvulsant, antispasmodic	Alters sodium channel receptor sites in CNS; may bind to GABA receptors; may modulate CNS neurotransmitters	Analgesic, sedative; anxiety and stress reduction	Severe hepatitis has been reported in a few humans—use whole herb only for short periods	Proportional to human dose
Licorice (*Glycyrrhiza glabra*, *Glycyrrhiza uralensis*)	Glycyrrhizin (saponins), flavonoids, polysaccharides, sterols, coumarins	Anti-inflammatory effects, choleretic, expectorant, antiviral effects; reduces carcinogenesis	Modulates activator protein 1 (AP-1, a transcription factor); may enhance leukocyte count and blastogenic responses to mitogens; may enhance interferon production	Gastritis, bronchitis, viral diseases	Hyperaldosteronism from prolonged use; hyperkalemia	Proportional to human dose
Maitake (*Grifola frondosa*)	Polysaccharides (beta 1,6 glucan)	Immune-modulating effects, antioxidant; reduces carcinogenesis	May activate T cells (CD4+), NK cells, and macrophages; may increase IL-1 production	Chronic infections, cancer, immunosuppression, diabetes, hyperlipidemias	None reported	Proportional to human dose

(*continued on next page*)

Table (continued)

Common name	Selected ingredients	Proposed mechanism of action	Proposed cellular effects	Traditional and potential uses	Adverse effects	Suggested dose
Milk thistle (*Silybum marianum*)	Bioflavanoid (silymarin)	Antioxidant, antihepatoxic effects, hypocholesterolemic effects	Reduces reactive oxygen species and glutathione depletion; may suppress NF-κB expression; may reduce hepatic fibrosis; may increase DNA synthesis of liver cells	Hepatitis, hepatic fibrosis, cholangio-hepatitis, hyper-lipidemias	Allergic reactions (rare)	Proportional to human dose
Nettle, stinging nettle (*Urtica dioica*)	Flavanoids, including quercitin, and amines (histamine, acetylcholine, serotonin)	Anti-inflammatory effects, diuretic, hypotensive, immune-modulating effects	May stimulate α-adrenergic receptors; may induce bradycardia; may promote nitric oxide release; may reduce cytokine expression; may reduce T cell response	Tonic, astringent. allergic rhinitis; rheumatoid arthritis; promotes diuresis	Contact with hairs causes inflammation due to histamine leukotriene and serotonin content	Proportional to human dose

Panax ginseng (Korean ginseng)	Triterpenoid saponins	Antioxidant, antistress effects; modulates blood pressure and immune function	May stimulate nitric oxide synthesis; may enhance cell differentiation and immune effects on macrophages; may improve gap junctional intercellular communication	Tonic, stimulant, cancer prevention, diabetes, reduce stress, performance enhancer	Insomnia, hypertension; irritability in high doses	Proportional to human dose
Passionflower (Passiflora incarnata)	Alkaloids, flavonoids, glycoside	Anxiolytic	May enhance CNS anxiolytic activity	Sedation, insomnia, reneral anxiety disorder	None reported	Proportional to human dose
Pau d'Arco (Tabebuia impestignosa); "lapacho" in Spanish	Bioflavonoids, quinones, lapachenole, carnosol, coenzyme Q10, saponins	Antimicrobial, immunostmulant, anti-inflammatory effects	May possess antinociceptive effects (blocking nonmyelin pain neuropathways)	Tonic, digestive aid, bacterial and fungal infections, chronic fatigue syndrome; folk remedy for cancer	GI upset, increased bleeding	Proportional to human dose
Peppermint (Mentha piperita)	Volatile oil (menthol), flavonoids, triterpenes	Antispasmadic	May modulate GI motility	Colitis, nausea, flatulence	GI "burning" sensation reported (rare)	Proportional to human dose
Psyllium (Plantago ovata)	Mucilage, fixed oil	Demulcent, bulk laxative, hypocholesterolemic effects; induces peristalsis	Induces peristalsis; may up-regulate bile acid synthesis	Constipation, fiber responsive GI disease, hypercholesterolemia	Increased fecal volume and frequency	As labeled (Vetasyl); as loose herb, ½–2 tsp sid–bid administer when necessary

(continued on next page)

Table (continued)

Common name	Selected ingredients	Proposed mechanism of action	Proposed cellular effects	Traditional and potential uses	Adverse effects	Suggested dose
Reishi (*Ganoderma lucidum*)	Polysaccharides, sterols, mannitol, ganoderic acids, triterpenoids	Immune-modulating effects, hepatoprotective effects	May induce cell cycle arrest and apoptosis in certain cancers; may block antigen-specific antibody production; may reduce fibrosis	Immunosuppression, cancer, liver disease	GI effects, long-term bleeding problems (rare)	Proportional to human dose; use of alcohol tincture or whole dried herb is preferred to teas
Saw palmetto (*Serenoa repens*)	Volatile oil, steroidal saponins, polysaccharides, tannins	Suppresses testosterone formation	5-α reductase inhibitor; may inhibit cell growth and COX-2 expression in prostatic tissue	Prostatic hypertrophy, urethral spasm	None reported	Proportional to human dose
Senna (*Cassia senna*, *Cassia angustifolia*)	Anthroquinone glycosides	Increases peristalsis and colonic fluid secretion	May stimulate nerve plexus in large colon	Constipation, stool softening, bowel evacuent	Avoid in young Animals; long-term use may lead to dependence and mitochondrial myopathy	Proportional to human dose
Slippery elm (*Ulmus fulva*)	Mucilage, tannins	Anti-inflammatory effects; insoluble and soluble fiber source (demulcent)	May reduce Peroxynitrite radicals	Urinary problems; traditional remedy for diarrhea, cough, bronchitis	None reported	Proportional to human dose

Shiitake (*Lentinus edodes*)	Polysaccharides (lentinan), amino acids, various vitamins	Immunostimulant, antimutagenic, antiviral effects	May increase IL-1 production and apoptosis monocytic cell line	Chemotherapy support, hepatitis, viral infections, cancer	None reported	Proportional to human dose
Schizandra (*Schizandra chinensis*) berries	Volatile oils, lignans (schizandrin), phytosterols, vitamin E and vitamin C	Antioxidant, antistress effects (adaptogen), hepatoprotective effects	May enhance hepatic mitochondrial glutathione redox	Liver aid, tonic	None reported	Proportional to human dose
St John's wort (*Hypericum perforatum*)	Volatile oils (hypericin, hyperforin), flavonoids	Antidepressant	Monoamine oxidase inhibition, GABA binding; may inhibit synaptosomal uptake of several CNS neurotransmitters	Depression, viral infection, analgesic	Do not use with other mood-altering drugs; may induce cytochrome P450 isoenzymes	Proportional to human dose; use 6 to 8 weeks for full effects
Tea tree (*Melaleuca alternifolia*)	Essential oils (alpha-pinene, alpha-terpineol, mimonene, aromadendrene, camphor)	Antifungal, antibacterial effects	May reduce histamine-induced skin inflammation; may alter the permeability of bacterial cytoplasmic and yeast plasma membranes	Disinfectant, wound aid, focal dermatophytosis	Topical use only (very toxic)—not for use in cats; dogs can be hypersensitive to undiluted essential oils	Topical; may dilute with vegetable oil 50:50

(continued on next page)

Table (continued)

Common name	Selected ingredients	Proposed mechanism of action	Proposed cellular effects	Traditional and potential uses	Adverse effects	Suggested dose
Turmeric (*Curcuma longa*)	Volatile oils (zingiberene, turmerone), curcumin, resin	Antioxidant, hematoprotective effects; prevents platelet aggregation and may inhibit carcinogenesis	May reduce NF-κB and mitogen-activated protein kinases (AP-1); may reduce COX-2 expression and leukotriene activity; may increase glutathione S-transferase activity	Cancer, hepatitis, HIV, circulation, hyperlipidemias, various inflammatory conditions	None reported	Proportional to human dose
Valerian (*Valeriana officinalis*)	Volatile oils (beta-caryphyllene, azulene, limonene, various others), beta carotene, iridoids (valepotriates), alkaloids	Sedative, relaxant, anti-anxiety effects	Modulates uptake and stimulates the release of GABA receptors	Insomnia, anxiety	Do not use with similar GABA-type sedatives	Proportional to human dose

Abbreviations: CNS, central nervous system; GABA, gamma-aminobutyric acid; GI, gastrointestinal; IL, interleukin; NF, necrosis factor; NK cells, natural killer cells; TNF, tumor necrosis factor.

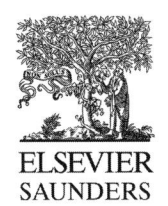

Index

Note: Page numbers of article titles are in **boldface** type.

A

AAFCO. *See* American Association of Feed Control Officials (AAFCO).

Adhesion molecules, 55–56

Aged dogs
  brains of
    oxidative damage in, 222

Aging
  cognitive dysfunction due to
    in dogs, 217–219
    nutrition effects on, 225–226
  immunity and, 238–240

Algae
  cellular effects of, 338

Alkaloid(s), 305–306
  pyrrolizidine
    toxicity of, 150

Aloe vera
  cellular effects of, 354

Alpha lipoic acid
  cellular effects of, 338

American Association of Feed Control Officials (AAFCO), 12–14

Amino acids
  branched chain
    cellular effects of, 339

Androstenedione
  cellular effects of, 338

Antioxidant(s)
  enzymatic, 81–82
  in reducing cognitive impairment in aged dogs, 223–224
  nonenzymatic
    soluble, 82–83
  nutritional, 222–223

Antioxidant enzymes, 221–222

Antioxidant systems
  hepatic, 81–83

Antioxidant vitamins
  for cancer, 262–263

Apoptosis, 57–59, 67–68

Arginine
  cellular effects of, 338
  in cancer patients, 255

Ashwagandha
  cellular effects of, 354

Aspirin
  chemical structure of, 295

Astragalus
  cellular effects of, 354

Astragalus membranaceus
  clinical effects of, 317–319

B

Berbamine
  chemical structure of, 308

Berberine
  chemical structure of, 308

Bilberry
  cellular effects of, 354

Bioflavonoids
  cellular effects of, 339

Black walnut
  cellular effects of, 355

Borage oil
  cellular effects of, 339

Boswellia
  cellular effects of, 355

Botanical(s)
  cellular effects of, **353–366**.
    See also specific types.

Branched chain amino acids
  cellular effects of, 339

C

Calendula
  cellular effects of, 355

Cancer
    metabolic alterations with, 250–253
        carbohydrate-related, 250–251
        fat-related, 252–253
        protein-related, 251–252
    nutritional profile for patients with, 253–259
        arginine, 255
        fat, 256–259
        fatty acids, 256–259
            omega-3, 256–259
        glutamine, 255–256
        protease inhibitors, 256
        protein, 255
        soluble carbohydrate and fiber, 253, 254
    treatment of
        nutraceuticals in, **249–269**. *See also Nutraceutical(s), in cancer therapy.*
        omega-3 fatty acids in clinical studies of, 259–262

Carbohydrate(s)
    metabolism of
        in cancer patients
            alterations in, 250–251
    soluble
        in cancer patients, 253, 254

Cardiac disease
    in dogs and cats
        treatment of, **187–216**
            carnitine in, 195
            current status of, 194–195
            taurine in, 195–198

Carnitine
    cardiac effects of, 207–213
    cellular effects of, 340

L-Carnitine, 141–146
    described, 207

Carnosine
    cellular effects of, 340

Carotenoid(s)
    cellular effects of, 341

Cartilage
    shark
        for cancer, 265–266

Cat(s)
    cardiac disease in
        treatment of, **187–216**. *See also Cardiac disease, in dogs and cats, treatment of.*

Catechin
    chemical structure of, 300

Catnip
    cellular effects of, 355

Cat's claw
    cellular effects of, 356

Cell(s)
    communication of, 46–48
    mitochondria, 43–45
    natural activities of, **39–66**
        free radical theory of, 40
    stellate, 70–71
    structures of, 40–43

Cell death, 57
    programmed, 57–59

Cell redox status
    mechanisms of defense involving, 80–81

Cellular inflammation
    mediators of, 51–52

Cellular injury, 50–51

Center for Food Safety and Applied Nutrition (CFSAN), 21

Center of Veterinary Medicine (CVM), 8

Cetyl myristolate
    cellular effects of, 341

CFSAN. *See Center for Food Safety and Applied Nutrition (CFSAN).*

Chamomile
    cellular effects of, 356

Chinese herbal medicines, 146–148

Cholestatic liver disease, 72–74

Choline
    cellular effects of, 342

Chondroitin
    cellular effects of, 340

Chondroitin sulfate, 279–280

Chondroprotectant(s)
    defined, 272–273
    during perioperative period, 285–286
    during physical rehabilitation, 285–286
    in osteoarthritic dogs and cats, **271–289**
    manufacturing of, 273
    mechanism of action of, 274
    mixed products, 280–281
    polysulfated glycosaminoglycan, 284–285
    quality control of, 273
    regulation of, 273

Chromium
    cellular effects of, 341

Clinical questions
  well-formulated, 2–4
    building clinical question, 2
    development of
      domain and element
        approach to, 2–3
      recommendations of
        quality of evidence
          and strength of, 3
        grades of, 3–4
      strength of, 4

Coenzyme Q10, 121–122
  cellular effects of, 341

Cognitive dysfunction
  aging and
    in dogs, 217–219
      nutrition effects on, 225–226
    biological basis of, 220
  in aged dogs
    reduction of
      antioxidants in, 223–224

Communication
  cell, 46–48
  intercellular, 48–50

Copper
  liver disease due to, 76–77

Cranberry
  cellular effects of, 356

Creatine
  cellular effects of, 341

Cytolytic cell death, 67–68

D

Dandelion
  cellular effects of, 356

Devil's claw
  cellular effects of, 357

DHA (docosahexaenoic acid)
  cellular effects of, 342

DHEA (dehydroepiandrosterone)
  cellular effects of, 342

Dietary supplement
  defined, 11–12

Diosgenin
  chemical structure of, 309

DMAE (dimethylaminoethanol)
  cellular effects of, 343

DMG (dimethylglycine)
  cellular effects of, 343

DMSO (dimethyl sulfoxide)
  cellular effects of, 342

Dog(s)
  aged
    brains of
      oxidative damage in, 222
  cardiac disease in
    treatment of, **187–216**. *See also*
      *Cardiac disease, in dogs
      and cats, treatment of.*

E

E. senticosus
  clinical effects of, 314–315

Echinacea
  cellular effects of, 357

Eleutherococcus spp.
  cellular effects of, 357

Eleutheroside B
  chemical structure of, 315

"Enforcement Strategy for Marketing
  Ingredients" (ESMI), 13

Enzymatic antioxidants, 81–82

Enzyme(s)
  antioxidant, 221–222
  cellular effects of, 344

EPA (eicopentaenoic acid)
  cellular effects of, 343

Ephedra
  cellular effects of, 357

ESMI. *See "Enforcement Strategy for
  Marketing Ingredients" (ESMI).*

Evidence-based medicine
  functional foods and, 176
  nephrology and, 173–176

Evidence-based medicine concepts, **1–6**
  defined, 1
  well-formulated clinical questions, 2–4

Evidence-based medicine practice
  literature appraisal in, 4–5

Exercise(s)
  immunity and, 237–238

F

Fat
  in cancer patients, 256–259

Fat metabolism
  in cancer patients
    alterations in, 252–253

Fatty acids
  in cancer patients, 256–259

Fatty (*continued*)
    omega-3, 283–284
        for cancer
            clinical studies of, 259–262
        polyunsaturated
            chronic kidney disease and,
                182–183
Federal Food, Drug, and Cosmetic Act
    (FDCA) of 1938, 8
Feeds
    regulatory issues of, **327–336**
Fiber
    in cancer patients, 253, 254
Fibrosis(es)
    hepatic, 71–72
5-HTP (5-hycroxytryptophan)
    cellular effects of, 344
Food(s)
    defined, 8
Food additives
    defined, 8–9
Food components
    biologically active, 292–294
Free radical homeostasis
    phytochemicals in, 299–301
Free radical scavengers, 282–283
Fructooligosaccharide(s)
    cellular effects of, 344
Functional foods
    chronic kidney disease and, 178–181
    evidence-based medicine and, 176
    regulatory issues of, **327–336**
    urinary tract effects of, **173–185.**
        *See also Urinary tract,
        functional foods and.*
    veterinary nephrology and, 176–178,
        183–184

G

GAGs (glucosamine HcL, glucosamine
    sulfate, chondroitin sulfate)
    cellular effects of, 345
Garlic
    cellular effects of, 358
    for cancer, 263–264
Ginger
    cellular effects of, 358
Ginkgo
    cellular effects of, 359

Glucosamine, 277–278
Glutamine
    cellular effects of, 345
    in cancer patients, 255–256
    in liver disease
        hazards related to, 135–139
        supplementation of
            hazards related to, 135–139
Glutathione, 83–90
    cellular effects of, 345
    functions of
        hepatocellular, 90–95
Glycosaminoglycan
    mixed products, 281–282
    polyunsaturated, 284–285
Glycoside(s)
    phenolytic, 294–297
Goldenseal
    cellular effects of, 359
Grape Seed
    cellular effects of, 359
Green tea
    cellular effects of, 360

H

Hamamelitanin
    chemical structure of, 299
Hawthorn
    cellular effects of, 360
Health claims, 331–332
Heart
    carnitine effects of, 207–213
    taurine effects on, 197–198
Hepatic antioxidant systems, 81–83
Hepatic fibrosis, 71–72
Hepatic macrophages
    resident, 69–70
Hepatic oxidative injury
    mitochondria and, 68–69
Hepatobiliary disorders. *See also Liver
    disease.*
    collateral oxidative/peroxidative
        organelle injury, 74–76
    management of, **67–172**
    metals and, 76–80
Hepatocellular death, 67–68
Hepatocellular glutathione functions, 90–95
Herb(s)
    adaptogenic activity of, 312–315

adverse effects of, 23–24
cellular effects of, **353–366**.
See also specific types.
clinical effects of, 312–315
drug interactions of, 25
hepatotoxicity of, 148–149

Herbal medicine
Chinese, 146–148

Homeostasis
free radical
phytochemicals in, 299–301

Horsetail
cellular effects of, 361

Human dietary supplements
defined, 10
laws pertaining to, 10–11

I

Ignorance
law of conservation of, 187–188

Immune response
dietary modulation of, 232–234
canine and feline
applications of, 234–237
modulation of
nutraceuticals in
implications in canine and
feline health, **229–247**

Immune system
cells of, 231
overview of, 230–232
reactive oxygen species of, 301–303

Immunity
aging and, 238–240
exercise and, 237–238

Inflammation
cellular
mediators of, 51–52

Ingredient(s). *See also* specific type
and ingredient.
novel. *See also* Novel ingredients.
fact and fiction of, **7–38**

Intercellular communication, 48–50

Ipriflavone
chemical structure of, 312

Iron
liver disease due to, 78–80

Ito cell, 70–71

J

Joint(s)
normal
structure and function of,
274–275

K

Kava kava
cellular effects of, 361

Kidney(s). *See also* Renal.

Kupffer cells, 69–70

L

Labeling
in novel ingredient evaluation, 15–21

Lactoferrin
cellular effects of, 345

Law of conservation of ignorance, 187–188

Leukotrienes, 52–53

Licorice
cellular effects of, 361

Lipid(s), 305

α-Lipoic acid, 108–110

Liver disease.
See also Hepatobiliary disorders.
cholestatic, 72–74
copper and, 76–77
glutamine for
hazards related to, 135–139
supplementation of
hazards related to, 135–139
iron and, 78–80
metals and, 76–80
probiotics for, 132–135

Lysine
cellular effects of, 346

M

Macrophage(s)
hepatic
resident, 69–70

Maitake
cellular effects of, 361

Matrix metalloproteinases (MMPs), 54–55

Melatonin
cellular effects of, 346

Metabolic alterations
cancer-related, 250–253. *See also*
Cancer, metabolic alterations with.

Metal(s)
    liver disease due to, 76–80
Methionine
    cellular effects of, 346
Methyl-sulfonyl-methane, 13
Milk thistle, 114–119
    cellular effects of, 362
Mitochondria, 43–45
    hepatic oxidative injury and, 68–69
Mitochondrial permeability transition (MPT), 45–46
MMPs. See *Matrix metalloproteinases (MMPs)*.
Molecule(s)
    adhesion, 55–56
MPT. See *Mitochondrial permeability transition (MPT)*.
MSM (methylsulfonylmethane)
    cellular effects of, 342
Myocardial failure
    taurine deficiency–induced, 198–207

N

NAC. See *N-acetylcysteine (NAC)*.
NAC (N-acetyl-L-cysteine), 95–99
    cellular effects of, 346
N-acetylcysteine (NAC), 95–99, 346
NADA. See *New Animal Drug Approval (NADA)*.
NASC. See *National Animal Supplement Council (NASC)*.
National Animal Supplement Council (NASC), 14
Natural food substances
    cellular effects of, **337–351**
        disclaimer for, 337
Necrosis, 57, 67–68
Nephrology
    evidence-based medicine and, 173–176
    veterinary
        functional foods and, 176–178, 183–184
Nettle
    cellular effects of, 362
Neutraceutical(s)
    cellular effects of, **337–351**
        disclaimer for, 337
        defined, 7–8
New Animal Drug Approval (NADA), 14
Nonenzymatic antioxidants
    soluble, 82–83
North American Veterinary Nutraceutical Council, 14
Novel ingredients
    adverse effects if, 23–30
    definitions related to, 7–15
    efficacy of, 30–34
    evaluation of, 15–21
        labeling in, 15–21
    fact and fiction of, **7–38**
    laws pertaining to use of, 7–15
    safety of, 21–30
Nutraceutical(s), 277–284
    cellular effects of
        disclaimer for, 353
    chondroitin sulfate, 279–280
    chronic kidney disease and, 181–182
    combination products, 280–281
    defined, 272–273
    free radical scavengers, 282–283
    glucosamine, 277–278
    in cancer therapy, **249–269**
        antioxidant vitamins, 262–263
        garlic, 263–264
        shark cartilage, 265–266
        tea polyphenols, 264
        trace minerals, 263
        vitamin A, 265
    in modulation of immune response
        implications in canine and feline health, **229–247**
    in osteoarthritic dogs and cats, **271–289**
    mechanism of action of, 274
    methyl-sulfonyl-methane, 283
    mixed products, 280–281
        glycosaminoglycan, 281–282
    omega-3 fatty acids, 283–284
    quality assurance of, 16–21
    regulatory issues of, **327–336**
    veterinary
        defined, 11
        laws pertaining to, 11–15
Nutrient content claims, 331
Nutrition
    as factor in cognitive effects of aging, 225–226
Nutritional antioxidants, 222–223
Nutritive cures for disease, 329–330

O

Oil
    borage
        cellular effects of, 339

Oligomeric procyanidins, 297–299

Omega-3 fatty acids, 283–284
    for cancer
        clinical studies of, 259–262
    in cancer patients, 256–259

Osteoarthritis
    in dogs and cats
        chondroprotectants in, **271–289**
        nutraceuticals for, **271–289**
    pathophysiology of, 275
    treatment of, 276–277

Oxidative damage
    in brains of aged dogs, 222
    reactive oxygen species and, 220–223

P

Panax ginseng
    cellular effects of, 363

Passionflower
    cellular effects of, 363

Pau d'Arco
    cellular effects of, 363

Peppermint
    cellular effects of, 363

Pharmacognosy, **291–326**

Phenol(s), 294–297

Phenolytic glycosides, 294–297

Phenylalanine
    cellular effects of, 347

Phospholipid(s)
    cellular effects of, 347

Physical rehabilitation
    chondroprotectants in, 285–286

Phytochemical(s), 292–294
    anti-inflammatory activity produced by, 303–305
    function in free radical homeostasis, 299–301

Phytoestrogen(s), 310–312

Phytomedicine(s), **291–326**

Polyenylphosphatidylcholine, 119–121

Polysulfated glycosaminoglycan, 284–285

Polyunsaturated fatty acids
    chronic kidney disease and, 182–183

Polyunsaturated phosphatidylcholine lecithin, 119–121

Pregnenolone
    cellular effects of, 347

Probiotic(s)
    for liver disease, 132–135

Procyanidin(s)
    oligomeric, 297–299

Programmed cell death, 57–59

Prostaglandin(s), 51–52

Protease inhibitors
    in cancer patients, 256

Protein
    in cancer patients, 255

Protein metabolism
    in cancer patients
        alterations in, 251–252

Psyllium
    cellular effects of, 363

Public policy process, **327–336**
    described, 327–329
    food–drug continuum in, 334–335
    labeling claims in, 331–334
        health claims, 331–332
        nutrient content claims, 331
        structure/function claims, 332–334
    rulemaking process in, 330–331

Pyrrolizidine alkaloids
    toxicity of, 150

Q

Quality assurance
    for novel ingredients, 16–21
    of nutraceuticals, 16–21

Quality control
    of chondroprotectants, 273

R

Reactive oxygen species, **39–66,** 301–303
    described, 221
    oxidative damage and, 220–223

Regulatory issues
    of functional foods, feeds, and nutraceuticals, **327–336**

Rehabilitation
    physical
        chondroprotectants in, 285–286

Reishi
  cellular effects of, 364
Renal disease
  chronic
    functional foods and, 178–181
    nutraceuticals and, 181–182
    polyunsaturated fatty acids and, 182–183
Rulemaking process, 330–331

S

S-adenosylmethionine (SAMe), 99–108
  pharmacologic applications of, 105–108
SAMe. *See S-adenosylmethionine (SAMe).*
SAM-e (S-adenosylmethionine)
  cellular effects of, 348
Saponins/phytosterols, 306–310
Saw palmetto
  cellular effects of, 364
Schisandra chinensis
  clinical effects of, 312–314
Schisandrin
  chemical structure of, 313
Schizandra
  cellular effects of, 365
Selenium, 126–127
  cellular effects of, 348
Senna
  cellular effects of, 364
Shark cartilage
  for cancer, 265–266
Shiitake
  cellular effects of, 365
Sho-saiko-to, 147–148
Silybin
  chemical structure of, 295
ß-Sitosterol
  chemical structure of, 309
Slicytic acid
  chemical structure of, 295
Slippery elm
  cellular effects of, 364
SOD (superoxide dismutase)
  cellular effects of, 349
Soluble nonenzymatic antioxidants, 82–83
St. John's wort
  cellular effects of, 365

Stellate cells, 70–71
Structure/function claims, 332–334

T

Tannic acid
  chemical structure of, 298
Tannin(s), 297–299
Taurine, 139–141
  cardiac effects of, 197–198
  cellular effects of, 349
  deficiency of
    myocardial failure due to, 198–207
  described, 195–196
  for cardiac disease in dogs and cats, 195–198
Tea polyphenols
  for cancer, 264
Tea tree
  cellular effects of, 365
Thioctic acid, 108–110
Thiol(s), 83
Thioredoxin, 93
Trace minerals
  for cancer, 263
Transfer factor
  cellular effects of, 349
Tumor necrosis factor, 53–54
Turmeric
  cellular effects of, 366

U

Ubiquinol, 121–122
Urinary tract
  functional foods and, **173–185**
Ursodeoxycholic acid, 122–126

V

Valerian
  cellular effects of, 366
Vanadium
  cellular effects of, 350
Veterinary nephrology
  functional foods and, 176–178, 183–184
Veterinary nutraceuticals
  defined, 11
  laws pertaining to, 11–15

Vitamin(s)
　A
　　for cancer, 265
　antioxidant
　　for cancer, 262–263
　C, 113–114
　　cellular effects of, 350
　E, 110–113
　　cellular effects of, 351

W

Witch doctor
　to real doctor
　　advances to, 189–194

Z

Zinc, 127–132
　cellular effects of, 351